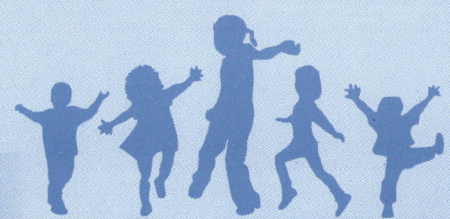

The Best of

Third Edition

Indian

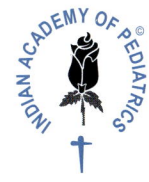

INDIAN ACADEMY OF PEDIATRICS

Pediatrics

W0230548

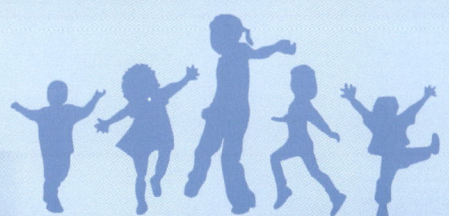

Editors' Choice

The Best of

Third Edition

Indian Pediatrics

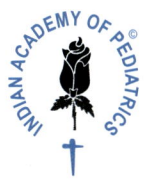

Devendra Mishra MD, ACME, FIAP
Managing Editor
Indian Pediatrics

Professor, Department of Pediatrics
Maulana Azad Medical College
Delhi

Dheeraj Shah MD, MNAMS, FIAP
Editor-in-Chief
Indian Pediatrics

Professor, Department of Pediatrics
University College of Medical Sciences
Delhi

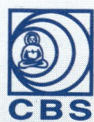

CBS Publishers & Distributors Pvt Ltd

New Delhi • Bengaluru • Chennai • Kochi • Kolkata • Mumbai
Bhopal • Bhubaneswar • Hyderabad • Jharkhand • Nagpur • Patna • Pune • Uttarakhand • Dhaka (Bangladesh)

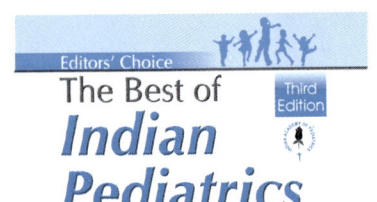

Notice: Research in treatment and drug therapy is continually in progress throughout the world. Recommendations and contraindications in dosage schedules require constant updating and change, both from year to year and country to country. Different drugs may have a similar name in other countries or the same drugs may be packed in different strengths. It is, therefore, advisable to consult the product information sheet provided with each drug, particularly in the case of new, foreign or rarely used drugs to ensure that changes have not been made in the recommended dosages.

Disclaimer
The view and opinions expressed in the articles are of the authors and not of the editors or of the journal.

ISBN: 978-93-88725-62-0

Published by Satish Kumar Jain and produced by Varun Jain for

CBS Publishers & Distributors Pvt Ltd
4819/XI Prahlad Street, 24 Ansari Road, Daryaganj, New Delhi 110 002, India.
Ph: 23289259, 23266861, 23266867 Website: www.cbspd.com
Fax: 011-23243014 e-mail: delhi@cbspd.com; cbspubs@airtelmail.in.

Corporate Office: 204 FIE, Industrial Area, Patparganj, Delhi 110 092
Ph: 4934 4934 Fax: 4934 4935 e-mail: publishing@cbspd.com; publicity@cbspd.com

Branches

- **Bengaluru:** Seema House 2975, 17th Cross, K.R. Road, Banasankari 2nd Stage, Bengaluru 560 070, Karnataka
  Ph: +91-80-26771678/79 Fax: +91-80-26771680 e-mail: bangalore@cbspd.com
- **Chennai:** 7, Subbaraya Street, Shenoy Nagar, Chennai 600 030, Tamil Nadu
  Ph: +91-44-26680620/26681266 Fax: +91-44-42032115 e-mail: chennai@cbspd.com
- **Kochi:** 42/1325, 1326, Power House Road, Opp KSEB, Power House, Ernakulam 682 018, Kochi, Kerala
  Ph: +91-484-4059061-65 Fax: +91-484-4059065 e-mail: kochi@cbspd.com
- **Kolkata:** 6/B, Ground Floor, Rameswar Shaw Road, Kolkata-700 014, West Bengal
  Ph: +91-33-22891126, 22891127, 22891128 e-mail: kolkata@cbspd.com
- **Mumbai:** 83-C, Dr E Moses Road, Worli, Mumbai-400018, Maharashtra
  Ph: +91-22-24902340/41 Fax: +91-22-24902342 e-mail: mumbai@cbspd.com

Representatives

• Bhopal	0-8319310552	• Bhubaneswar	0-9911037372	• Hyderabad	0-9885175004	• Jharkhand	0-9811541605
• Nagpur	0-9421945513	• Patna	0-9334159340	• Pune	0-9623451994	• Uttarakhand	0-9716462459
• Dhaka (Bangladesh)	01912-003485						

Printed at: India Binding House, Greater Noida, UP, India

Foreword

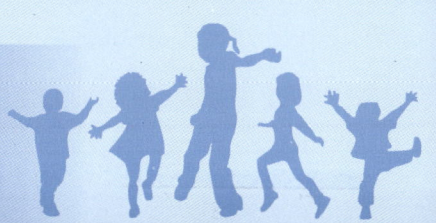

Indian Pediatrics, the official journal of our parent body Indian Academy of Pediatrics (IAP), regularly publishes articles and reviews of high scientific merit and wide clinical interest. In addition, it also publishes guidelines and recommendations of various IAP chapters and groups on management of common clinical conditions. A compendium of such stellar material is now in your hands, and is an important publishing milestone.

The 34 chapters of this book include reviews on important topics like surfactant therapy, metabolic liver diseases, inflammatory bowel disease, and subclinical hypothyroidism; IAP guidelines, including those of the Advisory committee on vaccines and immunization practices; Perspectives on issues of general interest; and Updates to the diagnosis and management of various conditions like epilepsy. The chapters on Prebiotics, Health drinks, and Media and children will be of both professional and personal interest to most readers. Such a well compiled publication will definitely prove to be useful to old reader as it can facilitate the revision of "old hits", and at the same time it will be useful to new reader to get updated with high quality scientific material.

Contributors to this compendium consist of both established 'experts' and also young and enthusiastic pediatricians, a veritable 'who's who' of the pediatric fraternity in India. They and the editors deserve kudos for compiling the material and presenting it in this pleasing format. I am sure the book will acquire a pride of place in the bookshelf of all practicing pediatricians, and will also assist the postgraduates in their studies as well as in the life ahead. I congratulate the team *Indian Pediatrics* led by Editor-in-Chief Dr. Dheeraj Shah for coming out with a very useful book.

Dr. Digant D Shastri
President
Indian Academy of Pediatrics 2019

Preface to the Third Edition

Following the tremendous response to the previous editions, especially from postgraduate students and practising pediatricians, we are pleased to present the third edition of this popular reference book. Containing guidelines and recommendations of various groups and chapters of the Indian Academy of Pediatrics, and state-of-the-art reviews and updates by subject experts; this compendium is likely to be of immense interest to all levels of pediatricians.

We place on record our thanks to the office bearers of various IAP chapters and committees for giving us an opportunity to present their work in this volume. We acknowledge the wholehearted support of Dr Digant Shastri (President IAP, 2019) and Dr Santosh Soans (President IAP, 2018) and all office-bearers of IAP 2018 and 2019. The editorial board members of Indian Pediatrics deserve special appreciation for their efforts in bringing this publication to its final form. The efforts of the editorial staff of the journal and publication team of CBS Publishers & Distributors Pvt. Ltd. are gratefully acknowledged. Finally, our authors and reviewers are the cornerstone of the consistently high-quality of the journal and this publication—our heartfelt thanks to them. Since the conception of this series and through its various editions, we have benefited greatly from the constant guidance of Prof Piyush Gupta, past editor-in-chief of Indian Pediatrics.

Readers' comments/suggestions are welcome at *jiap@nic.in, www.facebook.com/Indian Pediatrics, and www.indianpediatrics.net.*

Devendra Mishra
Dheeraj Shah

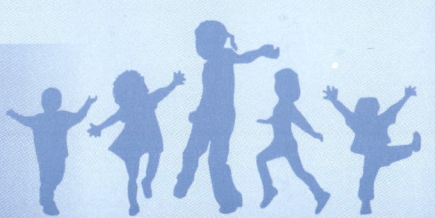

Preface to the First Edition

It gives us a great pleasure to place this volume in front of the readers. *Indian Pediatrics* regularly publishes topical reviews, guidelines and recommendations formulated by the Indian Academy of Pediatrics (IAP), its chapters, groups, and committees, and other national bodies. These publications are an important resource for guiding the practitioners in the management of various day-to-day pediatric problems. Though these articles are freely available on the *Indian Pediatrics* website, yet it was a long-standing demand of IAP members that a collection of these articles be published to facilitate their availability at one place for ready referral. The present compendium has been published by *Indian Pediatrics* in response to these suggestions.

We are overwhelmed with the pre-print orders for this volume and hope that it would receive a similar response after publication. We wish to thank the authors and experts who have contributed to these articles and guidelines for their time and effort. We are thankful to Dr Deepak Ugra (President, IAP), Dr Panna Choudhury (Immediate past-President) and Dr TU Sukumaran (President-elect) for their wholehearted support to this venture. We are thankful to the editiorial board of *Indian Pediatrics* for permission to bring out this volume, and plan to publish further volumes in the coming years. We are extremely thankful to Mr Pawan Nanda, Venus Printers and Publishers, who provided critical inputs at crucial junctures and unflinching support for this venture. Finally, we will be failing in our duty if do not thank the editorial staff of *Indian Pediatrics* who worked tirelessly behind the scene—Mr Santlal, Mr Mohan, Mr Ramgopal Bhardwaj and Mr Diwan to bring about this treatise.

We hope that this volume will serve the purpose it is intended for and help in practising standard treatment guidelines for disorders where consensus statements are in place.

Piyush Gupta
Devendra Mishra

Contributors

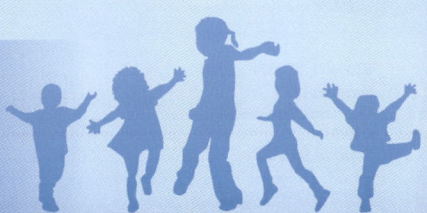

Abhay Shah
Advisory Committee on Vaccines and
Immunization Practices (ACVIP)
Indian Academy of Pediatrics, India

Abhijeet Saha
Department of Pediatrics
Lady Hardinge Medical College
New Delhi, India

Abraham Paul
Child Care Centre
Cochin Hospital

Akshay Kapoor
Department of Pediatric Gastroenterology
Apollo Centre for Advanced Pediatrics
Indraprastha Apollo Hospital
Sarita Vihar, New Delhi, India

Alice Cherian
Department of Pediatrics
Lakeshore Hospital
Kochi, Kerala, India

Anjan Bhattacharya
Apollo Gleneagles Hospital
Kolkata, India

Anupam Sachdeva
Sir Gangaram Hospital
New Delhi, India

Anupam Sibal
Department of Pediatric Gastroenterology
Apollo Centre for Advanced Pediatrics
Indraprastha Apollo Hospital
Sarita Vihar, New Delhi, India

Anuradha Khadilkar
Indian Academy of Pediatrics Guideline for
Vitamin D and Calcium in Children' Committee
Hirabai Cowasji Jehangir Medical Research Institute
Jehangir Hospital
Pune, India

Ashok Deorari
Departments of Pediatrics
AIIMS, New Delhi, India

Atul Kulkarni
Department of Pediatrics
Ashwini Medical College
Solapur, India

Aysu Turkmen Karaagac
Kartal Kobuyolu Research and Training Hospital
Pediatry, Istanbul, Turkey

B Resch
Research Unit for Neonatal Infectious Diseases and
Epidemiology
Division of Neonatology
Department of Paediatrics
Medical University of Graz
Austria

Bakul J Parekh
The Indian Academy of Pediatrics (IAP)
Advisory Committee on Vaccines and
Immunization Practices (ACVIP)
Mumbai, India

Baldev Prajapati
The Indian Academy of Pediatrics (IAP)
Advisory Committee on Vaccines and
Immunization Practices (ACVIP)
Mumbai, India.

Balraj S Yadav
IYCF Chapter of IAP

Bernhard Fassl
Department of Pediatrics
Division of Inpatient Medicine and Department of
Epidemiology and Biostatistics
University of Utah
Salt Lake City, UT, USA

Bikrant Bihari Lal
Department of Pediatric Hepatology
Institute of Liver and Biliary Sciences
New Delhi, India

Binita Shah
Departments of Emergency Medicine and
Pediatrics
SUNY Downstate Medical Center
Kings County Hospital Center
Brooklyn, NY, USA

Bonny Jasani
Department of Neonatology
King Edward Memorial Hospital
Parel, Mumbai, Maharashtra, India

Chandra Rath
Departments of Neonatology
Royal North Shore Hospital
Pacific High way, St Leonards
NSW, Australia

Chhaya Prasad
Max Super Speciality Hospital
Chandigarh, India

CR Banapurmath
The IYCF Chapter of IAP

D Narayanappa
Department of Pediatrics
JSS Medical College
JSS Univeristy, Mysuru

Devendra Mishra
Department of Pediatrics
Maulana Azad Medical College (University of Delhi)
and associated Lok Nayak Hospital
New Delhi, India

Dheeraj Shah
Department of Pediatrics
University College of Medical Sciences
Delhi, India

Digant Shastri
Advisory Committee on Vaccines and
Immunization Practices (ACVIP)
Indian Academy of Pediatrics, India

E Resch
Research Unit for Neonatal Infectious Diseases and
Epidemiology
Division of Neonatology
Department of Paediatrics
Medical University of Graz, Austria

Harish K Pemde
Advisory Committee on Vaccines and
Immunization Practices (ACVIP)
Indian Academy of Pediatrics, India

I Ray
Department of Human Physiology
Ramakrishna Mahavidyalaya
Tripura; India

Jagdish Chinnappa
Indian Academy of Pediatrics 'Guideline for
Vitamin D and Calcium in Children' Committee

Jagdish P Goyal
Department of Pediatrics
AIIMS, Rishikesh
Uttarakhand, India

Jaydeep Choudhary
The Indian Academy of Pediatrics (IAP)
Advisory Committee on Vaccines and
Immunization Practices (ACVIP)
Mumbai, India.

Jeeson Unni
Aster Medcity
Kochi, India

Kanya Mukhopadhyay
Neonatal Unit
Department of Pediatrics
PGIMER
Chandigarh, India

Ketan Bharadva
Indian Academy of Pediatrics

KK Agrawal
Indian Academy of Pediatrics Growth Charts
Committee

Lea Vodušek Reberšak
University Medical Centre, Ljubljana
University Children's Hospital, Ljubljana
Slovenia

Leena Shrivastava
Department of Pediatrics
Bharatiya Vidyapeeth Medical College and
Hospital
Pune, India

M Eibisberger
Research Unit for Neonatal Infectious Diseases and
Epidemiology
Division of Neonatology
Department of Paediatrics
Medical University of Graz
Austria

M Shriraam
Department of Pediatrics
Apollo Children's Hospital
Chennai, India

M Sridhar
Department of Pediatrics
Apollo Children's Hospital
Chennai, India

Madhulika Kabra
Division of Genetics
Department of Pediatrics
AIIMS, New Delhi, India

Mahesh Kamate
Department of Pediatrics
KLE University's JN Medical College
Belgaum

Marie Lozon
Department of Emergency Medicine
University of Michigan
Ann Arbor, MI, USA

MKC Nair
Kerala University
Thrissur, India
Monidipa Banerjee

MP Mohanta
Clinic Nua Sakala
Keonjhar, Odisha

Muralidharan Jayashree
Department of Pediatrics
Advanced Pediatrics Centre
PGIMER
Chandigarh, India

Nandini Mundkur
Centre for Child Development and Disabilities
Bangalore, India

Nandkishor Kabra
Department of Neonatology
King Edward Memorial Hospital
Parel, Mumbai, Maharashtra, India

Narendra Rai
Department of Pediatrics
Hind Institute of Medical Sciences
Lucknow, India

Narendra Rathi
Indian Academy of Pediatrics 'Guideline for
Vitamin D and Calcium in Children' Committee
Smile Healthcare, Rehabilitation and Research
Foundation
Smile Institute of Child Health, Ramdaspeth
Akola, India

Naveen Sankhyan
Division of Pediatric Neurology
Department of Pediatrics
PGIMER, Chandigarh, India

Neeraj Gupta
Departments of Pediatrics
AIIMS
Jodhpur, India

Neetu Sharma
Departments of Pediatrics
GR Medical College
Gwalior, MP, India

Neha Thakur
Department of Pediatrics
Hind Institute of Medical Sciences
Lucknow, India

Nidhi Bedi
Department of Pediatrics
Hamdard Institute of Medical Sciences and
Research
Delhi, India

Nisha Sharma
Department of Pediatrics
University College of Medical Sciences and
Guru Tegh Bahadur Hospital, Dilshad Garden,
Delhi, India

Nitin Trivedi
Department of Pediatrics
Mahatma Gandhi Medical College and Hospital
Jaipur, India

Pallab Chatterjee
Advisory Committee on Vaccines and
Immunization Practices (ACVIP)
Indian Academy of Pediatrics, India

Piyush Gupta
Department of Pediatrics
University College of Medical Sciences and
Guru Tegh Bahadur Hospital, Dilshad Garden,
Delhi, India

Pooja Dewan
University College of Medical Sciences and
Guru Tegh Bahadur Hospital, Dilshad Garden,
Delhi, India

Pradeep Suryawanshi
Bharati Vidyapeeth University Medical College
Pune, Maharastra, India

Pramod Jog
Indian Academy of Pediatrics 'Guideline for
Vitamin D and Calcium in Children' Committee
and
The Indian Academy of Pediatrics (IAP)
Advisory Committee on Vaccines and
Immunization Practices (ACVIP)
Mumbai, India.

Prashant Gangal
The IYCF Chapter of IAP

Prashant Mahajan
Departments of Emergency Medicine and
Pediatrics
University of Michigan (Ann Arbor, MI, USA)

Pratibha Singhi
Department of Pediatrics
PGIMER
Chandigarh, India

Praveen Kumar
Departments of Pediatrics
PGIMER
Chandigarh, India

Prerna Batra
Department of Pediatrics
University College of Medical Sciences and
Guru Tegh Bahadur Hospital, Dilshad Garden,
Delhi, India

R Dhinakaran
Department of Pediatrics
Maulana Azad Medical College (University of Delhi)
and associated Lok Nayak Hospital
New Delhi, India

Rajendra Bangal
Smt Kashibai Nawale Medical College
Pune, India

Rajesh Khadgawat
Indian Academy of Pediatrics 'Guideline for
Vitamin D and Calcium in Children' Committee

Ramesh Konanki
Departments of Pediatrics
Rainbow Hospital for Women and Children
Hyderabad, India

Reena Patel
Department of Pediatrics
Division of Inpatient Medicine
University of Utah
Salt Lake City, UT, USA

Remesh Kumar
Advisory Committee on Vaccines and
Immunization Practices (ACVIP)
Indian Academy of Pediatrics, India

RK Agrawal
The IYCF Chapter of IAP

Rockerfeller A Oteng
Department of Emergency Medicine
University of Michigan
Ann Arbor, MI, USA
and
Directorate of Emergency Medicine
KomfoAnokye Teaching Hospital
Kumasi, Ghana

Rok Orel
University Medical Centre, Ljubljana
University Children's Hospital, Ljubljana
Slovenia

Roopa Srinivasan
Ummeed Child Development Center
Mumbai, India

Ruchi Mishra
Departments of Pediatrics
ESI PGIMER
Basaidarapur, New Delhi, India

Ruchi Nanavati
Department of Neonatology
King Edward Memorial Hospital
Parel, Mumbai, Maharashtra, India

S Balasubramanian
Advisory Committee on Vaccines and
Immunization Practices (ACVIP)
Indian Academy of Pediatrics, India

S Shivananda
Advisory Committee on Vaccines and
Immunization Practices (ACVIP)
Indian Academy of Pediatrics, India

Sachidanand S Kamath
The Indian Academy of Pediatrics (IAP)
Advisory Committee on Vaccines and
Immunization Practices (ACVIP)
Mumbai, India.

Sagar Galwankar
Department of Emergency Medicine
University of Florida
Jacksonville, FL, USA

Samir Dalwai
New Horizons Group
Mumbai, India

Sangeeta Gupta
Gynecology and Obstetrics
MAMC and associated Lok Nayak Hospital
Delhi, India

Sangeeta Yadav
Indian Academy of Pediatrics Growth Charts
Committee
The Indian Academy of Pediatrics (IAP)
Advisory Committee on Vaccines and
Immunization Practices (ACVIP)
Mumbai, India.

Sanjay Srirampur
The Indian Academy of Pediatrics (IAP)
Advisory Committee on Vaccines and
Immunization Practices (ACVIP)
Mumbai, India.

Santosh Soans
Advisory Committee on Vaccines and
Immunization Practices (ACVIP)
Indian Academy of Pediatrics, India

Satinder Aneja
Department of Pediatrics
Lady Hardinge Medical College and
Associated Kalawati Saran Children's Hospital
New Delhi, India

Satish Tiwari
Indian Academy of Pediatrics
Indian Medico-Legal & Ethics Association
The IYCF Chapter of IAP

Satvik C Bansal
Department of Pediatrics
Pramukhswami Medical College

Seema Alam
Department of Pediatric Hepatology
Institute of Liver and Biliary Sciences
New Delhi, India

Seema Kapoor
Departments of Pediatrics

Shabina Ahmed
Assam Autism Foundation
Guwahati, India

Shalu Gupta
Department of Pediatrics
Advanced Pediatrics Centre
PGIMER
Chandigarh, India

Sharmila B Mukherjee
Department of Pediatrics
Lady Hardinge Medical College and
Associated Kalawati Saran Children's Hospital
New Delhi, India

Shiv Sajan Saini
Departments of Pediatrics
PGIMER
Chandigarh, India

Somashekhar M Nimbalkar
Department of Pediatrics
Central Research Services
Charutar Arogya Mandal
Karamsad, Gujarat, India

Srinivas Murki
Departments of Pediatrics
Fernandez Hospital
Hyderabad, India

SS Kamath
Welcare Hospital

Suchit Tamboli
Indian Academy of Pediatrics Growth Charts
Committee

Sudhir Mishra
Indian Academy of Pediatrics
Department of Pediatrics
Tata Main Hospital
Jamshedpur, Jharkhand, India

Sujata Kanhere
Department of Pediatrics and Neonatology
KJ Somaiya Medical College
Hospital and Research Centre
Mumbai, India

Sushma Malik
The IYCF Chapter of IAP

Suvasini Sharma
Departments of Pediatrics
Lady Hardinge Medical College
New Delhi, India

Ujjal Poddar
Department of Pediatric Gastroenterology
Sanjay Gandhi Postgraduate Institute of Medical
Sciences
Lucknow, Uttar Pradesh, India

Urmila Deshmukh
The IYCF Chapter of IAP

V Kumaravel
Alpha Hospital and Research Centre
Institute of Diabetes and Endocrinology
Madurai, India

V Mohan
Diabetes Research
Dr. Mohan's Diabetes Speciality Centre
Chennai, India

Vaman Khadilkar
Indian Academy of Pediatrics 'Guideline for
Vitamin D and Calcium in Children' Committee
Committee

Veena Kalra
Indraprastha Apollo Hospital
New Delhi, India

Vibha Krishnamurthy
Ummeed Child Development Center
Mumbai, India

Vidyut Bhatia
Department of Pediatric Gastroenterology
Apollo Centre for Advanced Pediatrics
Indraprastha Apollo Hospital
Sarita Vihar, New Delhi, India

Vijay Kumar Guduru
Advisory Committee on Vaccines and
Immunization Practices (ACVIP)
Indian Academy of Pediatrics, India

Vijay Yewale
Department of Human Physiology
Ramakrishna Mahavidyalaya
Tripura; India
Dr Yewale Multispeciality Hospital for Children
Navi Mumbai, India

Vipin M Vashishtha
The Indian Academy of Pediatrics (IAP)
Advisory Committee on Vaccines and
Immunization Practices (ACVIP)
Mumbai, India.

Vishesh Kumar
Indian Academy of Pediatrics

Vishesh Kumar
WHO Country Office of India
India

Vrajesh Udani
PD Hinduja Hospital
Mumba, India

Waheeda Pagakar
Audiovestibular Medicine
Hackney ARK and Royal National Throat
Nose and Ear Hospital
London

Zeeba Zaka-Ur-Rab
The IYCF Chapter of IAP

Contents

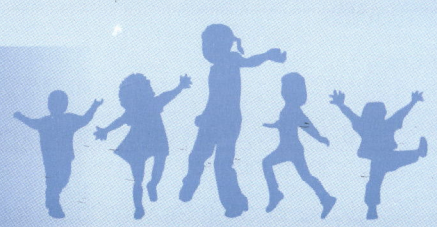

SECTION III: GUIDELINES/CONSENSUS STATEMENTS/RECOMMENDATIONS

SECTION IV: WHAT'S NEW

Initial Publication Details and Corresponding Authors of Chapters

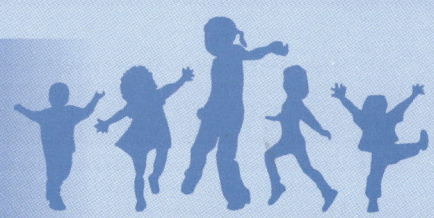

1. **Prenatal Screening: Perspective for the Pediatrician**
   Correspondence to: Dr Seema Kapoor, Division of Genetics, Department of Pediatrics, MAMC and associated Lok Nayak Hospital, New Delhi 110 002, India.
   drseemakapoor@gmail.com

2. **Incorporating Developmental Screening and Surveillance of Young Children in Office Practice**
   Correspondence to: Dr Sharmila B Mukherjee, Department of Pediatrics, Kalawati Saran Children's Hospital, Bangla Sahib Road, New Delhi 110 001, India.
   theshormi@gmail.com

3. **Growing Pains: Practitioners' Dilemma**
   Correspondence to: Dr Mahesh Prasad Mohanta, Practicing Pediatrician, Clinic Nua Sakala, Goudanibeda, PO Dhurpada, Dist Keonjhar, Odisha 758 013, India.
   mpmohanta@gmail.com

4. **Approach to Constipation in Children**
   Correspondence to: Dr Ujjal Poddar, Professor, Department of Pediatric Gastroenterology, SGPGIMS, Lucknow 226 014, Uttar Pradesh, India.
   ujjalpoddar@hotmail.com

5. **Organic Foods for Children: Health or Hype?**
   Correspondence to: Piyush Gupta, Professor in Pediatrics, Block R-6 A, Dilshad Garden, Delhi 110 095, India.
   prof.piyush.gupta@gmail.com

6. **Energy Drinks: Potions of Illusion**
   Correspondence to: Dr Piyush Gupta, Block R6A, Dilshad Garden, New Delhi 110 095, India.
   prof.piyush.gupta@gmail.com

7. **Undesirable Effects of Media on Children: Why Limitation is Necessary?**
   Correspondence to: Dr Aysu Turkmen Karaagac, Kartal Koþuyolu Research and Training Hospital, Denizer Cad., Cevizli Kavþaðý, No:2, 34846 Kartal/Istanbul,Turkey.
   ysukaraagac@gmail.com

8. **Surfactant Replacement Therapy in Extremely Low Gestational Age Newborns**
   Correspondence to: Prof. Dr. Bernhard Resch, Division of Neonatology, Department of Paediatrics, Medical University of Graz, Auenbruggerplatz 34/2, 8036 Graz, Austria.
   bernhard.resch@medunigraz.at

9. **Surfactant Replacement Therapy Beyond Respiratory Distress Syndrome**
   Correspondence to: Dr Bonny Jasani, Department of Neonatology, King Edward Memorial Hospital for Women. Perth, WA 6008.
   docbonny_2000@yahoo.com

10. **Continuous Positive Airway Pressure in Preterms Neonates**
    Correspondence to: Dr Praveen Kumar, Professor, Neonatal Unit, Department of Pediatrics, Advanced Pediatric Center, Post Graduate Institute of Medical Education and Research (PGIMER), Chandigarh 160 012, India.
    drpkumarpgi@gmail.com
    Received: September 30, 2014; Initial review: December 30, 2014; *Accepted:* January 29, 2015.

11. **Point of Care Neonatal Ultrasound — Head, Lung, Gut and Line Localization**
    Correspondence to: Dr Pradeep Suryawanshi, Professor and Head, Department of Neonatology, Bharati Vidyapeeth University Medical College, Pune-Satara Road, Pune, Maharastra 411 043, India.
    drpradeepsuryawanshi@gmail.com
    Received: July 25, 2015; Accepted: June 11, 2016.

12. **Hyperinsulinemic Hypoglycemia in Infancy**
    Correspondence to: Dr Shrenik Vora, Senior Staff Registrar, Department of Neonatology, KK Women's and Children's Hospital, 100, Bukit Timah Road, Singapore 229899.
    vora.shrenik@kkh.com.sg

13. **Subclinical Hypothyroidism in Children**
    Correspondence to: Dr M Sridhar, Consultant Pediatrician, Apollo children's Hospital, No. 15, Shafee Mohammed Road, Thousand Lights, Chennai 600 006, India.
    hemasridha@yahoo.co.uk

14. **Metabolic Liver Diseases Presenting as Acute Liver Failure in Children**
    Correspondence to: Prof Seema Alam, Professor and Head, Department of Pediatric Hepatology, Institute of Liver and Biliary Sciences, New Delhi 110 070, India.
    seema_alam@hotmail.com

15. **Pediatric Inflammatory Bowel Disease**
    Correspondence to: Dr Akshay Kapoor, Department of Pediatric Gastroenterology, Hepatology and Liver Transplantation, Indraprastha Apollo Hospital, Sarita Vihar, New Delhi, India.
    akshaydr80@yahoo.co.in

16. **Clinical Effects of Prebiotics in Pediatric Population**
    Correspondence to: Prof Rok Orel, University Children's Hospital, BohoriĀceva 20, 1000 Ljubljana, Slovenia.
    rok.orel@kclj.si

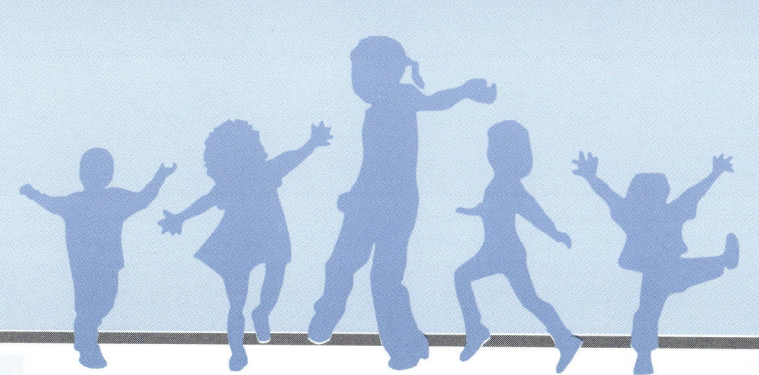

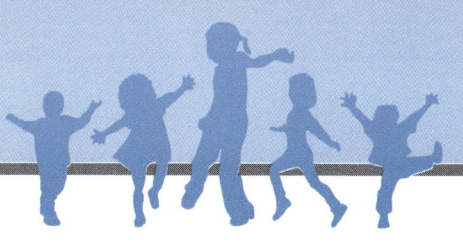

Prenatal Screening: Perspective for the Pediatrician

Seema Kapoor, Sangeeta Gupta, Madhulika Kabra

Births with Down syndrome and other aneuploidies continue to occur with a prevalence of 1 in 925.[1] Prenatal screening for fetal aneuploidies started early with triple test performed in the second trimester (a combination of alfa feto protein, conjugated estriol and beta human chorionic gonadotropin). In the last two decades, the focus of detection has shifted to the first trimester. Two serum markers (pregnancy associated plasma protein A and free beta human chorionic gonadotropin) and one marker assessed by ultrasound (nuchal translucency) are used to predict risk of aneuploidies. Prenatal screening has not been perceived as a health priority in developing countries. Chromosomal and certain common malformations pose additional financial and social constraints in developing countries. In addition, serum screening may also direct attention and resource allocation to high-risk pregnancies complicated by pre-eclampsia/eclampsia and intrauterine growth retardation (IUGR).[2]

DEFINITIONS

Aneuploidies refer to numerical chromosomal aberrations. Common aneuploidies include Trisomy 21 (Down syndrome), Trisomy 18 (Edward syndrome) and Trisomy 13 (Patau syndrome). Sex chromosomal aneupoidy

commonly screened for is Turner syndrome (XO). Risk ascertainment refers to the risk of having a child with any of the above mentioned aneuploidies. The likely risk computed in any pregnancy is illustrated in terms of a value for a given population having the same statistical measurements. Thus the risk computation of 1 in 150 means that if all demographic and biochemical parameters have the same statistical correlation, the likely possibility of a woman carrying a fetus with abnormality would be 1 in 150.

A *priori* risk means the baseline risk conferred on the woman either by age alone or as a result of biochemical screening. The risk increases as age increases due to a higher propensity for non-dysfunction. The risk of Trisomy 21 is 1 in 1667 at 20 years of age and increases to 1 in 385 at 35 years of age, and 1 in 30 at 45 years of age.[3] The risk calculation takes into account the gestational age at sampling, the status of the fetus-singleton/twinning, maternal weight, maternal diabetes, maternal smoking, and previous history of baby with Trisomy 21. Incorporation of values of biochemical analytes along with the demographic data into a designated software generates a risk. Individual values of any analyte or factor are less predictive individually compared to the entire risk computed in a statistical manner incorporating all these factors.

Triple test and Quadruple test (addition of inhibin A) are used to compute risk of aneuploidies in the second trimester (16–20 weeks).[4] Screening has now shifted to the first trimester and uses both serum and ultrasound markers. Nuchal translucency (NT) refers to the measurement of skin at the nape of the neck in the fetus in sagittal plane.[5] Integrated screening is the term used for assessing the risk in the first trimester followed by using this generated risk as *a prori* risk for the second trimester. The results of the first trimester are not disclosed before the final risk is generated. Contingent screening indicates that second trimester screening is subject (or contingent to) to risk generated in the first trimester.[6] Table 1.1 presents the performance characteristics of these tests.[7–9]

Like any other screening technique, confirmatory testing is required to evaluate the risk generated in the first trimester. Women demonstrating a high risk in the first trimester are offered chorionic villus sampling (CVS) and those demonstrating high risk in the second trimester are offered amniotic fluid sampling. In the integrated screening modality, those demonstrating high risk in the first trimester are offered CVS while those with low risk are asked to report later for screening of neural tube defects.[10] The risk cut-offs are carefully weighed against the risk of fetal loss due to amniocentesis and chorionic villus sampling.[11] Even the best modalities are limited in sensitivity and specificity for a confirmed diagnosis of aneuploidies. Table 1.2 depicts the timing and the procedures as an option for any parent.

A large number of these analytes are also being evaluated as potential tools for adverse pregnancy outcome such as pre-eclampsia, IUGR and intrauterine demise.[12] More recently, noninvasive prenatal diagnosis as a screening test using next generation sequencing technology has been found to be highly accurate with sensitivity and specificity of up to 98–99%.[13] Despite the accuracy, the cost of the test presently is prohibitive as a screening test.

TABLE 1.1: Performance characteristics of prenatal screening modalities

Test	Timing (wks)	Sensitivity	False positive rate
Triple	15–20	72–74%	5%
Quadruple	15–20	79–81%	5%
Serum integrated	10–13 & 15–19	86–89%	5%
Fully integrated with Nuchal translucency	Same as above 10–12	93–95%	5%

TABLE 1.2: Prenatal screening tests

Test/procedure	First trimester screening	Integrated prenatal screening	Serum integrated prenatal screening
First blood sample	9–13 wks	9–13 wks	11–14 wks
Nuchal translucency ultrasound	11–14 wks	11–14 wks	None
Second blood sample	None	15–18 wks	15–18 wks
Results available	12–19 wks	15–19 wks	15–19 wks
Detection rate (accuracy)	80–85%	85–90%	80–90%
False positive rate	3.9%	2–4%	2–7%
Diagnostic test (if screen positive)	CVS 11–13 wks	Amniocentesis	Amniocentesis

CVS: Chorionic villous sampling

IMPORTANCE FOR THE PEDIATRICIAN

Pediatricians often face the responsibility of revealing the diagnosis to the parents and dealing with the emotional overture. They also have to deal with complications in the neonatal period (IUGR, congenital anomalies) and various comorbidities (hypothyroidism, recurrent otitis media, atlanatoaxial instability, transient myeloproliferative disorders). The problems encountered in a child with Down syndrome are complex and require that the pediatrician liaises with a multidisciplinary team to adequately follow-up every child. Education regarding preventive strategies that reduce the burden of this disorder is of paramount importance.

CURRENT SCENARIO

Prenatal screening is common in developed countries. The biggest challenge in developing countries is late registration of pregnancy missing the opportunity of first trimester screening. Another challenge is the lack of correct recall of maternal age which forms the basis of ascertaining *a priori* risk of screening. With multiple birth orders and large family sizes, mothers tend to forget the date and at times even the year of their birth. A proportion of these women also do not remember the exact date of last menstrual period necessitating a dating scan for correct risk assignment. Since they do not register in the first trimester, this itself is a challenge. Even when women are registered in the first trimester of pregnancy, feasibility and availability of tests are important issues. Inclusion of nuchal translucency and nasal bone parameters improve detection rates and lower false positive rates in first trimester. However, these measurements require expertise and commitment.

The integrated mode of the screening is likely to pose even a bigger challenge because of the attrition between the first and second trimesters. The second trimester is an opportune window for screening not only neural tube defects but also a wider spectrum of malformations.[14] It is very important for the pediatrician to stress upon the availability of the screening modality to fellow obstetricians as it is ultimately the pediatrician who has to deal with a child having disabilities.

The indecisiveness of families to opt for invasive testing after positive screening test is another hurdle delaying the test beyond the permissible time frame of the Prenatal diagnostic techniques (PNDT) act.

THE WAY FORWARD

Mandatory registration of births and deaths may help us overcome certain challenges. However, this is likely to take some time till the current birth cohort registered by workers grows up to become sexually productive. Prenatal involvement of male partner is associated with beneficial outcomes such as higher first trimester antenatal visits, and abstinence from smoking and alcohol consumption.[15,16] This practice must be encouraged at least until female literacy and empowerment improve.

Gynecologists posted at primary and secondary level of care should be trained in methods of correct ascertainment of gestational age. Radiologists should also be roped in for encouraging early scanning and helping the gynecologists to effectively date the pregnancy. In our setting, the strategy should be to encourage early registration, improve availability of an early scan for gestational age assessment, provide serum screening to all who register within the stipulated period, and offer nuchal translucency and nasal bone measurement in screen positive group. A contingent approach in the first trimester is likely to be more feasible, but is unlikely to become universal due to limited care-seeking during this period.

Resource allocation for such a program is justified by the excellent predictability of first trimester markers to predict adverse pregnancy outcomes. Apart from reducing the financial and social burden from the birth of a child with Down syndrome, it would help gynecologists to identify the subset of women who require closer surveillance and are at a greater risk of developing pre-eclampsia, preterm birth, fetal demise and IUGR. These may also be selected for expert ultrasonic surveillance, both in first and second trimesters. If we take the example of Delhi, approximately 3.6 lakh deliveries take place every year; 63% of these are institutional deliveries.[17] Further, the proportion of women who receive at least one antenatal care visit was 74.4%.[17] Considering this, approximately 75% of pregnant women would be accessible in the second trimester, a time when triple test coupled with a genetic sonogram would pick up more than 70% aneuplodies and a large number of structural defects. Taking Delhi as a model—by implementing screening strategies, approximately 245 births with Trisomy 21 could be prevented every year. We suggest that facilities for collection of samples for triple test should be available at most health facilities. Genetic sonograms currently should be offered in screen positive population, the high risk group and the affordable group. This is probably a trade-off of the limited resources to ensure the best possible yield.

Our second suggestion is implementation of first trimester screening in tertiary-care hospitals. The newer techniques in place can utilize dried blood spots which can be collected at any place and transported across without degradation of biochemical analytes. So the cost of machinery, personnel and expertise need not be duplicated, and the samples collected can be sent to a few centers that are committed and motivated to take up the task of screening. Nuchal translucency and nasal bone parameters can then be used in a contingent manner in the screen positive and high risk group. Preparedness to implement preventive strategies is important today for a better tomorrow.

REFERENCES

1. Kaur G, Srivastav J, Kaur A, Huria A, Goel P, Kaur R, et al. Maternal serum second trimester screening for chromosomal disorders and neural tube defects in a government hospital of North India. Prenat Diagn. 2012;32:1192–6.

2. Saruhan Z, Ozekinci M, Simsek M, Mendilcioglu I. Association of first trimester low PAPP-A levels with adverse pregnancy outcomes. Clin Exp Obstet Gynecol. 2012;39:225–8.

3. Penrose LS. Mongolian idiocy (mongolism) and maternal age. Ann NY Acad Sci. 1954:15;57: 494–502.

4. Benn PA, Fang M, Egan JF, Horne D, Collins R. Incorporation of inhibin-A in second-trimester screening for Down syndrome. Obstet Gynecol. 2003;101:451–4.

5. Hafner E, Schuchter K, Philipp K. Screening for chromosomal abnormalities in an unselected population by fetal nuchal translucency. Ultrasound Obstet Gynecol. 1995;6:330–3.

6. Benn PA. Advances in prenatal screening for Down syndrome: II First trimester testing, integrated testing, and future directions. Clin Chim Act. 2002;324:1–11.

7. Ball RH, Caughey AB, Malone FD, Nyberg DA, Comstock CH, Saade GR, et al. First- and second-trimester evaluation of risk for Down syndrome. Obstet Gynecol. 2007;110:10–7.

8. Wald NJ, Rodeck C, Hackshaw AK, Rudnicka A. SURUSS in perspective. Semin Perinatol. 2005; 29:225–35.

9. Malone FD, Canick JA, Ball RH, Nyberg DA, Comstock CH, Bukowski R, et al. First-trimester or second-trimester screening, or both, for Down's syndrome. N Engl J Med. 2005;353:2001–11.

10. Spencer K. Screening for Down syndrome. Scand J Clin Lab Invest Suppl. 2014;74:41–7.

11. Palomaki GE, Haddow JE. Maternal serum alpha-fetoprotein, age, and Down syndrome risk. Am J Obstet Gynecol. 1987;156:460–3.

12. Dane B, Dane C, Kiray M, Cetin A, Koldas M, Erginbas M. Correlation between first-trimester maternal serum markers, second-trimester uterine artery doppler indices and pregnancy outcome. Gynecol Obstet Invest. 2010;70:126–31

13. Chan YM , Leung TY, Chan OK, Cheng YK, Sahota DS. Patient's choice between a non invasive prenatal test and invasive prenatal diagnosis based on test accuracy. Fetal Diagn Ther. 2014; 35:193–8.

14. Renna MD, Pisani P, Conversano F, Perrone E, Casciaro E, Renzo GC, *et al.* Sonographic markers for early diagnosis of fetal malformations. World J Radiol. 2013;28:356–71.

15. Tweheyo R, Konde-Lule J, Tumwesigye NM, Sekandi JN. Male partner attendance of skilled antenatal care in peri-urban Gulu district, Northern Uganda. BMC Pregnancy Childbirth. 2010; 10:53.

16. Redshaw M , Henderson J. Fathers' engagement in pregnancy and childbirth: Evidence from a national survey. BMC Pregnancy Childbirth. 2013;20:13:70.

17. National Family Health Survey (NFHS-3), India, 2005-06 Mumbai: International Institute for Population Sciences (IIPS) and Macro International; 2009 Available from: *http://www.rchiips.org/nfhs/ NFHS-3%20Data/Delhi_printed_version_ for_website.pdf*. Accessed September 7, 2014.

Incorporating Developmental Screening and Surveillance of Young Children in Office Practice

Sharmila B Mukherjee, Satinder Aneja, Vibha Krishnamurthy, Roopa Srinivasan

Development is a continuous process that occurs normally in childhood, wherein skills are acquired in various inter-related developmental domains. It is intricately influenced by a combination of genetic, biological and psycho-social factors.[1] Pediatricians frequently face parental concerns regarding development and/or behavior.[2] Some of these issues may be transient and easily rectifiable but a small but significant proportion may actually be harbingers of neuro-developmental disorders.

The global prevalence of developmental delay in children is reported as 1–3%, while World Health Organization (WHO) estimates that 15% of the world's population lives with some form of disability.[3,4] There is a paucity of community-based data from lower and middle income countries (LMIC), but a similar or higher prevalence is expected.[5] Due to improving maternal and child health care and better neonatal and child survival, there is now a large group of children at high risk for developmental delay in these countries. In addition, the proportion of children experiencing poverty, ill-health, malnutrition and lack of early stimulation–factors that adversely affect attaining optimum developmental potential–are much more in comparison to high income countries.[1]

One of the main reasons for lack of community-based data from India is the absence of routine developmental screening and surveillance. Developmental surveillance is the longitudinal process of identification and monitoring of newborns and children at high risk.[6] This comprises of eliciting parental concerns, acquiring developmental history, identifying risk and protective factors, evaluation, and maintenance of records.[7] Screening is the brief cross-sectional process of evaluating children by screening tools with good psychometric qualities (sensitivity and specificity >70–80%), that have been norm-referenced and standardized on populations representative of the target population.[5–7] In developed countries, both strategies are core components of the health, education and social care systems.[8] The American Academy of Pediatrics (AAP) recommends developmental surveillance of high-risk children at each health visit from birth to 3 years, and routine screening of low-risk children at 9, 18, and 24/30 months or earlier if concerns are elicited.[7] Screening for behavioral disorders and academic/learning disorders is also recommended.[9] Hix-Small, *et al.*[10] reported an increase in screening in USA after these guidelines were framed, though it is still far from ideal. Lack of screening means delay in detection, initiation of intervention, increased morbidity and parental anguish, more health service utilization and poorer prognosis.[11]

Routine developmental screening in India

In India, there are multiple challenges to practice of universal developmental surveillance and screening. Parents are unaware of the existence and need of these services. Health care seeking is prioritized for acute illnesses which are not appropriate opportunities for screening. A heterogeneous population of doctors with variable proficiency caters to the health needs of Indian children. If parents express concerns, they are often given false assurances without proper appraisal. Well-child visits are primarily for immunization with a few perfunctory questions asked about development, if at all. This was documented in a study of perceptions and practices of 90 pediatricians from Gujarat.[12] Most participants (97.3%) reported parents expressing developmental concerns but only 13.6% used structured tools for evaluation. Reasons cited by those relying on informal assessment were time constraints (72%), non-availability of treatment or referral options (45%), and inability to use screening tools (28%). Contrary to this common misconception, informal evaluation has been proved unreliable in detecting developmental delay. Recognition is difficult in early childhood unless specifically looked for in a structured way, since changes in development are rapid, there is intra-domain overlap, and early indicators are often subtle.

At present, exposure and training in formal developmental screening and assessment is lacking in the post-graduate pediatric curriculum. Pediatricians may be cognitively aware but lack the necessary psycho-motor and communication skills to screen effectively. There is a scarcity of developmental pediatricians. Available assessment tools are mostly of international origin, which are expensive, not easily available, and require training and accreditation. Recommendations for developmental screening by the Indian Academy of Pediatrics (IAP) are yet to be formulated. Although the 'Persons with Disabilities Act, 1995' states that 'children should be screened annually to detect high risk cases', the process is not outlined.[13] In 2013, the '*Rashtriya Bal Swasthya Karyakram (RBSK)*' was launched by the Government of India, which aims at screening for defects at birth, diseases, deficiencies and development delays including disabilities (4 D's) in children between 0 to 18 years.[14] It is envisioned that pre-school children will be screened by *Anganwadi* workers using age-appropriate developmental checklists in the periphery and the positive cases will be re-assessed by trained personnel at the secondary and tertiary care levels. Once this swings into action there will naturally be an upsurge of pediatric consultations by concerned parents, which will need to be tackled responsibly. Reviews of screening tools that may be used in LMICs are available but are hampered by lack of clear guidelines or practice algorithms.[5,15,16]

This article aims at sensitizing pediatricians, reviewing certain general (not domain-specific) developmental screening and monitoring tools validated for use in Indian under-five children, and proposes an office practice paradigm.

DEVELOPMENTAL SCREENING TOOLS IN USE IN INDIA

Screening tools currently in use in India include those developed and validated in high-income countries, translations of the above in Indian languages, and indigenously developed tools. Each type has its own problems. In addition to the drawbacks outlined earlier, internationally acclaimed tools may not be suitable for our populations due to presence of items that are culturally alien or which lose context after translation. They also require validation on large reference groups comprising of healthy children of the target population without conditions averse to development like iron-deficiency anemia, malnutrition, poverty, and decreased stimulation.[17] Translations may be understandable but still face the aforementioned drawbacks, unless validated. Indian tools are language and culturally suitable, have been validated but may not have optimal psychometric properties since most were originally developed largely for community surveys by health workers. Taking these aspects into consideration, a list of screening tools for developmental delay popularly in use or validated in Indian settings was compiled and those that could be administered by pediatricians in any office setting were reviewed. Tools screening for behavior problems or specific domains or overt disability were not included.

Comparing Development Screening Tools

To be able to compare tools qualitatively, it is essential to understand their characteristics. Table 2.1 outlines the definitions and acceptable standards of commonly used psychometric parameters. These are important for making educated decisions regarding quality. If screening tools are not used for their intended purpose (i.e. screening tools being used for diagnosis or in children outside the intended age range), reliability gets compromised. Choice of tools also differs according to level of risk for developmental delay; high-risk

children being those with biological and/or environmental risk factors. Constituent items of tools may be historically based (milestones, opportunity-based skills), performance-based or both. In contrast to developed counties, parental interviews are not as reliable in LMICs due to poorer literacy levels, unawareness of milestones and possibility of socially acceptable responses being given due to associated social stigma.[5,15,16] Interpretation of a screening result as pass or fail is done by comparing with scores derived from standardized population norm-references or pre-decided performance criterion.

Tool Best Suited for Indian Children

Hypothetically, an ideal screening tool for Indian children is a brief, inexpensive tool with good psychometric properties, available in Indian languages, comprising of purely developmental/culturally-adapted items, that has been validated on representative healthy Indian children and requiring minimal training.[17] Such a designer tool does not exist in reality; so each pediatrician has to make an educated choice best suited for individual practice. Developmental tools of International origin are compared in Table 2.2. Only two of these have been validated in Indian children.

TABLE 2.1: Definitions and acceptable standards of development tool-related psychometric properties

Term	Description	Acceptable standard
Standardization	The uniformity of procedure in administering and scoring the test exactly as outlined by the developer of the tool.	On representative population
Validity	The ability of a tool to assess what it is intended to assess in comparison with a gold standard diagnostic tool	70%
Sensitivity	Percentage of children with delay/problem who are correctly identified by the screening test	70–80%
Specificity	Percentage of children without delay/problem who are correctly identified by the screening test	≥80%
Positive predictive value	Percentage of children identified with delay/problem by the screening test who do indeed have the delay/problem	30–50%
Negative predictive value	Percentage of children identified as normally developing by the screening test who are indeed developing normally	+5–7 lines
Reliability Inter-rater Test-retest	How consistently similar results are obtained repeatedly Result variability if test given by different interviewers Result variability when repeated later	High/strong-coefficients >0.60

TABLE 2.2: Comparison of developmental screening tools of International origin

Factors	Denver developmental screening test II (DDST)	Bayley infant neuro-developmental screen (BINS)	Parents evaluation of developmental status (PEDS)	Ages and stages questionnaire (ASQ)	Developmental* Profile II/III (DP)
Age	0–6 years	3–24 month	0–8 years	1–66/3–66 m	0–9 y/12 y 11 m
Format	Directly-administered	Directly-administered	Parent-report	Parent-report	Parent-report
Screens/domains	Expressive and receptive language, gross motor, fine motor, personal, social	Neurological processes, expressive and receptive functions and cognitive	Cognitive, expressive and receptive language fine and gross motor, social-emotional, behavior, self-help and school	Communication, gross motor, fine motor, problem-solving, and personal adaptive skills	Physical, self-help/ adaptive, social/ social-emotional, academic/cognitive and communication
Items	125	11–13	10	22–36	186/180
Scoring/result	Risk category: normal/ abnormal/ questionable	Risk category: high/low moderate	Risk category: low/ medium/high	Pass/fail scores	Total score gives domain wise age equivalents
Time	10–20 min	10 min	2–10 min	10–15 min	10 /20–40 min
Language	English, Spanish	English	English	English, Hindi	English
Psychometric properties	Sensitivity 0.56–0.83 Specificity 0.43–0.80	Sensitivity 0.75–0.86 Specificity 0.75–0.86	Sensitivity 0.74–0.79 Specificity 0.70–0.80	Sensitivity 0.70–0.90 Specificity 0.76–0.91	Validity coefficients* 0.52–0.72
Validated in India	Not validated	Not validated	Sensitivity 62% Specificity 65%	Sensitivity 83.3% Specificity 75.4%	Not validated but used extensively
Cost	$111	$325	$30	$249	$240
Access site	http://www.denverii. com/	www.pearsonassess ments.com	www.pedstest.com	www.brookespub lishing.com/asq	www.wps publish.com

*Internal consistency: 0.89–0.97 and Test-retest reliability: 0.81–0.92

The Denver Developmental Screening Test (DDST) is a very popular and frequently used International screening test.[18–20] However, its low specificity (43%) leads to over identification of false positives, parental apprehension, and burden on the system for diagnosis and intervention. Hence, it is no longer considered appropriate for the purpose of screening. The Bayley Infant Neuro-developmental Screen (BINS) has been used for monitoring children at moderate to severe high risk.[21,22] Though psychometric properties are acceptable, its drawbacks are lack of validation in Indian children and inability to screen children beyond 2 years of age. The Ages and Stages Questionnaire (ASQ) is a parent-completed questionnaire with acceptable properties.[23] In a study by Juneja, *et al.*,[24] ASQ was validated against the Developmental Scale for Assessment of Indian Infants. After being translated into Hindi and substitution of a few culturally inappropriate items, this version of ASQ was administered to parents by an interviewer to screen children aged 4, 10, 18 and 24 months with both high and low risk. The overall sensitivity in detecting developmental delay was 83.3% (higher for the high-risk children), specificity 75.4% and negative predictive value 84.6%. ASQ has the potential to be used in India after being translated into local languages, if interviewer–administration replaces parent-completion when required.

Studies in the West have shown that asking parents about development concerns is reliable for assessment.[25] Parent Evaluation of Developmental Status (PEDS) considers concerns as either 'not predictive' or 'predictive' of developmental disabilities. The latter categorizes children as having high, moderate or Low risk of developmental disabilities. Each is linked with related management protocols: referral, more screening or continued surveillance, respectively. PEDS has been found reliable in other developing countries; however, there is limited literature from India.[19,26,27] The only available study from India was by Malhi, *et al.*[28] in which it was compared with Developmental Profile II (DP II) and Vineland Social Maturity Scale. Psychometric properties were found to be sub-optimal. The authors suggested that PEDS could be used to identify children requiring in-depth screening in situations involving time constraints. The limitations of this study were use of another screening tool as gold standard and a small sample size. Further research is warranted before its value in the Indian context is clarified.[5,15] Developmental Profile III (DP III) is an updated version of DP II that screens for developmental delay in five key areas.[29,30] Its norms are based on a large representative sample of typically developing American children. Although used in India frequently in numerous research studies, it is yet to be validated in Indian children.

These are some Indian screening tools that were designed for community surveys but can be used for office practice. These are easy to perform and interpret, inexpensive, and have been norm-referenced and standardized in representative populations. The main drawback is less than acceptable psychometric properties. Normative data of both Baroda Developmental Screening Test (BDST) and Trivandrum Developmental Screening Chart (TDSC) are derived from the Bayley Scales of Infant Development (BSID) which has not been re-validated since its inception more than 20 years ago.[31] The same drawback lies in the Indian Council Medical Research Psychosocial Developmental Screening Test (ICMR-PDST).[32,33] In the TDSC validation study, the gold standard that was used was not a diagnostic tool but DDST (no longer considered suitable): so the results may be considered questionable until re-validated against a more robust gold standard.[34] These tools are compared in Table 2.3.

Development Screening Tools of the Future

Two promising screening tools may become available for use in the near future. The first– Guide for Monitoring Child Development

TABLE 2.3: Comparison of Indian developmental screening tools

Factors	Baroda developmental screening test (BDST)[24]	Trivandrum developmental screening chart (TDSC)[25]	ICMR psychosocial developmental screening test[27, 28]
Developed from	Bayley scales of infant development, normative data from Indian children	Bayley scales of infant development (Baroda Norms)	Programme for estimating Age-related gentiles using piece-wise polynomials* normative data from Indian children
Age	0–30 m	0–24 m	0–6 y
Format	Directly-administered 54 items	Directly-administered 17 items	Parent interview 66 items
Domains	Motor and cognitive	Mental and motor	Gross motor, vision and fine motor, hearing, language and concept development, self-help and social skills
Scoring/result	Age equivalent and developmental quotient calculated	Within age range	3rd, 5th, 25th, 50th, 75th, 95th and 97th centiles given significant delay <3rd centile (2 SD)
Training	Minimal training	Minimal training	None
Setting	Community/office	Community/office	Community/office
Time taken	10 min	5 min	Minimal
Psychometric properties	Sensitivity: 65–93%, Specificity: 77.4–94.4% PPV: 6.67–34.37%	Sensitivity: 66.8%, Specificity: 78.8%	Not given
Access site and cost	Promila Phatak, Department of Child Development, University of Baroda, India Inexpensive	MKC Nair, Child Developmental Centre Trivandrum, Kerala, India. Inexpensive	ICMR, free

ICMR: Indian Council of Medical Research, PPV: Positive Predictive value; * Child Health and Development, Maternal and Child Health and Family Planning, Geneva, 1992.

(GMCD)—is a parental report-based development monitoring tool for children between 0 to 3.5 years originally developed in Turkey.[8] It comprises of 7 items pertaining to developmental concerns, and takes 5–10 minutes to administer. The sensitivity and specificity are 86% and 93%, respectively. It also has an intervention package that helps in supporting normal development and managing developmental difficulties. A five-year project 'Development of International guide for monitoring child development' is currently underway in India, Turkey, Argentina and South Africa since 2010.[5] The aim of this project is to standardize GMCD for universal use in children irrespective of demographic, cultural or linguistic considerations. The project also aims at examining an approach in which monitoring is done at community health clinics by trained personnel.

The second new kid-on-the-block is the INCLEN Neurodevelopmental Screening Test (NDST) that was developed by the composite efforts of a team of neuro-developmental experts from India and abroad. It screens for 10 neurodevelopmental disorders (NDD): Autism Spectrum Disorders, Learning Disorder, Attention Deficit and Hyperactivity Disorder, Vision Impairment, Hearing Impairment, Intellectual Disability, Speech and Language Disorders, Epilepsy, Cerebral Palsy and other Neuro-Muscular Disorders.

Diagnostic criteria (Consensus Clinical Criteria) have been developed for establishing each diagnosis which are sequentially applied according to an algorithm when the screening test is positive.[35] Application of the NDST in a recently concluded multi-centric validation study in rural, urban, hilly and tribal areas revealed that the prevalence of ≥1 NDD in children aged 2–9 years ranged between 7.5–18.5%.[36]

DEVELOPMENTAL SCREENING IN OFFICE PRACTICE

Setting up routine screening practice involves creating parental awareness and demand, finding the right opportunity, tool selection, acquisition and training in administration, scoring, interpreting results and counseling. This entails planning when, where, and how screenings will be accomplished, devising a method for documenting observations and maintaining records, communicating results to parents, referring to experts for further evaluation when required and scheduling future screenings. Parents can be sensitized by information pamphlets and office displays. Since visits for acute illnesses are not appropriate opportunities; a practical option would be to club screening with pre-existing scheduled visits like immunization and vitamin A prophylaxis. A system needs to be devised to document results, maintain and update records at subsequent visits. Comparison with previous records helps to recognize potential developmental problems or regression, deviancy or dissociation. Experience from other countries has shown that time actually gets saved since it takes the same time that would otherwise have been spent in unstructured questioning and answering other parental queries. Ultimately evaluation time becomes predictable, detection rate increases, parent and provider satisfaction level increases and office attendance increases as parents start appreciating the monitoring process.

An Algorithmic Approach to Developmental Screening

Based on the advantages and drawbacks of the tabulated tools and until consensus statements are formulated by expert groups, the authors suggest a potential practice paradigm for pediatricians based on degree of risk of developmental delay (Fig. 2.1). Preliminary steps involve creating awareness, procuring tools according to the type of patients encountered (low-risk, high-risk or both), and achieving competency in administration, scoring and interpretation. The schedule of screening and follow up monitoring will differ according to level of risk.

Discussing Parental Concerns and Test Outcomes

Parental concerns should always be asked. In the initial visit, if the parent of a low-risk child expresses developmental concerns, the pediatrician is expected to discuss these with the parents and offer options of more frequent and earlier monitoring (as in the high-risk group) or referral for an in-depth evaluation even if the screen is negative. If the parents opt for the former and the concerns persist at the next visit, immediate referral is warranted. If not, monitoring should continue as for the high-risk group, in this group, the first visit recommended by AAP is 4–6 months (coinciding with the 2nd or 3rd immunization visit). The corresponding immunization visit in India would be at 3.5 months. At this age, a small proportion of infants display transient benign tone abnormalities that may be mistaken as pathological. In these instances, the pediatrician should make a note in the child's records and schedule a repeat visit after a month, without unduly alarming the parents. If it persists, in-depth evaluation would be required.

Once screening is complete, it is important to properly convey the significance of the results. If negative, parents should be reassured that development is currently appropriate, anticipatory guidance should be

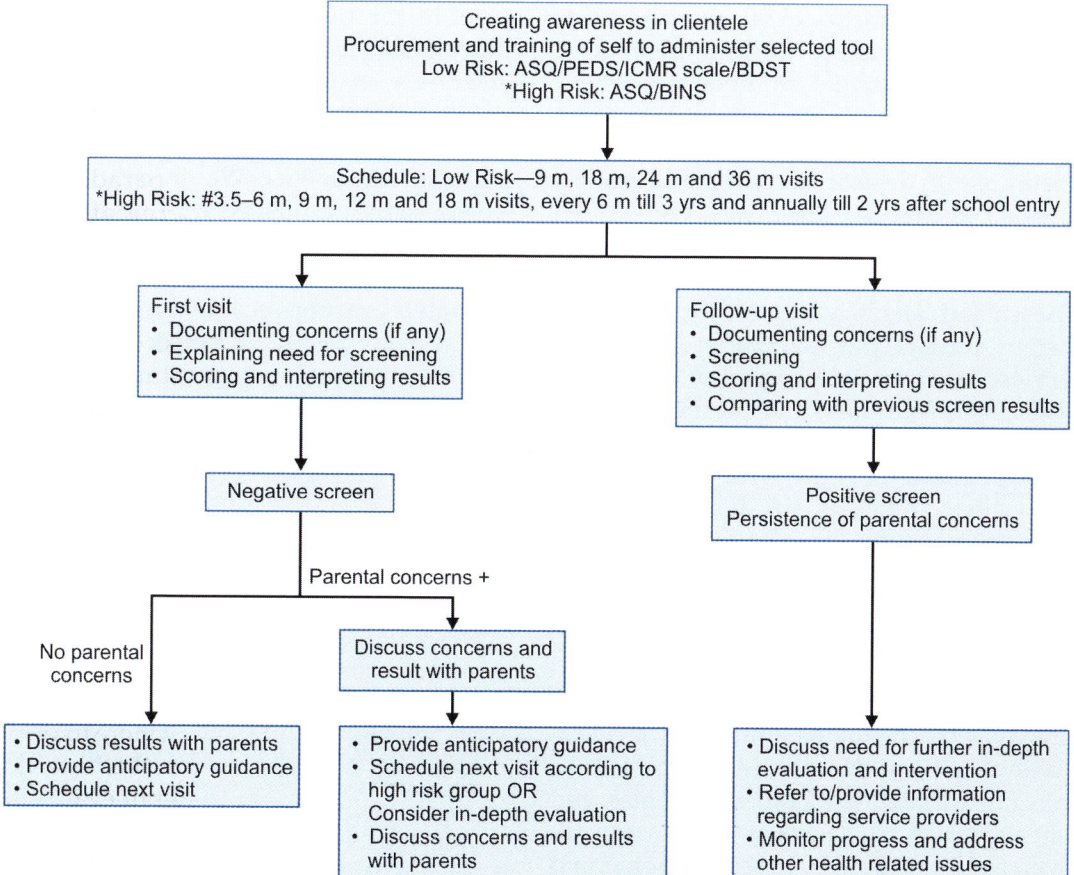

Neonates, infants or children with ≥1 high-risk factors viz., Genetic: positive family history of illness associated with neuro-developmental morbidity; Biological: acute and chronic illnesses, nutritional (macro and micro) deprivation; Environmental: exposure to poverty, violence, neglect, teratogens, arsenic, lead, drugs, etc.; Psycho-social: illiteracy, lack of stimulation, learning opportunities, poor parenting skills, parental illness or substance abuse, maternal depression, etc.; Presence of any parental concerns regarding development. #Abnormality present at 3.5 months: refer to text (discussing parental concerns and test outcomes).

PEDS: Parent evaluation of developmental status; BDST: Baroda developmental screening test; ASQ: Ages and stages questionnaire; BINS: Bayley infant neuro-developmental scren; ICMR: Indian Council of Medical Research.

Fig. 2.1: Proposed schema of office based developmental screening and surveillance

given about expected milestones and the necessity of returning for the next screening visit should be explained and scheduled. If positive, the implications need to be discussed in depth with the parents, and they should be counseled about the need of diagnostic evaluation and start of stimulation or intervention as indicated post evaluation. Since parents have intrinsic faith in us as health care providers of their children, it is our moral responsibility to be instrumental in arranging referrals (by providing contact details or direct communication) as well as providing continual medical help and moral support. It is good practice to develop a two-way communication system with service providers to instill confidence in parents regarding management issues.

Screening should be considered the initial step of intervention services.[37] Unfortunately, it is a common practice to falsely reassure or delay referral to alleviate parental anxiety. Actual practice should be 'Refer not defer.' Failing to refer for diagnosis and intervention after detection on screening is considered unethical.[38] In developed countries, a referral rate of 1/6 children screened is considered optimal.[39] It is important to understand that starting multi-disciplinary intervention (speech and language therapy, occupational therapy, physical therapy, special educational services, etc.) should proceed in parallel to diagnosis establishment and not afterwards. In addition to formal intervention, pediatricians must become familiar with home-based intervention strategies that should be shared with the parents. Development oriented packages have been combined with tools like 'Integrated Management of Child Illnesses–Care for Development' (WHO/UNICEF), GMCD, TDSC and Developmental Assessment Tool for Anganwadis (DATA) or are already in practice at the community level via National Rural Health Mission, RBSK, Integrated Child Development Schemes, and other agencies, the details of which are available, can be practiced by parents at home, and have been proven to be beneficial.[8,14,34,40–45]

CONCLUSION

Many parents and children struggle in their daily lives due to problems arising from undetected development delay. Considering the widespread prevalence of developmental problems, the pediatrician must remain vigilant. By adopting developmental screening and surveillance, one can ensure a systematic approach to children with developmental concerns and help improve their future. Both strategies are integral parts of child healthcare, benefit the individual child and society, and also protect the doctor from possible future litigation. In this review, an attempt has been made to sensitize colleagues to the importance of screening and surveillance, compare existing screening tools and propose those

suitable for Indian children along with strategies for incorporation into office practice. There is a strongly felt need to develop more culturally appropriate, norm-based, valid and reliable Indian developmental screening instruments. We strongly urge that a consensus be formulated at the National level by experts on appropriate developmental surveillance and screening recommendations. Ultimately, earlier recognition of developmental delay results in better inclusion of affected individuals in society, establishment of prevalence data, educated health policy decisions, and resource allocation at the Government level.

REFERENCES

1. Grantham-Mc Gregor S, Cheung YB, Cueto S, Glewwe P, Richter L, Strupp B, *et al*. Child development in developing countries: Developmental potential in the first 5 years for children in developing countries. Lancet. 2007; 369:60–70.

2. Lynch TR, Wildman BG, Smucker WD. Parental disclosure of child psychosocial concerns: relationship to physician identification and management. J Fam Pract. 1997;44:273–80.

3. Bellman M, Byrne O, Sege R. Developmental assessment of children. BMJ: 2013: 346;e8687.

4. World Health Organization, World Bank. World report on disability. Geneva, World Health Organization, 2011. Available from: URL:*http:// www.who.int/disabilities/world_report/2011.* Accessed January 15, 2014.

5. Krishnamurthy V, Srinivasan R. In: Childhood Disability Screening Tools: The South East Asian Perspective. A Review for the WHO Office of the South East Asian Region. Mumbai. WHO, 2011.

6. Dworkin PH. British and American recommendations for developmental monitoring: the role of surveillance. Pediatrics. 1989;84:1000–10.

7. Council on Children with Disabilities, Section on Developmental Behavioral Pediatrics, Bright Futures Steering Committee, Medical Home Initiatives for Children with Special Needs Project Advisory Committee. Identifying infants and young children with developmental disorders in the medical home: an algorithm for developmental surveillance and screening. Pediatrics. 2006;118:405-20.

8. Ertem IO, Dogan DG, Gok CG, Kizilates SU, Caliskan C, Atay G, *et al*. A guide for monitoring child development in low- and middle-income countries. Pediatrics. 2008;121:e581–89.

9. Macias MM, Lipkin PH. Developmental surveillance and screening: refining principles, refining practice. How you can implement the AAP's new policy statement. Contemp Pediatr. 2009;26:72–76.

10. Hix-Small H, Marks K, Squires J, Nickel R. Impact of implementing developmental screening at 12 and 24 months in a pediatric practice. Pediatrics. 2007;120:381–9.

11. Radecki L, Sand-Loud N, O'Connor KG, Sharp S, Olson LM. Trends in the use of standardized tools for developmental screening in early childhood: 2002-2009. Pediatrics. 2011;128:214–19.

12. Desai PP, Mohite P. An exploratory study of early intervention in Gujrat State, India: Pediatricians' perspectives. J Dev Behav Pediatr. 2011;32:69–74.

13. Persons with Disabilities (equal opportunities, protection of rights and full participation) Act, 1995. Part II, section 1 of the Extraordinary Gazette of India, Ministry of Law, Justice and Company affairs (legislative department). Available from: URL: *http://socialjustice.nic.in.* Accessed December 27, 2013.

14. National Rural health mission, Ministry of Health and Family Welfare, Government of India. Rashtriya Bal Swasthya Karyakram (RBSK) Child Health Screening and Early Intervention Services Under NRHM: Operational Guidelines. Nirman Bhavan, New Delhi. 2013.

15. Robertson J, Hatton C, Emerson E. The identification of children with or at significant risk of intellectual disabilities in low and middle income countries: a review. CeDR Research Report. 2009:3.

16. Fernald LCH, Kariger P, Engle P, Raikes A. Examining Early Child Development in Low Income countries: A Toolkit for the Assessment of Children in the First Five Years of Life. World Bank Human Development Group. 2009

17. Lansdown RG. Culturally appropriate measures for monitoring child development at family and community level: A WHO collaborative study. Bull World Health Organ. 1996;74:283 90.

18. Glascoe FP, Byrne KE, Ashford LG, Johnson KL, Chang B, Strickland B. Accuracy of Denver II in development screening. Pediatrics. 1992;89:1221–5.

19. Glascoe FP, Byrne KE. The accuracy of three developmental screening tests. JEI 1993; 17:268–379.

20. Frankenburg WK, Dodds J, Archer P, Shapiro H, Bresnick PB. Denver II: A major revision of re-standardization of Denver Developmental Screening Tool. Pediatrics 1992; 89:91–7.

21. Aylward GP. The Bayley Infant Neuro-developmental Screener. San Antonia, Tex: Psychological Corporation 1995.

22. Macias MM, Saylor CF, Greer MK, Charles Jm, Bell N, Katikaneni LD. Infant screening: the usefulness of the Bayley Infant Neurodevelopmental Screener and the Clinical Adaptive Test/Clinical Linguistic Auditory Milestone Scale. J Dev Behav Pediatr. 1998;19:155–61.

23. Bricker D, Squires J, Potter L. Revision of a parent completed screening tool: Ages and Stages Questionnaires. J Pediatr Psychol. 1997;32:313–28.

24. Juneja M, Mohanty M, Jain R, Ramji S. Ages and Stages Questionnaire as a screening tool for developmental delay in Indian children. Indian Pediatr. 2012;49:457–61.

25. Majnemer A, Rosenblatt B. Reliability of parental recall of developmental milestones. Pediatr Neurol. 1994;10:304–8.

26. Glascoe FP. Parents concerns about children's development: pre-screening technique or screening test. Pediatrics. 1997;99:522–8.

27. Pritchard MA, Colditz PB, Beller EM. Parents evaluation of developmental status in children with a birthweight of 1250 gm or less. J Paediatr Child Health. 2005;41:191–6.

28. Malhi P, Singhi P. Role of Parents Evaluation of Developmental Status in detecting developmental delay in young children. Indian Pediatr. 2002;39:271–5.

29. Alpern G, Boll T, Shearer M. Developmental Profile II (DP II). Los Angeles: Western Psychological Services; 1986.

30. Developmental Profile 3rd Ed. Revised and updated. An Accurate and an Efficient Means to Screen for Development delays. Los Angeles: Western Psychological Services; 2004.

31. Phatak AT, Khurana B. Barado Developmental Screening Test for infants. Indian Pediatr. 1991; 28:31–7.

32. Vazir S, Naidu AN, Vidyasagar P, Landsdown RG, Reddy V. Screening Test for Psychosocial development. Indian Pediatr. 1994;31:1465–75.

33. Malik M, Pradhan SK, Prasuna JG. Screening for psychosocial development among infants in an urban slum of Delhi. Indian J Pediatr. 2007; 74:841–5.

34. Nair MK, George B, Lakshmi S, Haran J, Sathy N. Trivandrum developmental screening Chart. Indian Pediatr. 1991;28:869–72.

35. Gulati S, Aneja S, Juneja M, Mukherjee S, Deshmukh V, Silberberg D, *et al*. INCLEN diagnostic tool for neuro-motor impairments (INDT-NMI) for primary care physicians: Development and validation. Indian Pediatr. 2014;51: 613–9.

36. Silberberg D, Arora N, Bhutani V, Durkin M, Gulati S. Neuro-developmental disorders in India–An INCLEN study. Neurology. 2013; 80:IN6-2.001.

37. Early Headstart National resource Centre. Developmental Screening, Assessment and Evaluation: Key Elements for Individualizing Curricula in Early Headstart Programs. Available from *http://www.zerotothree.org*. Accessed Dec. 27, 2013.

38. Perrin E. Ethical questions about screening. J Dev Behav Pediatr. 1998;19:350–2.

39. Glascoe FP. Screening for developmental and behavioral problems. Dev Disabil Res Rev. 2005; 11:173–9.

40. Department of Child and Adolescent Health Department, WHO. IMCI Care for Development. Available from: *http://www.who.int/maternal_child_adolescenthealth*. Accessed November 19, 2013.

41. Nair MKC, Russell PS, Rekha RS, Lakshmi MA, Latha S, Rajee K, *et al*. Validation of Developmental assessment Tool for Anganwadis (DATA). Indian Pediatr. 2009;46:S27–35.

42. Landis D, Bennett JM, Bennett MJ, (Eds) Handbook of Intercultural Training. 3rd ed. Thousand Oaks, CA: Sage Publications; 2004.

43. Nair MKC. Early stimulation CDC Trivandrum Model. Indian J Pediatr. 1992;59:662–7.

44. Nair MKC. Early Child Development–Kerala Model. Global Forum for Health research, Forum 3 Geneva: WHO 1999.

45. World Health Organization, UNICEF. Counsel the Family on Child Development-Counseling Cards. Available from: *http://www.unicef.org/early childhood*. Accessed December 27, 2013.

Growing Pains: Practitioners' Dilemma

MP Mohanta

Most pediatricians and general practitioners – in their day-to-day office practice–often come across children complaining of pain in their legs. These pains may sometimes point to serious underlying conditions such as malignancies, infections or injuries. However, majority of the cases may be due to 'growing pains', that have a benign and self-limiting course.[1]

Growing pains, though considered benign, can cause considerable anxiety in the parents. Sometimes, the child wakes up in the middle of night with extreme agony, complaining of severe pain in the legs. There are no symptoms in the morning and pediatrician finds no abnormality on physical examination.[2] The pediatrician may be in a dilemma; should parents be simply reassured or the child has to be investigated thoroughly?

This article reviews the current knowledge regarding the diagnosis, etiopathogenesis and management of this fairly common but perturbing condition.

DIAGNOSIS

Growing pains are typically intermittent, nocturnal and poorly localized, usually occurring once or twice per week–though there is never a regular pattern. Children suffering from 'growing pains' are charac-teristically well without any physical problems, despite severe pain experienced in the night. Night awakenings are common but not an essential feature. The usual age group is 4–14 years with equal gender preponderance.[1–3] The diagnostic criteria given by Naish and Apley[4] are: intermittent lower limb pains for at least 3 months duration, not specifically located in the joints, and of sufficient severity to interrupt sleep. The definition provided by Peterson[5] guides clinicians better, and has several inclusion as well as exclusion criteria (Table 3.1). Growing pains is essentially a clinical diagnosis and laboratory investigations or X-rays are unnecessary.[2,6,7]

DIFFERENTIAL DIAGNOSIS

Though diagnosis of growing pain seems easy; there may be a danger of over-diagnosis, if leg pains due to other conditions are not kept in mind.[5,7,8] Entities mimicking growing pains may be grouped under five broad headings (Box 3.1) as follows:

Injury-related leg pains: History is obvious, if there is any trauma, and usually the pain is localized. However, history may not be that obvious in cases of non-accidental trauma or battered child syndrome; presence of injuries of different ages and their inappropriate

TABLE 3.1: Diagnostic criteria for growing pains

Characteristics of pain	Inclusion criteria	Exclusion criteria
Frequency and duration	Intermittent pains once or twice per week, rarely daily, totally pain free in between the episodes; individual episodes lasting for 30 min to 2 hours	Pain, that is persisting or increasing in severity with time
Site	Usually in the muscles of calf, sometimes anterior thigh muscles, shins and popliteal fossa and affects both limbs	a. Pain involving joints b. Pain occurring only in one limb
Time	In the evening and nights	Daytime pain and nocturnal pain that persists till next morning
Physical examination	Normal	Signs of inflammation

explanation may be the clue. Osgood-Schlatter disease is characterized by pain over the tibial tubercle, usually in athletes and more common in boys between ages 10–15 years. Chondromalacia patella or idiopathic adolescent anterior knee pain syndrome (also known as Runner's knee), on the other hand, commonly affects adolescent girl athletes doing a lots of running.[8]

Box 3.1: Differential diagnosis of growing pains

Injury-related
Inflammation of soft-tissue or bone due to sports injuries or accidental injuries or battered child syndrome, Osgood-Schlatter disease, chondromalacia patella

Infections
Osteomyelitis, septic arthritis, cellulitis and soft tissue abscess

Tumors
Benign: Osteoid osteoma, unicameral cyst, fibrous dysplasia, aneurismal bone cyst, gaint cell tumor, histiocytosis X and osteochondroma
Malignant: Osteosarcoma, Ewing's sarcoma, leukemia and neuroblastoma

Developmental and congenital
Slipped capital femoral epiphysis, hypermobile joints, limb deformities such as genu valgum, flat foot, discoid lateral meniscus, patellar subluxation

Others
Legg-Calve-Perthes disease, osteochondritis dissecans, sickle cell crisis, amplified musculoskeletal pain syndromes, restless leg syndrome, juvenile idiopathic arthritis

Infections: There are usually systemic features such as fever and toxicity. Localized tenderness, swelling and erythema at the site of pain may be found on examination.

Tumors: Benign tumors, which produce pain in leg, are usually associated with swelling and are well localized. Pain in Osteoid osteoma can cause night awakening, but it is persistent and gradually increasing in severity as opposed to intermittent painful nights in growing pains.[9]

Malignant tumors that can cause leg pain are associated with systemic features such as fever and weight loss. Osteosarcoma can present with deep bone pain with night awakening, but there is usually a palpable mass.[8]

Slipped capital femoral epiphysis may present as knee pain due to referred pain along the course of obturator nerve. Usually, patients with this disorder have some limp and have externally rotated lower limb and restriction of movements at hip.[9]

Hypermobile joints can produce knee pain, that is worse after activity and relieved by rest. Hypermobile joints have abnormally increased range of motions and may be assessed with the Beighton scale.[8]

Legg-Calve-Perthes disease may present as referred pain in knee, but there is usually associated limp and restriction of movements in hip. Osteochondritis dissecans often presents with vague knee pain. However, localized tenderness over medial femoral condyle may be elicited on careful examination. The leg pain in sickle cell anemia is persistent in nature. Other characteristic features of sickle cell anemia will be difficult to miss by careful history and physical examination.

There are two major forms of amplified musculoskeletal pain syndromes (AMPS); diffuse AMPS and localized AMPS.[8] Diffuse AMPS, also known as juvenile primary fibromyalgia syndrome (JPFS), reveals well defined tender points, and usually affects older child or adolescent with a female preponderance. These children look debilitated; have disturbed personality and daytime symptoms.[8] Localized AMPS, also known as complex regional pain syndrome (CRPS), is characterized by ongoing burning pain in leg subsequent to an injury or other noxious event. Other characteristic features include allodynia, hyperalgesia and autonomic dysfunction.[8]

Restless leg syndrome (RLL) may sometimes be confused with growing pains as both these conditions tend to manifest during the evening hours and are related to discomfort in the legs. However, the uncomfortable feeling in the legs in RLL is associated with an irresistible urge to move the legs, worsened by rest and relieved by movements such as walking or stretching (only as long as motion continues).[10,11] Juvenile idiopathic arthritis may present as leg pains initially, where minimal joint involvement may be missed. The key here is the persistent nature of pain and morning symptoms.[9]

Presence of red flag signs in a child with leg pain should alert a clinician for further investigations (Box 3.2).[8,9]

Box 3.2: Red flag signs in a child with leg pain

  i. Involvement of joints,
 ii. Systemic involvement,
iii. Persistent pain or daytime pain or pain that is localized, and
 iv. Limping.

PREVALENCE AND NATURAL HISTORY

It is believed that growing pains affect about 10–20% of children.[1] Estimated prevalence ranges from 2.6% to 36.9%. This is mainly due to different and unspecified sample sizes, different age ranges in the literature, and lack of objective diagnostic criteria adopted in different studies.[4,12,13]

Abu-Arafeh and Russell determined the prevalence rate to be 2.6%, among school children aged 5–15 years.[14] Evans, et al.[12] estimated the prevalence of growing pains among children aged 4–6 years to be 36.9%, in a well-designed sample using a validated questionnaire. A relatively recent study by Kaspiris and Zafiropoulou[15] reported a prevalence of 24.5% among 532 children of age 4–12 years.

Growing pains is the most common cause of recurrent musculoskeletal pain in children.[1] Two recent studies reported that most of cases of unexplained recurrent limb pains in children could be classified as growing pains.[16,17]

Usually, there is a gradual decline in the frequency of pain episodes over a period of 1 to 2 years and most cases of growing pains resolve by adolescence.[18] Uziel, et al.[19] reported persistence of growing pains in 18 out of 35 cases in 5-year follow up, though the episodes became less frequent and milder. However, more recently, Pavone, et al.[20] reported resolution of all pain episodes of growing pains after 1 year, in all 30 cases.

TERMINOLOGY

The terminology growing pains is being used since 1823, since the condition was first described in medical literature by French physician Marcel Duchamp as *Maladies de la Croissance* (pains of growth).[21] Many authors have raised objections and questioned the validity and rationale of the term.[5] Clearly, these pains cannot be attributed to growth. Peak age for growing pains (4–8 years) corresponds to the relatively slower growth period of childhood. Moreover, the sites of pain (diaphyses) do not match the site of maximal growth (epiphyses).[4] Besides, no difference of rate is seen between the children with and without growing pains.[13] Thus the term growing pains appears to be a misnomer; there is no evidence that growth *per se* can cause pain. Alternate terms such as 'paroxysmal nocturnal pains'[4] and 'recurrent limb pains in childhood'[14] have been suggested. However, these terms are non-specific and describe the disorder incompletely. The terminology benign idiopathic paroxysmal nocturnal limb pains of childhood[9] perhaps describes the condition properly, but sounds too long and inconvenient for general use. On the other hand, the term growing pains has the advantage of emphasizing the benign nature of the disease and indicates that the pain occurs in the growing children, and not after growth is complete.[5] Thus, despite the controversy, the term growing pains enjoys wide acceptance and popularity.[22]

ETIOPATHOGENESIS

In the 19th century, at the time when the term growing pain was coined, growth was considered to be the causative agent of nearly all pains during the childhood.[7] By early 20th century, medical community believed that growing pains were actually a sub-acute form of rheumatic fever.[7,23] Studies of Sheldon in 1936 and thereafter Hawksley in 1939 proved that growing pains are not associated with rheumatic fever.[24,25]

The exact mechanisms, by which these pains occur, are still poorly understood. Some of the theories, put forward to explain the etiology of 'growing pains', are summarized below.[2,3]

Anatomical/mechanical theory: Hawksley observed that growing pains were often associated with postural or orthopedic defects such as flat foot, knock-knee, scoliosis or bad

stance.[25] Mechanical instability such as flexible flat feet with hind foot valgus had been suggested as a cause of growing pains.[20] A small controlled study reported that shoe inserts were effective in reducing the frequency and severity of growing pains.[26] However, subsequent study by the same author did not found any association between foot posture and growing pains.[27] A cross sectional study[28] reported a statistically significant association between joint hypermobility and growing pains. Some cases of growing pains occurring after increased activity may be explained by hypermobile joints. However, due to absence of universally reliable and valid assessment tool for hypermobility in children, the notion of hypermobility causing growing pains remains largely unproved.[3]

Fatigue theory: It was observed that bone strength (based on speed of ultrasound in tibia), in children with growing pains, was significantly lesser than in controls.[2] Often episodes of growing pains are reported on days of increased activity and during the latter part of a day. These observations probably signify that growing pains represent, a *local overuse syndrome* leading to bone fatigue.[7]

Psychological theory: John Apley (1951) found emotional disturbance and family stress to be associated with 'growing pains'.[4] His famous saying *"physical growth is not painful, but emotional growth can hurt like hell"* often gets quoted.[29] Oster (1972) also showed that psychogenic abdominal pains and nervous headaches are more often found in children with growing pains than in other healthy children.[13]

Lower pain threshold: Haskes, *et al.*[30] have recently shown that children with growing pain have decreased pain threshold when compared with the age- and sex-matched controls. They suggested that 'growing pains' may represent a form of non-inflammatory pain amplification syndrome. This was further supported by the findings of Uziel, et al.[19] in a 5-year follow-up study of growing pains. They found a correlation between persistence of symptoms and lower pain threshold. Pathirana, et al.[31] also demonstrated a lower threshold of pain response to cold, vibration and deep pressure in cases of growing pains than in controls.

Other associations: A positive family history associated in some cases of growing pains suggests that there may be a genetic component playing role in the pathogenesis.[3] Some cases of growing pain may be actually having childhood onset, e.g. restless leg syndrome.[11] Children with growing pains may also represent a parasomnia such as sleep walking and sleep terrors.[32] A study found hair of children with growing pain contained increased levels of lead and zinc and decreased levels of copper and magnesium.[33] However, the usefulness of the analysis in the pathogenesis is not validated.[3] In a recent study–Golding, et al.[34] could not find any role of dietary omega-3 fatty acids in the development of growing pains.[34]

Thus growing pains may be caused by lower extremity overuse, in children having lower pain threshold or decreased bone strength.[2,20] The negative psychosocial environment may also be a contributing factor.

MANAGEMENT

The most important component of management is proper explanation regarding the benign nature of growing pains. The family may be reassured that these pains will be resolved in time and will not progress to any serious organic disease.[35] The parents may be advised to use analgesics as well as non-pharmacologic measures to relieve pain such as leg massages, rubbing, and hot fomentation. But it remains unclear whether these interventions actually help to resolve the attack, as the pain episodes are self-limiting. Considering the intermittent nature of pain, use of analgesics on regular or long-term basis can be harmful, and should not be advised.[8]

In this era of evidence-based medicine, treatment modalities proven with randomized controlled trials are the gold standards for management. A randomized controlled trial[36] involving treatment of growing pains described efficacy of a muscle stretching program (involving the quadriceps, hamstrings, and gastrosoleus muscle groups) in faster decline of pain episodes. These exercises may be taught to the parents and done at home twice-a-day for 10 minutes in the morning and at night. This treatment modality has further advantage of providing an extra attention of the parent, fulfilling the psychological needs of the children.[22]

Evans[26] reported use of in-shoe devices such as tri-plane wedges and orthoses was effective in children with pronated foot posture. However, the study involved single-case experimental design, which is much lower in evidence hierarchy.[26] These in-shoe devices may be helpful in selected cases with postural defect.

Widespread vitamin D deficiency is being reported among population at large, and vitamin D may affect body's endocrine system, immune system, cardiovascular system, neuro-psychological functioning and neuro-muscular performance.[37] Thus, it is interesting to know whether vitamin D has any role in management of growing pains. A recent study reported insufficient vitamin D levels in majority of cases with growing pains.[38] However, the study does not mention, if the children without growing pains had different vitamin D levels. Efficacy of vitamin D supplementation in growing pains has not been studied. Currently, there is insufficient evidence to use vitamin D for the management of growing pains. Use of vitamin C, calcium or magnesium etc. have no scientific basis and should not be advocated.

REFERENCES

1. Anthony K, Schanberg L. Musculoskeletal Pain Syndromes. *In*: Kliegman R,Stanton B,Geme III J, Schor N, Behrman R, *editors*. Nelson Textbook of Pediatrics. 19th ed. Philadelphia: Saunders; 2011. *P*. 878.

2. Uziel Y, Hashkes PJ. Growing pains in children. Pediatr Rheumatol Online J. 2007;5:5. Available From: URL: *http://www.ped-rheum.com/content/5/1/5*. Accessed October 10, 2013.

3. Evans AM. Growing pains: contemporary knowledge and recommended practice. J Foot Ankle Res. 2008;1:4.

4. Naish JM, Apley J. 'Growing pains': A clinical study of non-arthritic limb pains in children. Arch Dis Child. 1951;26:134–40.

5. Petersen H. Growing pains. Pediatr Clin North Am. 1986;33:1365–72.

6. Asadi-Pooya AA, Bordbar MR. Are laboratory tests necessary in making the diagnosis of limb pains typical for growing pains in children? Pediatr Int. 2007; 49:833–5.

7. Lowe RM, Hashkes PJ. Growing pains: a non-inflammatory pain syndrome of early childhood. Nat Clin Pract Rheumatol. 2008;4:542–9.

8. Weiser P. Approach to the patient with non-inflammatory musculoskeletal pain. Pediatr Clin North Am. 2012;59:471–92.

9. Foster HE, Boyd D, Jandial S. Growing Pains: A Practical Guide for Primary Care. Arthritis Research UK. Available from URL: http://www.arthritisresearchuk.org/health-professionals-and-students/reports/hands-on/hands-on-autumn-2008.aspx. Accessed December 21, 2013.

10. Brindani F, Francesca, Franco G. Restless leg syndrome: differential diagnosis and management with pramipexole. Clin Interv Ageing. 2009; 4:305–13.

11. Rajaram SS, Walters AS, England SJ, Mehta D, Nizam F. Some children with growing pain may actually have restless leg syndrome. Sleep. 2004;27:767–73.

12. Evans AM, Scutter SD. Prevalence of "growing pains" in young children. J Pediatr. 2004;145: 255–8.

13. Oster J, Neilsen A. Growing pains: clinical investigation of a school population. Acta Pediatr Scand. 1972;61:329–34.

14. Abu-Arafeh I, Russel G. Recurrent limb pain in school children. Arch Dis Child. 1996;74:336–9.

15. Kaspiris A, Zafiropoulou C. Growing pains in children: Epidemiological analysis in a Mediterranean population. Joint Bone Spine. 2009; 76:486–90.

16. De Piano LPA, Golmia RP, Golmia APF, Sallum AME, Nukumizu LA, Castro DG, *et al*. Diagnosis of growing pains in a Brazilian pediatric population: a prospective investigation. Einstein. 2010; 8:430–2.

17. Saha SK, Modak A, Chowdhury K, Uddin MS, Ghosh D, Al-Mamun MA. Diagnosis of growing pain in Bangladeshi pediatric population. J Shaheed Suhrawardy Med Coll. 2013;5:46–8.

18. El-Metwally A, Salminen JJ, Auvinen A, Kautiainen H, Mikkelsson M. Lower limb pain in a preadolescent population: prognosis and risk factors for chronicity–a prospective 1- and 4 –year follow-up study. Pediatrics. 2005;116:673–81.

19. Uziel Y, Chapnick G, Jaber L, Nemet D, Hashkes PJ. Five-year outcome of children with growing pains: Correlation with pain threshold. J Pediatr. 2010;156:838–40.

20. Pavone V, Lionetti E, Gargano V, Evola F, Costarella L, Sessa G. Growing Pains: A study of 30 cases and a review of literature. J Pediatr Orthop. 2011; 31:606–9.

21. Duchamp M. Maladies de la Croissance. *In*: Levrault FG, *editor*. Mémoires de médecine practique. Paris: Jean-Frédéric Lobstein; 1823.

22. Leung A, Robson W. Growing pains. Can Fam Physician. 1991;37:1463–7.

23. Bennie PB. Growing pains. Arch Pediatr. 1894; 11:337–47.

24. Sheldon, W. *In*: Diseases of Infancy and Childhood, London: Churchill; 1936.

25. Hawksley JC. The nature of growing pains and their relation to rheumatism in children and adolescents. BMJ.1939;1:155–7.

26. Evans AM. Relationship between growing pain and foot posture in children: single case experimental design in clinical practice. J Am Pediatr Med Assoc. 2003;93:111–7.

27. Evans AM, Scutter SD. Are foot postures and functional health different in children with growing pains? Pediatr Int. 2007;49:991–6.

28. Viswanathan V, Khubchandani RP. Joint hypermobility and growing pains in school children. Clin Exp Rheumatol. 2008;26:962–6.

29. Apley J. Clinical Canutes. A philosophy of paediatrics. Proc R Soc Med. 1970; 63:479–84.

30. Haskesh PJ, Friedland O, Jaber L, Cohen A, Wolach B, Uziel Y. Decreased pain threshold in

children with growing pains. J Rheumatol. 2004; 31:610–3.

31. Pathirana S, Champion D, Jaaniste T, Yee A, Chapman C. Somatosensory test responses in children with growing pains. J Pain Res. 2011; 4:393–400.

32. Aeschlimann FA, Werner H, Jenni OG, Saurenmann RK. Are growing pains a parasomnia. Pediatr Rheumatol. 2012;10:A78.

33. Lech T. Lead, copper, zinc, and magnesium levels in hair of children and young people with some disorders of the osteomuscular articular system. Biological Trace Element Res. 2002;89:111–25.

34. Golding J, Northstone K, Emmett, Steer C. Do ω-3 or other fatty acids influence the development of growing pains? A pre-birth cohort study. BMJ Open. 2012;2:e001370.

35. Goodyear-Smith F, Arrol B. Growing pains. parents and children need reassuring about this self-limiting condition of unknown cause. BMJ. 2006;333:456–7.

36. Baxter MP, Dulberg C. Growing Pains in childhood—A proposal for treatment. J Pediatr Orthop.1988;8:402–6.

37. Rathi N, Rathi A. Vitamin D and child health in the 21st century. Indian Pediatr. 2011;48:619–25.

38. Qamar S, Akbani S, Shamim S, Khan G. Vitamin D levels in children with growing pains. J Coll Physicians Surg Pak. 2011;21:284–7.

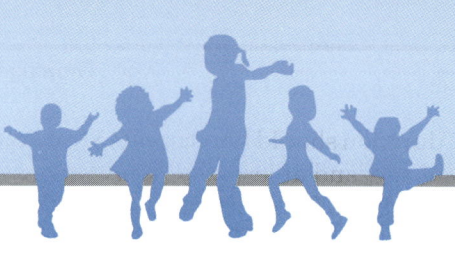

Approach to Constipation in Children

Ujjal Poddar

Constipation is a common problem in children and it accounts for 3% of visits to general pediatric clinics and as many as 30% of visits to pediatric gastroenterologists in developed countries.[1] There is very little information about its prevalence from developing countries. However, some recent reports from South Asia have suggested that it is not uncommon in Asia.[2–4] The common perception in South Asia is that functional constipation is uncommon as diet here is rich in fiber. Hence, many children with constipation are subjected to detailed investigations to rule out Hirschsprung disease. However, whatever limited information we have from Asia shows that functional constipation is the commonest type of constipation in Asia as well.[2–4] The prevalence, etiology, pathogenesis, assessment and management of constipation in children is discussed in this review.

decreased significantly at 3 months of age to 2 (0–6) per day. Moreover, there was a significant difference in stool frequency between breastfed and formula-fed babies at 1 month of age [4 (0–9) *vs.* 1 (0–5) per day, respectively, $P<0.01$] but there was no difference at 3 months of age [2 (0–6) *vs.* 1 (0–5) per day].[5,6] Another study from Turkey in 911 children aged 0 to 24 months has shown that the median defecation frequency at 1 month of age was 6 per day and by 4–6 months of age it became 1 per day. The most interesting observation of this study is that the stool frequency was <1 per day (once in 2–3 days but soft stool) in 39.3% babies in 2–6 months of age.[7] Hence, while considering constipation we should remember the normal variations of stool frequency and consistency in healthy infants and variations as per their feeding pattern (breastfed *versus* bottlefed).

STOOL PATTERN OF NORMAL INFANTS

Normal variation in stool frequency and consistency often leads to over-diagnosis of constipation especially in infants. Two recent studies from the Europe (12,984 healthy children, 1–42 months from UK[5] and 600 healthy infants from Netherlands[2]) have shown that the median stool frequency at 1 month of age was 3 (0–9) per day and it

DEFINITION OF CONSTIPATION

In view of wide variations in stool frequency and consistency in normal healthy children, ROME III criteria[8,9] have included other variables besides frequency of stool to define constipation in children. As per ROME III criteria, functional constipation is defined as presence of two or more of the following in absence of any organic pathology and the duration should be at least 1 month in <4 years of age, and at least once per week for at least 2 months in ≥4 years of age; (i) two or less defecations per week, (ii) at least one episode of fecal incontinence per week, (iii) history of retentive posture or stool withholding maneuver, (iv) history of painful or hard bowel movement, (v) presence of large fecal mass in the rectum, (vi) history of large-diameter stools that may obstruct the toilet. In children <4 years of age, the history of retentive posture or stool withholding maneuver is being replaced by history of excessive stool retention as retentive posture is difficult to assess in younger children.

PREVALENCE

Constipation is a common problem in children and an estimated prevalence of functional constipation is 3% worldwide.[1,10,11] Though, we do not have any prevalence data from Asia, in a study from our center we reported 138 cases of constipation diagnosed over a period of 6 years and 85% of them were functional.[2] In next 8 years (2007 to 2014), we managed another set of 330 children with constipation and the proportion of functional constipation was 82% (270 of 330) (unpublished data). Hence, constipation is not uncommon in the Indian subcontinent. It is commonly seen among toddlers and preschool children, and in 17% to 40% of cases, constipation starts in first year of life.[12,13]

ETIOLOGY

The common perception in South Asia is that functional constipation is uncommon as diet in South Asia is rich in fiber. In our study,[2] we have shown that this perception is incorrect. Constipation is quite common in India and functional constipation is the commonest cause. Common causes of constipation in children are given in Box 4.1. In fact 95% cases are due to functional and only 5% are due to some organic causes.[14] Among the organic

Box 4.1: Causes of constipation in children

- Functional constipation of childhood
- Motility related: Hirschsprung disease, myopathy
- Congenital anomalies: Anal stenosis, anteriorly located anus, spinal cord anomalies (meningo-myelocele, myelomalacia, spina bifida)
- Neurological: Cerebral palsy, mental retardation
- Endocrine/metabolic: Hypothyroidism, renal tubular acidosis, diabetes insipidus, hypercalcemia
- Drugs: Anticonvulsants, antipsychotic, codein containing anti-diarrheal

causes, Hirschsprung disease is the most common and important cause.[2]

Pathogenesis of Functional Constipation (Fig. 4.1)

The initiating event in functional constipation is a painful bowel movement which leads to voluntary withholding of stools by the child who wants to avoid unpleasant defecation.[15] Events that lead to initial painful defecation are change in routine like timing of defecation or diet, stressful events, inter-current illness, non-availability of toilets (travel etc.), child's postponing defecation because he or she is too busy (morning school), and forceful toilet training (too early). All these events give rise to large, hard stool and passage of such stool leads to stretching of the pain sensitive anal canal, and that frightens the child. As a result of which the child fearfully determines to avoid defecation by all of means. Such children respond to the urge to defecate by contracting their external anal sphincter and gluteal muscles, in an attempt to withhold stool. Withholding of feces leads to prolonged fecal stasis in the rectum, with resultant absorption of fluids and harder stools. Successive retention of stools in rectum make them larger. As the cycle is repeated, successively greater amounts of larger and harder stools are built up in the rectum and passed with even greater pain accompanied by severe "stool with-holding maneuvers". Thus a vicious cycle sets-in (Fig. 4.1). These children develop a "stool-withholding maneuver" or retentive posture

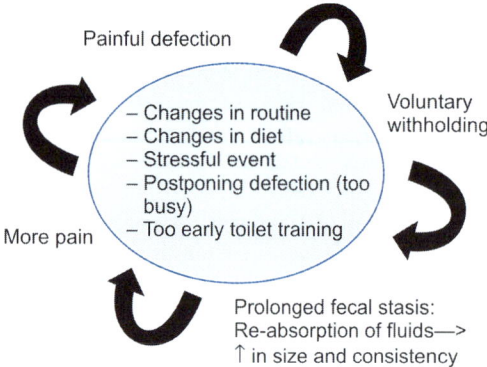

Painful defection

Voluntary withholding

– Changes in routine
– Changes in diet
– Stressful event
– Postponing defecation (too busy)
– Too early toilet training

More pain

Prolonged fecal stasis: Re-absorption of fluids—> ↑ in size and consistency

Fig. 4.1: Pathogenesis of functional constipation

which parents erroneously think it as an attempt to defecate. They feel that the child is trying hard (straining) in an attempt to pass stool when the child is actually trying his best to stop it. In response to the urge, they refuse to sit on the toilet, rather rise on their toes, hold their legs and buttocks stiffly and often rock back and forth, holding on to a furniture, scream, turn red until a bowel movement finally takes place. With time, such retentive behavior becomes an automatic reaction. They often perform this while hiding in a corner. Eventually, liquid stool from the proximal colon may percolate around hard retained stool and pass per rectum involuntarily (fecal incontinence). Sometimes, this fecal incontinence is mistaken as diarrhea. In fact almost 30% children with functional constipation develop fecal incontinence.[12] Eventually, with more and more stasis, the rectum becomes dilated and redundant, and the sensitivity of the defecation reflex and the effectiveness of peristaltic contractions of rectal muscles decrease. This is the stage when it becomes more difficult to have a normal defecation due to fecal impaction.

ASSESSMENT OF A CHILD WITH CONSTIPATION

A careful history and thorough physical examination (including digital rectal examination) are all that is required to diagnose functional constipation provided, there are no "red flags" like fever, vomiting, bloody

diarrhea, failure to thrive, anal stenosis, and tight empty rectum.[16] Abnormal physical findings, which help to distinguish organic causes of constipation from functional, are failure to thrive, lack of lumbo-sacral curve, sacral agenesis, flat buttock, anteriorly displaced anus, tight and empty rectum, gush of liquid stool and air on withdrawal of finger, absent anal wink and cremasteric reflex. Features which differentiate Hirschsprung disease from functional constipation are given in Table 4.1. The most important features in the history, which help to distinguish Hirschsprung disease from functional constipation, are onset in first month of life and delayed passage of meconium beyond 48 hours and the most important examination finding is empty rectum on digital rectal examination. It has been shown that 99% healthy, term neonates and 50% babies with Hirschsprung disease pass meconium in first 48 hours of life.[17,18] In fact, in a classical case of functional constipation, no investigation is required to make the diagnosis. There is no need to do barium enema in all cases of constipation to rule out Hirschsprung disease. If the clinical suspicion of Hirschsprung disease is strong (based on history of delayed passage of meconium and empty rectum on digital rectal examination) then only one may consider getting barium enema done.

TABLE 4.1: Differences between functional constipation and Hirschsprung disease

Features	Functional constipation	Hirschsprung disease
Delayed passage of meconium	None	Common
Onset	After 2 years	At birth
Fecal incontinence	Common	Very rare
History of fissure	Common	Rare
Failure to thrive	Uncommon	Possible
Enterocolitis	None	Possible
Abdominal distension	Rare	Common
Rectal examination	Stool	Empty
Malnutrition	None	Possible

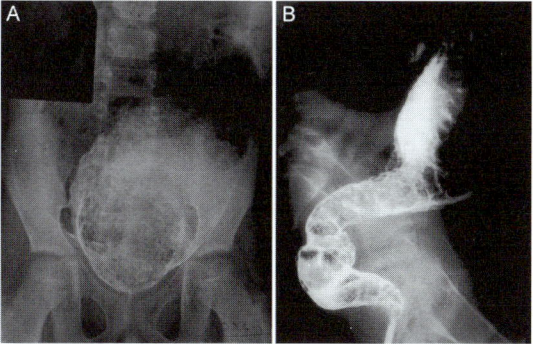

Fig. 4.2: (A) Barium enema (delayed film) of functional constipation; (B) Barium enema of a patient with Hirschsprung disease

However, to diagnose Hirschsprung disease, rectal biopsy is a must. The common mistake that leads to further confusion is delayed film (24 hours) showing retention of barium which is a common finding in functional constipation as well. The interpretation of barium enema should be on the basis of reversal of recto-sigmoid ratio (sigmoid becomes more dilated than rectum) and documentation of transition zone and not on mere presence of barium in rectum after 24 hours (Fig. 4.2).

MANAGEMENT

Most children with functional constipation get benefited from a precise, well-organized treatment plan, which includes cleaning of fecal retention, prevention of further retention and promotion of regular bowel habits. The general approach includes the following steps: (a) determine whether fecal impaction is present, and treat the impaction if present, (b) initiate maintenance treatment with oral laxative, dietary modification, toilet training, and (c) close follow-up and medication adjustment as necessary.[16] Suggested approach to constipation is given in Fig. 4.3.

Disimpaction

First step in the management of constipation is to decide whether the child has fecal impaction or not. This can be accomplished by abdominal examination (in half of the cases hard fecal mass or fecalith is palpable in the lower abdomen),[19] by digital rectal examination (rectum is usually loaded with hard stools), or rarely by abdominal X-ray. Routinely abdominal X-ray is not required to detect fecal

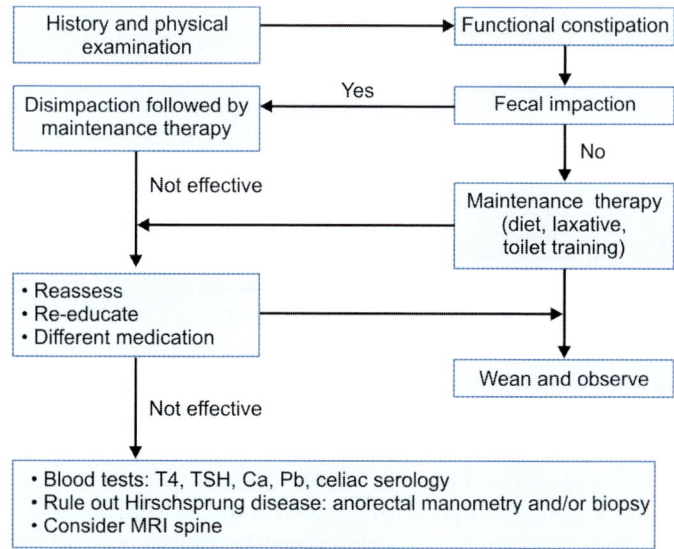

Fig. 4.3: Suggested approach to functional constipation. Modified from ESPGHAN recommendations

impaction. However, if the child refuses rectal examination, if he/she is obese, or if there is a doubt about the diagnosis of constipation then only an abdominal X-ray is required to document excess fecal matter in the colon.

If there is fecal impaction (most of the children with functional constipation do have), then the first step in the management is disimpaction, means clearing or removal of retention from the rectum. This can be achieved by oral or by rectal route. Oral route is non-invasive, gives a sense of power to the child but compliance is a problem. Poly-ethylene glycol (PEG) lavage solution is given orally (1–1.5 g/kg/day for 3–6 days) or by nasogastric tube (25 mL/kg/h, reconstituted PEG solution) until clear fluid is excreted through anus. Adequate disimpaction means both output (stool) and input (lavage solution) should be of same color in case of nasogastric tube disimpaction.[16] Successful disimpaction for home-based regimen (3–6 days) is defined as either empty or a small amount of soft stool on rectal examination and resolution of the left lower quadrant mass if it was there.[20, 21]

Rectal approach (enema) is faster but invasive, likely to add fear and discomfort that the child already has in relation to defecation. This may aggravate defecation avoidance or retention behavior and usually not preferred. However, if PEG is not available then enema can be used for disimpaction [sodium phosphate enema (proctoclysis): 2.5 mL/kg, maximum 133 ml/dose for 3–6 days].[16] In a retrospective chart review of 223 children, Guest, et al.[22] have shown that 97% children treated with PEG were successfully dis-impacted compared to 73% of those who received enemas and suppositories (*P* <0.001). In a randomized-controlled trial, Bekkali, et al.[20] have compared 6 days enemas with dioctyl sodium sulfosuccinate (60 mL in <6 years and 120 mL in ≥6 years) in 46 children with PEG in 44 children and showed that both were equally effective for disimpaction. However, two retrospective studies have shown that the reimpaction rate after initial

disimpaction with enemas was much more than that with PEG.[22,23] For infants, glycerine suppositories are to be used for disimpaction as enemas and lavage solution are not indicated in them.[16]

Maintenance Therapy

To prevent re-accumulation after removing impaction maintenance therapy in the form of dietary modification, toilet training and laxatives needs to be started immediately after disimpaction or if there is no impaction, then as a first step.

Dietary modification: The diet of most children with functional constipation lacks fiber. Many of them are predominantly on milk with very little complementary food. The children with functional constipation should be encouraged to take more fluids, absorbable and non-absorbable carbohydrate as a method to soften stools. Non-absorbable carbohydrate (sorbitol) is found in some fruit juices like apple, pear and prune juices. A balanced diet that includes whole grains, fruits and vegetables is advised. The recommended daily fiber intake is age (in years) + 5 in g/day. In our practice, where most children are predominantly on milk diet, we counsel the parents to restrict milk so that the child starts eating solid foods. Though cow milk protein allergy (CMPA) was proposed as one the common causes of constipation,[24] subsequent studies[16,25] and our experience did not substantiate that claim.

Toilet training: It should be imparted after 2 to 3 years of age. Too early and vigorous toilet training may be detrimental for the child. The child is encouraged to sit on the toilet for 5 to 10 minutes, 3 to 4 times a day immediately after major meals for initial months.[26] The gastro-colic reflex, which goes into effect shortly after a meal, should be used to advantage.[27] Children are encouraged to maintain a daily record (*stool diary*) of bowel movements, fecal soiling, pain or discomfort, consistency of stool and the laxative dose. This helps to monitor compliance and to make appropriate adjustment in the treatment program. Parents are instructed to follow a reward system. Children should be rewarded for not soiling and for regular sitting on the toilet. This acts as a positive reinforcement for the child.

Laxatives: Doses and side effects of various laxatives are presented in Table 4.2.[28] It has been shown that lactulose, sorbitol, milk of magnesia (magnesium hydroxide), and mineral oil (castor oil), all are equally effective in children. Milk of magnesia and mineral oil are unpalatable and due to the risk of lipoid pneumonia mineral oil is contraindicated in infants. The commonly used laxative in children so far was lactulose, until the introduction of PEG. The study by Loening-Baucke[26] has shown that low volume (0.5 to 1 g/kg/day) polyethylene glycol (PEG) without electrolytes is as effective as milk of magnesia in the long-term treatment of constipation in children. Low volume PEG has been compared with lactulose in the treatment of childhood functional constipation and a meta-analysis of five RCTs comprising of 519 children has shown that PEG was more effective than lactulose with equal tolerability

and fewer side effects.[29] Side effects, especially bloating and pain are less with PEG. With long term use, lactulose loses its efficacy due to change in gut flora but PEG does not.[30] The dose of laxative should be adjusted to have one or two soft stools/day without any pain or soiling. Once this target is achieved, the same dose should be continued for at least 3 months to help the distended bowel to regain its function. Point to be remembered here is that laxative needs to be continued for several months and sometimes years at the right dose. Early and rapid withdrawal is the commonest cause for recurrence. Stimulant laxatives (senna, bisacodyl) are not used routinely and are contraindicated in infants. They may be used for a short course in refractory cases as a rescue therapy.[16]

Follow-up Schedule

A close and regular follow-up is a key to the success of treatment of functional constipation. Initial follow-up should be monthly till a regular bowel movement is achieved. After that it should be 3 monthly for 2 years and then yearly.[26] On each visit, by reviewing stool records and repeating abdominal and (if

TABLE 4.2: Laxatives–dosage and side effects (modified from NASPGHAN position statement)[28]

Drugs	Dose	Side effects
Lactulose	1–2 g/kg, 1–2 doses	Bloating, abdominal cramps
Sorbitol	1–3 mL/kg/d, 1–2 doses	Same as lactulose
Milk of Magnesia	1–3 mL/kg/d, 1–2 doses	Excess use leads to hypocalcemia, hypermagnesemia, hypophosphatemia
PEG		
for disimpaction	25 mL/kg/hr (R/T) or 1–1.5 g/kg for 3–6 d	Nausea, bloating, cramps, vomiting
for maintenance	5–10 mL/kg/d or 0.4 to 0.8 g/kg/d	
Mineral oil		
for disimpaction	15–30 mL/y of age (max. 240 mL)	Lipoid pneumonia, interference with absorption of fat soluble vitamins
for maintenance	1–3 mL/kg/d	
Senna	2–6 y: 2.5–7.5 mL/d (8.8 mg/5 mL) 6–12 y: 5–15 mL/d	Melanosis coli, hepatitis, hypertrophic osteoarthropathy, neuropathy
Bisacodyl	0.5–1 suppository (10 mg)1–3 tabs/dose (5 mg)	Abdominal pain, diarrhea, hypokalemia

PEG: Polyethylene glycol; R/T: Ryle's tube

required) rectal examination, progress should be assessed. If necessary, dosage adjustment is to be made. Once a regular bowel habit is established, the laxative dosage is to be decreased gradually before stopping.

Outcome

In a long-term follow up study [mean (SD), 6.9 2.7 years] on 90 children, who were <4 years at diagnosis, Loening-Baucke[31] showed that 63% had recovery but symptoms of chronic constipation persisted in one-third of cases 3 to 12 years after initial evaluation and treatment. In another study, it has been shown that 50% of patients were off laxative at 1 year, another 20% at 2 years and the remaining 30% were on laxative for many years.[14] von Ginkel, et al.[32] in a long-term follow-up (mean 5 years) study on 418 cases have also shown that 60% were successfully treated at 1 year but 30% of cases in the 16 years or older age group continued to have constipation. They found that age at onset of constipation (<4 years) and associated fecal incontinence were poor prognostic factors. In a large study on 300 children, Clayden[33] has shown that 22% required laxative for <6 months, 44% for <12 months and 56% for >12 months. By summarizing all these studies it can be said that half to two-thirds of children with functional constipation had successful outcome with laxative therapy for 6 to 12 months but the remaining one-thirds require long-term therapy and they may continue to have constipation as an adult. Recurrence of constipation after initial recovery is common (50% may have relapse within a year of stopping therapy) but they respond well to retreatment.[12] Poor prognostic factors are; early onset (<4 years), associated with fecal incontinence, and longer duration of symptoms (>6 months).[16]

REFRACTORY CONSTIPATION

A case of constipation is labeled as refractory when there is no response to optimal conventional treatment for at least 3 months.[6]

The prevalence of refractory constipation is said to be 20–30%[16, 34] but the prevalence is much higher in India at primary care pediatrician level due to lack of awareness about optimal conventional treatment. At primary care level, disimpaction is hardly practiced and as a result of which the response of laxative therapy is not optimal. The second important reason is early discontinuation of therapy which leads to refractoriness of constipation. The true refractory constipation is extremely uncommon in primary care set up. Even at tertiary care centers, refractory constipation is uncommon.[2]

Besides organic causes of constipation, motility disorders (like slow transit constipation), disorders of stool expulsion like dyssynergic defecation, internal anal sphincter achalasia and sphincter dysfunction in children with Hirschsprung disease which persist after surgery are important causes of refractory constipation.[34] While approaching refractory constipation common organic causes like Hirschsprung disease, hypothyroidism, celiac disease, hypercalcemia, spinal cord abnormalities should be ruled out first and then motility studies [like colon transit time (CTT), anorectal manometry with balloon expulsion test, colonic manometry] to be done to find out motility disorders.[34,35] The simplest and the most informative of all these tests is colon transit time (CTT) study which can be done by radio-opaque markers and by radionuclide scintigraphy (NTS or nuclear transit studies).[34] In radiographic CTT study, a capsule containing 20 radio-opaque markers (different shape in different days) are given daily for 3 days and plain X-ray abdomen is taken on day 4 and if required on day 7 (when all markers are retained on day 4). From X-ray, markers are counted in right colon, left colon and recto-sigmoid regions and the mean segmental time is calculated. Slow transit constipation is defined as retention of markers for 62 hours or more.[36,37] As per the CTT study, constipation can be divided into three categories; (i) normal transit constipation,

(ii) functional outlet obstruction or dys-synergic defecation (retention of markers in rectosigmoid region) and (iii) slow transit constipation (retained markers are distributed all over) (Figs 4A and B). In a study of 225 children (135 pediatric constipation, 56 non-retentive fecal incontinence and 24 recurrent abdominal pain) Benninga, *et al*.[36,37] have shown that 56% of constipated children had normal CTT, 24% had functional outlet obstruction and just 20% had slow transit constipation. In another study on 85 children with functional constipation with rectal fecal impaction by Bekkali, *et al*.[20] have shown that 93% had delayed CTT and as expected majority (83.5%) of them had delayed rectosigmoid segment CTT. As the basic pathophysiology of functional constipation is voluntary withholding of feces, it is expected that most children with functional constipation will have either functional outlet obstruction/dyssynergic defecation or normal transit constipation.

In normal defecation there is synchronized relaxation of puborectalis muscle (makes ano-rectal angle straight) and external anal sphincter along with generation of propulsive force through contraction of colon and increased in intra-abdominal pressure, which propels stools out of rectum. In dyssynergic defecation, there is paradoxical contraction or failure of relaxation of external anal sphincter and puborectalis muscle with or without increased rectal pressure (propulsive force).[38] These features are detected on anorectal manometry. Therapeutic option of refractory constipation due to dyssynergic defecation is biofeedback (to restore the normal pattern of defecation) and for slow transit constipation is to enhance colonic transit with newer drugs like colon-specific prokinetics like prucalo-pride (5HT4 agonist)[39] and intestinal secretagogue (lubiprostone),[40] which increases intestinal chloride secretion and accelerates small intestinal and colonic transit. Antegrade continence enema helps in refractory slow transit constipation cases.[41]

Most reports of slow transit constipation in children are from Australia and the clinical presentations of this subset of patients are different from functional constipation (Box 4.2). In a study of 100 children with slow transit

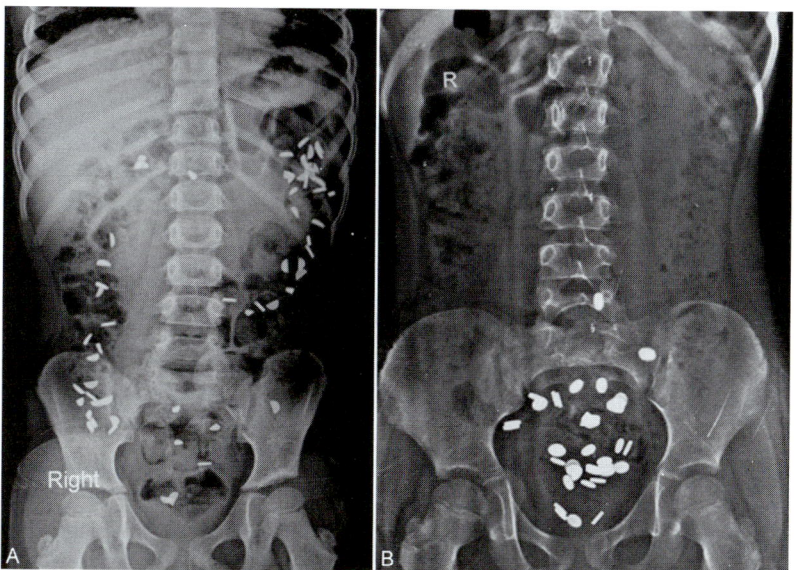

Fig. 4.4: (A) Colon transit time (CTT) study by radio-opaque markers showing slow transit constipation; (B) Functional outlet obstruction

- High frequency of delayed passage of meconium
- Onset of symptoms early in first year and/or failure to toilet training
- Feces soft rather than rock hard
- Failure of high fiber diets (they tend to make symptoms worse)
- Global delay in colonic transit on transit study.

constipation, Hutson, *et al.*[42,43] have shown that a history of delayed passage of meconium was seen in 30% of cases, onset of severe constipation in infancy in 63% and half (52%) of those presenting after 2 years of age had history of soiling (fecal incontinence) and failure of toilet training, and the majority (90%) had no hard fecal mass in rectosigmoid area. The management of slow transit constipation is quite difficult as they do not respond to conventional laxative therapy and the main concern is soiling. Fiber therapy is contraindicated (as the motility is slow), the newer drugs like colon-specific prokinetics like prucalopride[39] and chloride channel activator (lubiprostone)[40] are still investigational drugs in children. The only effective therapy for this subset of patients is antegrade continence enema. Here, appendix is used as conduit to insert cecostomy button (Chait trapdoor button) to give enema.[44,45] It has minimal scar and just a button at right iliac fossa which is used in the morning to give antegrade enema and the whole day patient remains dry (no soiling). In a recent study on 203 cases (median age 10 years, follow-up 5.5 years, 62% due to refractory chronic idiopathic constipation) of this modality, Randall, *et al.*[41] showed good result in 93%, soiling prevented in 75% and symptoms resolved (no longer on antegrade continence enema) in 26% (81% of them were chronic idiopathic constipation).

Colonic manometry plays an important role in guiding both medical and surgical treatment in refractory constipation. In fact, it has been shown that the success of antegrade continence enema procedure depends on colonic manometry results.[46] If there is generalized colonic dysmotility [absence of high-amplitude propagating contraction [HAPC] in the entire colon] then there is no point in putting cecostomy catheter. Similarly, colonic manometry results can dictate the type of surgery following colonic diversion; subtotal colectomy if small bowel motility is normal but whole colonic motility is abnormal, left hemicolectomy if only left colonic motility is abnormal and reanastomosis if colonic motility is normal.[47]

A relatively less common but important cause of refractory constipation is internal anal sphincter achalasia. In a study of 332 patients with severe constipation, De Caluwe, *et al.*[48] have reported this as a cause in just 4.5% of cases. This subset of patients usually present with severe constipation (99.7%) which often associated with fecal incontinence (46%) and are diagnosed by absence of anorectal inhibitory reflex (ARIR) on anorectal manometry along with presence of ganglion cell on rectal biopsy.[49] The treatment options for internal anal sphincter achalasia are posterior anal sphincter myectomy and intrasphincteric botulinum toxin injection. In a recent meta-analysis, it has been shown that former is better.[49]

CONCLUSION

Constipation is quite common in Asia, and most often of functional origin. Detailed history and proper physical examination, including digital rectal examination, can easily differentiate functional from organic constipation. There is no need to do any investigation before starting treatment in functional constipation. Disimpaction with oral polyethylene glycol is the main step in the management and skipping this step leads to refractoriness of constipation. Polyethylene glycol is shown to be superior to lactulose in the management of constipation. In most cases, prolonged (months to years) laxative therapy is required and early withdrawal leads to recurrence.

Radiological colon transit time study plays an important role in the management of refractory constipation. Slow transit constipation is altogether a different entity and antegrade continence enema helps in this subset of patients.

REFERENCES

1. Van den Berg MM, Benninga MA, Di Lorenzo C. Epidemiology of childhood constipation: a systematic review. Am J Gastroenterol 2006; 101:2401–9.

2. Khanna V, Poddar U, Yachha SK. Constipation in Indian children: need for knowledge not the knife. Indian Pediatr. 2010;47:1025–30.

3. Rajindrajith S, Devanaryana NM, Adhikari C, Pannala W, Benninga MA. Constipation in children: an epidemiological study in Sri Lanka using Rome III criteria. Arch Dis Child. 2012; 97:43–5.

4. Aziz S, Fakih HAM, Di Lorenzo C. Bowel habits and toilet training in rural and urban dwelling children in a developing country. J Pediatr. 2011; 158:784–8.

5. Steer CD, Emond AM, Golding J, Sandhu B. The variation in stool patterns from 1 to 42 months: a population bases observational study. Arch Dis Child. 2009;94:231–4.

6. den Hertog J, van Leengoed E, Kolk F, van den Broek L, Kramer E, Bakker E, et al. The defecation pattern of healthy term infants up to the age of 3 months. Arch Dis Child Fetal Neonatal Ed. 2012;97:F465–F470.

7. Tunc VT, Camurdan AD, Ilhan MN, Sahin F, Beyazova U. Factors associated with defecation patterns in 0 to 24 months old children. Eur J Pediatr. 2008;167:1357–62.

8. Hyman PE, Milla PJ, Benninga MA, Davidson GP, Fleisher DF, Taminiau J. Childhood functional gastrointestinal disorders: neonate/toddler. Gastroenterology. 2006;130:1519–26.

9. Rasquin A, Di Lorenzo C, Forbes D, Guiraldes E, Hyams JS, Staiano A. Childhood functional gastrointestinal disorders: child/adolescents. Gastroenterol. 2006; 130:1527–37.

10. Levine MD. Children with encopresis: a descriptive analysis. Pediatrics. 1975;56:412–6.

11. Taitz LS, Water JKH, Urwin OM, Molnar D. Factors associated with outcome in management of defecation disorders. Arch Dis Child. 1986; 61:472–7.

12. Amendola S, De-Angelis P, Dall'Oglio L, Di Abriola GF, Di Lorenzo M. Combined approach to functional constipation in children. J Pediatr Surg. 2003;38:819–23.

13. Loening-Baucke V. Constipation in early childhood: Patient characteristics, treatment and long-term follow up. Gut. 1993;34:1400–4.

14. Loening-Baucke V. Chronic constipation in children. Gastroenterol. 1993;105:1557–64.

15. Partin JC, Hamill SK, Fischel JE, Partin JS. Painful defecation and fecal soiling in children. Pediatrics. 1992;89:1007–9.

16. Tabbers MM, Di Lorenzo C, Berger MY, Faure C, Langendam MW, Nurko S, et al. Evaluation and treatment of functional constipation in infants and children: evidence-based recommendations from ESPGHAN and NASPGHAN. J Pediatr Gastroenterol Nutr. 2014;58:258–74.

17. Metaj M, Laroia N, Lawrence RA, Ryan RM. Comparison of breast- and formula-fed normal new born in time to first stool and urine. J Perinatol. 2003;23 624–8.

18. Jung PM. Hirschsprung's disease: one surgeon's experience in one institution. J Pediatr Surg. 1995;30:646–51.

19. Loening-Baucke V. Factors determining outcome in children with chronic constipation and fecal soiling. Gut. 1989;30 999–1006.

20. Bekkali N, van den Berg MM, Dijkgraaf MGW, van Wijk MP, Bongers MEJ, Liem D, et al. Rectal fecal impaction treatment in childhood constipation: enemas versus high doses oral PEG. Pediatric. 2009;124:e1108–e15.

21. Youssef NN, Peters JM, Henderson W, Shultz-Peters S, Lockhart DK, Di Lorenzo C. Dose response of PEG 3350 for the treatment of childhood fecal impaction. J Pediatr. 2002;141: 410–4.

22. Guest JF, Candy DC, Clegg JP, Edwards D, Helter MT, Dale AK, et al. Clinical and economical impact of using macrogol 3350 plus electrolytes in an outpatient setting compared to enemas and suppositories and manual evacuation to treat pediatric fecal impaction based on actual clinical practice in England and Wales. Curr Med Res Opin. 2007;23:2213–25.

23. Freedman SB, Thull-Freedman J, Rumantir M, Eltorki M, Schuh S. Pediatric constipation in the emergency department: evaluation, treatment and outcomes. J Pediatr Gastroenterol Nutr. 2014;59:327–33.

24. Iacono G, Cavataio F, Montalto G, Florena A, Tumminello M, Soresi M, et al. Intolerance of

cow's milk and chronic constipation in children. N Engl J Med. 1998;339:1100–4.

25. Simeone D, Miele E, Boccia G, Marino A, Troncone R, Staiano A. Prevalence of atopy in children with chronic constipation. Arch Dis Child. 2008;93:1044–7.

26. Loening-Baucke V. Polyethylene glycol without electrolytes for children with constipation and encopresis. J Pediatr Gastroenterol Nutr. 2002; 34:372–7.

27. Lowery SP, Srour JW, Whitehead WE, Schuster MM. Habit training as treatment of encopresis secondary to chronic constipation. J Pediatr Gastroenterol Nutr. 1985;4:397–401.

28. Baker SS, Liptak GS, Colletti RB, Croffie JM, Di Lorenzo C, Ector W, et al. Clinical practice guideline: Evaluation and treatment of constipation in infants and children: recommendations of the North American Society of Pediatric Gastroenterology and Nutrition. J Pediatr Gastroenterol Nutr. 2006;43:e1–e13.

29. Candy D, Belsey J. Macrogol (polyethylene glycol) laxatives in children with functional constipation and fecal impaction: a systematic review. Arch Dis Child. 2009;94:156–60.

30. Candelli M, Nista EC, Zocco MA, Gasbarrini A. Idiopathic chronic constipation; pathophysiology, diagnosis and treatment. Hepatogastroenterol 2001;48:1050–7.

31. Loening-Baucke V. Constipation in early childhood: patient characteristics, treatment and long-term follow-up. Gut. 1993;34:1400–4.

32. van Ginkel R, Reitsma JB, Buller HA, van Wijk MP, Taminiau JA, Benninga MA. Childhood constipation: longitudinal follow-up beyond puberty. Gastroenterology 2003;125:357–63.

33. Clayden GS. Management of chronic constipation. Arch Dis Child. 1992;67:340–4.

34. Southwell BR, King SK, Hutson JM. Chronic constipation in children: organic disorders are a major cause. J Pediatr Child Health. 2005;41:1–15.

35. Kwshtgar A, Ward HC, Clayden GS. Diagnosis and management of children with intractable constipation. Semin Pediatr Surg. 2004;13:300–9.

36. Benninga MA, Voskuijl WP, Akkerhuis GW, Taminiau JA, Buller HA. Colonic transit times and behavior profiles in children with defecation disorders. Arch Dis Child. 2004;89:13–6.

37. Benninga MA, Buller HA, Staalman CR, Gubler FM, Bossuyt PM, van der Plas RN, et al. Defecation disorders in children, colonic transit times versus the Barr-score. Eur J Pediatr. 1995; 154:277–84.

38. Rao SS. Dyssynergic defecation and biofeedback therapy. Gastroenterol Clin North Am. 2008; 37:569–86.

39. Winter HS, Di Lorenzo C, Benninga MA, Gilger MA, Kearns GL, Hyman PE, et al. Oral prucalopride in children with functional constipation. J Pediatr Gastroenterol Nutr. 2013; 57:197–203.

40. Hyman PE, Di Lorenzo C, Prestridge LL, Youssef NN, Ueno R. Lubiprostone for the treatment of functional constipation in children. J Pediatr Gastroenterol Nutr. 2014;58:283–91.

41. Randall J, Coyne P, Jaffray B. Follow up of children undergoing antegrade continent enema: experience of over two hundred cases. J Pediatr Surg. 2014;49:1405–8.

42. Hutson JM, McNamara J, Gibb S, Shin YM. Slow transit constipation in children. J Pediatr Child Health. 2001;37:426–30.

43. Wheatley JM, Hutson JM, Chow CW, Oliver M, Hurley MR. Slow transit constipation in childhood. J Pediatr Surg. 1999;34:829–33.

44. Malone PS, Ransley PG, Kiely EM. Preliminary report: the antegrade continence enema. Lancet. 1990;336:1217–8.

45. Chait PG, Shandling B, Richards HF. The cecostomy button. J Pediatr Surg. 1997;32;849–51.

46. Van den Berg MM, Hogan M, Caniano DA, Di Lorenzo C, Benninga MA, Mousa HM. Colonic manometry as predictor of cecostomy success in children with defecation disorders. J Pediatr Surg. 2006;41:730–6.

47. Villarreal J, Sood M, Zangen T, Flores A, Michel R, Reddy N, et al. Colonic diversion for intractable constipation in children: colonic manometry helps guide clinical decisions. J Pediatr Gastroenterol Nutr. 2001;33:588–91.

48. De Caluwe D, Yoneda A, Akl U, Puri P. Internal anal sphincter achalasia: outcome after internal sphincter myectomy. J Pediatr Surg. 2001;36:736–8.

49. Florian F, Puri P. Comparison of posterior internal anal sphincter myectomy and intrasphincteric botulinum toxin injection for treatment of internal anal sphincter achalasia: A meta-analysis. Pediatr Surg Int. 2012;28:765–71.

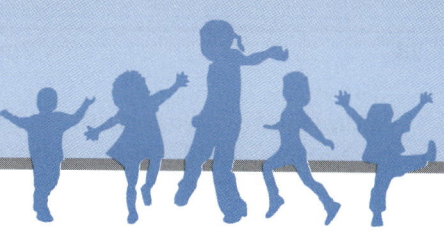

Organic Foods for Children: Health or Hype?

Prerna Batra, Nisha Sharma, Piyush Gupta

Concerns regarding quality of food are on the rise. A surge in diseases like cancers and atopic disorders has motivated health professionals, consumers, and policymakers to look for safe and healthy lifestyle measures. Organically grown foods are being promoted as a promising alternative by their manufacturers and certain activists and lobbies concerned with human health, environment and animal welfare.[1] As a result, the market is flooded with a variety of organic foods, including fruits, vegetables, cereals, dairy products and baby foods. Nutrition and safety are two important aspects that prompt the consumers to prefer organic over conventional foods. We intend to probe the status of organic foods, regulations governing their production, marketing and advertising, and whether these foods really hold an edge over the conventional foods, especially for the children in India.

PRODUCTION (ORGANIC FARMING AND REARING)

National Organic Program (NOP) was implemented in 2000—by United States Department of Agriculture (USDA) to enforce regulations for certifying a food product as organic. National Program for Organic Production (NPOP) under the aegis of Ministry of Commerce and Industry, India released its recommendations in 2000, to provide standards for organic production to farmers, producers and traders. The certification scheme was initiated in 2002, with its logo of 'India Organic'. It defines organic farming as the process of developing a viable and sustainable agro-ecosystem where the foods are grown without application of synthetic fertilizers, pesticides, fumigants (containing nitrogen or other heavy metals), human excreta, growth hormones or genetically engineered techniques.[2,3] The land has to be free of any of these substances for at least 3 years, before organic crop is grown. Organic production increases with suitable crop rotations, green manure, early and pre-drilling seed bed preparation, mulching, physical or mechanical control of pest and weeds, and disturbing the developmental cycles of the pest.[2]

Organic animal products (milk, egg, chicken, meat, etc.) are produced from animals fed on 100% organic food for at least 12 months.[2] For organic animal rearing, biological needs (food, shelter, reproduction) of these animals should be met naturally, and in time. Diseased animals should be promptly and adequately treated. Antibiotics, synthetic growth promoters, hormones for heat induction, and genetically engineered vaccines to increase the yield are prohibited.[2, 3]

Natural food is often confused with organic food. Natural food refers to minimally processed foods free of synthetic preservatives, artificial sweetener, colors, flavors, additives, and stabilizers. Natural foods can be prepared through conventional means but are preserved with minimal artificial techniques. On the other hand, organic foods are prepared, processed, and preserved in natural environment.[4]

THE GROWING MARKET FOR ORGANIC FOOD

Global organic food market has shown a boom over the last two decades; United States, Germany, France, and Australia are the major consumers. The domestic market for organic foods in India was estimated to be of one billion rupees (2007–2008), and export market approximately 100 million USD.[5]

According to the status report of National Program on Organic Production, 5.2 million hectares of land in India is currently undergoing organic farming, of which 0.5 million hectares is certified. More than 6,00,000 farmers are involved in organic farming. India's primary organic produce include cereals, pulses, oil seeds, spices, fruits and vegetables, nuts and dry fruits, sugar, honey, milk and milk products, poultry, and other animal products.[5] The major buyers are supermarkets, embassies, five-star hotels, hospitals, and Ayurveda clinics. The availability and consumption of organic products is primarily urban. Advertising and marketing strategies are evolving.

ORGANIC FOOD PRODUCTS FOR CHILDREN IN INDIA

There is a scope for a large market for organic food products meant specifically for infants and toddlers. These products include baby cereals, smoothie fruits, yogurts, toddler meals, biscuits, nibbles, cereal flakes, which are specially produced, flavored and packaged keeping in view the needs of children of different ages. A few of these products are available in the Indian market, mostly through online purchase. Most manufacturers are international. No Indian company, to the best of our market survey, is producing and marketing organic baby foods for the local consumer. India, due to its largest birth cohort in the world, is a luring proposition for the corporate world dealing in organic products. The need of the hour is therefore to be prepared for the onslaught, and have a clear-cut policy or guideline on the utility and consumption of organic foods by children in India. Parental education programs will also need to be developed accordingly.

Due to rigorous procedures required for organic farming and rearing, the price of organic foods is much higher than the conventional foods. Production cost is high because of requirements of farmer training, post-harvest handling, pesticide-free storage, segregated marketing and high retailer margin.[6] Additionally, organic foods have a shorter shelf-life. High cost of organic food is visualized as a major barrier for its widespread use. On the flip side, the higher cost is also perceived to be a marker of higher quality (in terms of nutritive value); but is it really true?

NUTRITIVE VALUE

Organic food is considered to be of higher nutritional value despite lack of high-quality scientific evidence. Most of the research is observational; there is a lack of controlled trials on their health benefits. Organic foods are said to be rich in antioxidants, phenolics, vitamins A, C and E, potassium, phosphorus, and nitrates. Omega-3 fatty acids, and alpha linoleic acid (ALA) are also claimed to be in higher amount in the organic foods.[7] Worthington reported higher levels of vitamin C, iron, magnesium and phosphorus, lower quantities of proteins (though of better quality), lesser nitrates and lesser amount of heavy metals in crops produced by organic farming system.[8] A recent meta-analysis documented higher concentrations of protein, ALA, total omega-3 fatty acid, cis-9, trans-11 conjugated linoleic acid, trans-11 vaccenic acid, eicosapentanoic acid, and docosapentanoic acid in organic dairy products.[9] Rist, et al.[10] compared the levels of conjugated linolenic acid isomers (CLA) and trans-vaccenic acid (TVA) between breastmilk of mothers consuming organic or conventional foods. CLA is suggested to have anti-carcinogenic, anti-atherosclerotic, anti-diabetic and immune-modulating properties in animal models. It is also known to modify bone mass composition.[11] Rumenic acid–the most common isomer of CLA–and TVA were significantly higher in mothers on organic diet.[10] In a recent observational study, Vrèek, et al.[12] demonstrated lower levels of protein, calcium, manganese, and iron in organically grown wheat flour, in comparison to conventional one. The protein digestibility and levels of potassium, zinc, and molybdenum were significantly higher. Lombardi-Boccia, et al.[13] compared the composition of organic yellow plums with conventional plums. The authors found only marginal differences in levels of macronutrients, whereas antioxidant vitamins like vitamin C, vitamin E, β-carotene, and phenolic compounds showed significant differences. Interestingly, the levels also differed with the type of organic cultivation used.

An important nutritional advantage of organically produced foods is their anti-oxidant effect. It is hypothesized that organically grown foods develop the capability to produce more antioxidants than conventionally grown foods, as an adaptive response to fight insect and fungal attacks. However, Caris-Veyrat, et al.[14] failed to demonstrate significant difference in two major anti-oxidants, namely, vitamin C and lycopene, *in vivo*, in organically grown tomatoes.

Table 5.1 presents a comparison of macro-nutrient contents of commonly consumed foods (organic *vs.* conventional) as available in the Indian market. There is hardly any difference between the calorie and protein content of organic and conventional foods. However, the fat content of baby food and egg appear to be somewhat lower than their conventional counterparts.

TABLE 5.1: Macronutrient content and cost (per 100 g) of organic and conventional food items

Food item (per 100 grams)	Calories (kcal)	Protein (grams)	Fat (grams)	Cost* (INR)
Chicken				
Organic	134	29.1	17	35
Conventional	119	21.4	3.1	23
Corn flakes				
Organic	383	8	1	66
Conventional	357	7.1	0	30
Mixed whole grain baby food				
Organic	393	14.3	5.4	156
Conventional	393	14.3	10.7	43
Mustard oil#				
Organic	884	0	100	28
Conventional	884	0	100	11
Poultry egg				
Organic	123	10.6	7.0	15
Conventional	135	11.4	9.0	10
Regular basmati rice				
Organic	345	6.8	0.5	18
Conventional	333	6.7	0	5
Toor dal				
Organic	335	22.3	1.7	16.5
Conventional	365	21.9	1.7	10
Wheat flour				
Organic	347	20.1	1.5	6
Conventional	380	20	0	3
Whole wheat bread				
Organic	225	10	2.5	16
Conventional	224	7.6	1.6	7
Ghee (cow's)#				
Organic	900	0	100	74
Conventional	900	0	100	30

*Costs are approximate costs in Indian market, and may vary with brands. Nutritive content is based on a market survey by the authors that recorded the display on packaged foods by the manufacturer; this may again vary with different brands. #per 100 mL.

HEALTH BENEFITS

A large number of studies have compared organic and conventional produces with respect to macro- and micro-nutrient composition, and their potentially harmful effects, but not many studies have evaluated the direct health benefits of organic foods on humans. Chabbra, et al.[15] used fruitfly (*Drosophila melanogaster*) model to assess the overall health benefits of organic fruits, and demonstrated improved fertility and longevity of the fly on organic diet.

We could identify only one study evaluating organic *vs* conventional food in children. This questionnaire-based study from Netherlands conducted on a birth cohort of 2764 infants concluded that the risk of eczema was lowered (OR 0.64, 95% CI 0.44–0.93) in infants less than 2 years of age consuming organic dairy products.[16] However, the study could not demonstrate any association between consumption of organic meat, fruits and vegetables, eggs, or proportion of organic products within the total diet, with developing eczema, wheeze or atopic sensitization. Authors were uncertain whether their findings represented a true association and recommended further studies for confirmation.

Most of the International health authorities are silent on issues regarding benefits of organic food. American Academy of Pediatrics reviewed the scientific evidence available on the merits and demerits of organic produces with the aim to provide a recommendation for pediatricians and parents. In the absence of well-planned human studies showing any direct health benefit of organic foods, the report[17] supports incorporation of a wide variety of foods to provide a balanced nutrition to the children, which need not necessarily be organic. Facts about composition, pesticide residues, health benefits, and cost of organic foods should be widely available to parents.[17]

ORGANIC FOODS: ARE THEY REALLY PESTICIDE-FREE?

Pesticide exposure and use of synthetic chemicals are a major concern with conventional farming. However, Gonzalez, et al.[18] reported contamination of organically grown crops of tomatoes with organochlorine pesticide (OCP) residues which were never used in these farms. Similar results were also reported by Baker, et al.[19], though less (one-third) often than conventional foods. The possible causes include previously contaminated fields, wind dispersion, surface run-off and volatilization. Interestingly, the levels in the crops grown by both conventional and organic methods are well below the safe limit of pesticide residues.[20] Recently, 61 commercially available brands of cheese were evaluated for OCPs and polychlorinated biphenyls (PCB) in Spain. The authors reported OCP levels to be lower than recommended total dietary intake (TDI) in both types of products, though the levels of PCBs were in the higher centile range of TDI.[21] Lu, et al.[22] in an interventional study, reported that urinary excretion of metabolites of commonly used organophosphorus pesticides (malathion and chloropyrifos) were immediately and greatly reduced when the child switched from conventional to organic diets.[22]

POTENTIAL RISKS OF ORGANIC FOODS

Microbiological safety of the organic animal foods is a questionable domain, the reason being prohibited use of antimicrobials. Cui, et al.[23] analyzed organic and conventional chicken samples for prevalence and antimicrobial resistance of *Campylobacter* and *Salmonella*. They found organic chicken to be more contaminated with these organisms, although the pathogen isolated from organic chicken were more susceptible to some antimicrobials. In a contradictory study, foods from conventional farms isolated *Salmonella* more frequently with higher level of resistance to streptomycin and sulphamethoxazole.[24] Contamination by mycotoxins has also been reported with organic farming.[25,26]

CERTIFICATION

United States Department of Agriculture (USDA) certifies any food as '100% Organic', if it has 100% organically-produced ingredients and processing aids, and 'Organic', if it fulfills 95% of the above criteria. Remaining 5% should be non-agricultural substances approved in their national list. Another category with 70% organic components can use the label reading 'Made with organic ingredients', but cannot use USDA logo.[27] EU Oganic is the certification given to products with more than 95% organic ingredients by European countries. 'India Organic' certification is provided to the organic products complying with the USDA standards by INDOCERT, the nationally and internationally operating certification body by NPOP. The certificate is valid for 3 years and needs to be renewed every 3 years.[2] Guidelines are available for ingredients, additives, processing, packaging, labeling, storage and transport to ensure the quality of products. The certification is liable to suspension or termination in the event of violation.

THE ROAD AHEAD

With the dramatic increase in the growth of organic food market globally, issues regarding nutritive value and safety need to be answered. The consumer is willing to pay a higher price for a healthier option. The literature shows that there are few qualitative differences between organic and conventional foods, but whether they actually produce a beneficial effect on human health is currently not known. Evidence available till date is insufficient to promote or refute the use of organic foods over conventional foods, with particular consideration of high cost involved. There is a need for controlled trials to study the actual health benefits with organic foods,

and efforts to reduce the cost by working on organic farming techniques.

American Academy of Pediatrics issued its report on health and environmental advantages and disadvantages of organic foods. The report gives the guidelines to pediatricians for the purpose of guiding the parents. Despite the increasing market of organic produces in India, Indian Academy of Pediatrics (IAP) has not formulated any guidelines for their use in children. The brands available in India should provide exact details of the composition of the product, to enable the consumers to compare and chose the option best suited to their pocket. Manufacturers should abide by the guidelines for factual display of contents in advertising, and not just use it merely to lure the consumers; IAP can play an important role in this regard.

REFERENCES

1. Magnusson MK, Arvola A, Hursti UK, Aberg L, Sjoden PO. Choice of organic foods is related to perceived consequences for human health and environmentally friendly behavior. Appetite. 2003;40:109–17.
2. National Programme for Organic Production. New Delhi; Department of Commerce, Ministry of Commerce and Industry; 2000. p. 21–35.
3. Winter CK, Davis SF. Organic foods. J Food Sci. 2006;71:R117–24.
4. FMI Backgrounder. Natural and Organic Foods. Available from *http://www.fda.gov/ohrms/dockets/dockets/06p0094/06p-0094-cp00001-05-Tab-04-Food-Marketing-Institute-vol1.pdf*. Accessed January 16, 2014.
5. Organic Products-APEDA. Available from http://www. apeda.gov.in/apedawebsite/organic/organic_products.htm. Accessed January 15, 2014.
6. Organic agriculture: Why is organic food more expensive than conventional food? Available from *http://www.fao. org/organicag/oa-faq/oa-faq5/en/*. Accessed January 15, 2014.
7. State of Science Review: Nutritional Superiority of Organic Foods. Available from *http://www. organic-center.org/reportfiles/5367_Nutrient_Content_SSR_ FINAL_V2.pdf*. Accessed January 15, 2014.

8. Worthington V. Nutritional quality of organic versus conventional fruits, vegetables, and grains. J Altern Complement Med. 2001;7: 161–73.

9. Palupi E, Jayanegara A, Ploeger A, Kahl J. Comparison of nutritional quality between conventional and organic dairy products: a meta-analysis. J Sci Food Agric. 2012; 92:2774–81.

10. Rist L, Mueller A, Barthel C, Snijders B, Jansen M, Simões-Wüst AP, *et al*. Influence of organic diet on the amount of conjugated linoleic acids in breastmilk of lactating women in Netherlands. Br J Nutr. 2007;97:735–43.

11. Banu J, Bhattacharya A, Rahman M, Fernandes G. Beneficial effects of conjugated linoleic acid and exercise on bone of middle-aged female mice. J Bone Mineral Metabol. 2008;2:436–45.

12. Vrcek IV, Cepo DV, Rašic D, Meraica M, Zuntar I, Bojic M, *et al*. A comparison of the nutritional value and safety of organically and conventionally produced wheat flours. Food Chemistry. 2014;143:522–9.

13. Lombardi-Boccia G, Lucarini M, Lanzi S, Aguzzi A, Cappelloni M. Nutrients and antioxidant molecules in yellow plums (*Prunus domestica* L.) from conventional and organic productions: a comparative study. J Agric Food Chem. 2004; 52:90–4.

14. Caris-Veyrat C, Amiot MJ, Tyssandier V, Grasselly D, Buret M, Mikolajczak M, *et al*. Influence of organic versus conventional agricultural practice on the antioxidant microconstituent content of tomatoes and derived purees; consequences on antioxidant plasma status in humans. J Agric Food Chem. 2004;52:6503–9.

15. Chhabra R, Kolli S, Bauer JH. Organically grown food provides health benefits to *Drosophila melanogaster*. PLoS One. 2013; 8: e52988.

16. Kummeling I, Thijs C, Huber M, van de Vijver LP, Snijders BE, Penders J, *et al*. Consumption of organic foods and risk of atopic disease during the first 2 years of life in the Netherlands. Br J Nutr. 2008;99:598–605.

17. Forman J, Silverstein J. Committee on Nutrition; Council on Environmental Health; American Academy of Pediatrics. Organic foods: health and environmental advantages and disadvantages. Pediatrics. 2012;130:e1406–15.

18. Gonzalez M, Miglioranza KS, Aizpún de Moreno JE, Moreno VJ. Occurrence and distribution of organochlorine pesticides (OCPs) in tomato (*Lycopersicon esculentum*) crops from organic production. J Agric Food Chem. 2003;51:1353–9.

19. Baker BP, Benbrook CM, Groth E 3rd, Lutz Benbrook K. Pesticide residues in conventional, integrated pest management (IPM)-grown and organic foods: insights from three US data sets. Food Addit Contam. 2002;19: 427–46.

20. Tsatsakis AM, Tsakiris IN, Tzatzarakis MN, Agourakis ZB, Tutudaki M, Alegakis AK. Three-year study of fenthion and dimethoate pesticides in olive oil from organic and conventional cultivation. Food Addit Contam. 2003;20:553–9.

21. Almeida-González M, Luzardo OP, Zumbado M, Rodríguez-Hernández A, Ruiz-Suárez N, Sangil M, *et al*. Levels of organochlorine contaminants in organic and conventional cheeses and their impact on the health of consumers: an independent study in the Canary Islands (Spain). Food Chem Toxicol. 2012;50:4325–32.

22. Lu C, Toepel K, Irish R, Fenske RA, Barr DB, Bravo R. Organic diets significantly lower children's dietary exposure to organophosphorus pesticides. Environ Health Perspect. 2006; 114:260–3.

23. Cui S, Ge B, Zheng J, Meng J. Prevalence and antimicrobial resistance of Campylobacter spp and Salmonella serovars in organic chickens from Maryland retail stores. Appl Env Microbiol. 2005;71:4108–11.

24. Ray KA, Warnick LD, Mitchell RM, Kaneene JB, Ruegg PL, Wells SJ, *et al*. Antimicrobial susceptibility of Salmonella from organic and conventional dairy farms. J Dairy Sci. 2006;89:2038–50.

25. Tosun H, Arslan R. Determination of aflatoxin B1 levels in organic spices and herbs. Scientific World J. 2013;26:1–4.

26. Serrano AB, Font G, Mañes J, Ferrer E. Emerging Fusarium mycotoxins in organic and conventional pasta collected in Spain. Food Chem Toxicol. 2013;51:259–66.

27. Indocert. Available from *http://www.indocert.org/ new/index.php/en/*. Accessed January 15, 2014.

Energy Drinks: Potions of Illusion

Nidhi Bedi, Pooja Dewan, Piyush Gupta

In a competitive world–where achieving targets rules the roost–more energy is a desirable virtue. Some adolescents are naturally energetic, while others look for commercially available stamina boosters to provide instant energy. Energy drinks seem to be just the solution this group is looking for.

Energy drinks are non-alcoholic beverages containing stimulants like caffeine, herbal extracts (*guarana, ginseng, yerba mate, ginkgobiloba*), glucuronolactone, taurine, inositol, L-carnitine and B-vitamins as the main ingredients to enhance physical and mental endurance.[1] In addition, these drinks may contain carbonated water. Energy shots are a specialized form of energy drinks which contain the same amount of caffeine in a small amount of liquid, typically 60–90 mL small bottles or cans. These may be considered as concentrated energy drinks with lesser calories and lower sugar content.[2] Energy drinks/ energy shots are consumed to improve the stamina and energy levels before and during exercise, to rehydrate the body, to keep awake in demanding situations, to compensate for loss of sleep especially during examinations, or to get a kick as a mood elevator by mixing it with alcohol. Natural caffeinated beverages including coffee, cocoa, tea, and cola drinks are not regarded as energy drinks. Energy drinks should not be confused with sports drinks that contain carbohydrates, minerals, electrolytes, and flavoring agents. These are intended to replenish water and electrolytes lost through sweating during exercise. Unlike energy drinks, sports drinks do not contain any stimulants.[3]

GROWING DEMAND

Energy drinks were introduced to the world in 1949 by the name of 'Dr Enuf' in US; these were fortified with vitamins and projected as a better alternative to sugar sodas. Subsequently, these became available in Europe and Asia in 1960s.[4] Lipovate D, an energy drink that still dominates the Japanese market, was launched in 1962. Later, several companies introduced similar drinks but none could make a mark till 1997, when 'Red Bull' was introduced by an Austrian entrepreneur.[4] This brought a boom to the industry and ever since the market for energy drinks is growing exponentially. More than 300 variants of energy drinks are available in the US market alone. India, China, and Brazil are considered as the growing markets. Red Bull was launched in India in 2003. With a 75% market share, it is presently leading the Indian market of energy drinks. The energy drink market in

India was pegged at ₹ 700 crore in 2013; comprising of 5% of the total soft drinks market dominated by colas, fruit juices, and flavored milk (5), compared to 8–9% in global market.

Manufacturers have now shifted their focus from athletes–the primary target for energy drinks–to teenagers and young adults. According to an estimate, about 71% of adolescents in urban centers of India consume energy drinks.[6] Despite the cost factor, youth do not mind spending money on energy drinks due to their much advertised perceived benefits on endurance, attention, and stamina.

CONSTITUENTS OF ENERGY DRINKS

The main constituent of energy drinks is caffeine. In non-alcoholic energy drinks, caffeine content varies between 75 mg and 150 mg per can[1] compared to 80–120 mg and 60 mg in a cup (250 mL) of coffee and tea, respectively.[7] Maximum recommended intake of caffeine per day, varies from 2.5 mg/kg/day to 6 mg /kg/day in children, 100 mg/day in adolescents and up to 400 mg/day in adults.[8]

Caffeine attaches to the adenosine receptor due to its similar chemical structure as that of adenosine. Due to this, the adenosine effect to promote sleep is stopped by competitive inhibition resulting in speeding up of neurons. Caffeine also improves the physical and mental performance by increasing epinephrine secretion. Once ingested, caffeine is rapidly absorbed from the gastrointestinal tract where it is demethylated to form paraxanthine (84%), theobromine (12%), and theophylline (4%). Caffeine intake leads to increased energy utilization and thereby better performance. It has also been found to enhance mood and alertness. In addition, it has been found to decrease food intake and promote lipolysis [9].

Guarana (also called guaranine, *Paullinia-cupana*, and *Sapindaceae*)–another ingredient of energy drinks–is a plant extract containing large amounts of caffeine with small amounts of theobromine, theophylline, saponins, flavonoids, and tannins. The seeds contain about twice the concentration of caffeine found in coffee beans. One gram of guarana is equal to approximately 40 mg of caffeine.[9] Consumption of guarana increases energy, enhances physical performance, and promotes weight loss. These effects are largely contributed to the high caffeine content of guarana.

Ginseng (*Panax ginseng*) is a herbal supplement; root being its most important part. Athletes use ginseng for its alleged performance-enhancing attributes; however, no scientific evidence is there till date to support its performance-enhancing claims.[9]

Yerba mate, obtained from *Ilex paraguariensis* is known for its anti-inflammatory, anti-diabetic, and anti-oxidative properties. It is a central nervous system stimulant due to its high caffeine concentration (78 mg in 1 cup of yerba mate tea).[9]

L-carnitine, D-glucuronolactone, taurine, and inositol are other ingredients of energy drinks. Data remain insufficient regarding their safe use and claims to increase endurance.[6,9,10] Certain other ingredients like milk thistle, ginkgo, acai berry, L-theanine and creatine have bioactive properties for which they are sometimes added to energy drinks.[9]

POTENTIAL ADVERSE EFFECTS

When consumed in moderation, most energy drinks are considered safe. Over-consumption is fraught with potential adverse effects attributed to the high caffeine content.

Caffeine tolerance varies between individuals, though most people would develop toxic symptoms in doses of 200 mg (1 mg = 4 ppm). Some of the energy drinks may contain caffeine as high as 300–500 mg per can.[1] Table 6.1 shows the caffeine content of commonly available energy drinks in the Indian market. Symptoms of caffeine intoxication include palpitations, anxiety, insomnia, nausea, vomiting, restlessness, and tremors.[1] The risk increases if multiple drinks are

TABLE 6.1: Caffeine content of commercially available energy drinks in the Indian market

Brand	Amount (mL)	Cost (₹)	Caffeine content declared by manufacturer (ppm)	Caffeine content as tested by CSE (ppm)
Red Bull	250	95	320 (80 mg/250 mL)	310.08
Tzinga	250	25	300 (75 mg/250 mL)	258.37
Triple X	250	75	100	117.14
Cloud 9	250	85	Not given	142.25
Burn	300	75	320	291.73

Source: CSE (Centre for Science and Environment)

consumed in a short period of time. A cocktail of energy drinks when mixed with alcohol decreases the awareness of the amount of intoxication, leading to a higher risk of alcohol-related injuries.[11] The combination might also increase the risk of arrhythmia if there is an underlying heart disease. Teens are shown to mix their energy drinks with alcohol.[12] This can be potentially dangerous cocktail as the drinkers will be unaware of the amount of alcohol they have actually consumed. Caffeine content of beverages consumed by adolescents has also been linked to high blood pressure.[13]

Caffeine, taken in large amounts over an extended period of time, leads to caffeinism characterized by nervousness, increased risk of addiction, irritability, anxiety, tremulousness, muscle twitching, insomnia, headache, respiratory alkalosis, and palpitations.[1] The Diagnostic and Statistical Manual of Mental Disorders (Fourth Edition) recognizes four caffeine-induced psychiatric disorders: caffeine intoxication, caffeine-induced anxiety disorder, caffeine-induced sleep disorder, and caffeine-related disorder. Studies in adult twins have shown a significant positive association between major depression, generalized anxiety disorder, panic disorder, antisocial personality disorder, alcohol dependence, and cannabis and cocaine abuse/dependence; with lifetime caffeine intake, caffeine toxicity, and caffeine dependence.[14]

Another demerit of caffeine is its ability to foster dependence. Genetic factors have also been found to play some role in caffeine intoxication, dependence, and withdrawal.[14].

Ginseng has been associated with adverse effects like hypotension, edema, palpitations, tachycardia, cerebral arteritis, insomnia, mania, and cholestatic hepatitis but they are not noted at levels found in energy drinks. Studies are insufficient to prove its safety.[15]

Most energy drinks contain a lot of sugar or artificial sweeteners to mask the bitterness of caffeine. The sugar content in energy drinks ranges from 21 g to 34 g per 8 oz. Sugars in energy drinks may be in the form of sucrose, glucose, or high fructose corn syrup. Their intake poses a risk for obesity and diabetes in children.

Most sports and energy drinks have citric acid, which lowers their pH in the acidic range (pH 3–4). A pH this low is associated with enamel demineralization and dental problems.

ENERGY DRINKS AND MEDICAL CONDITIONS

- Energy drinks if taken by children being treated for attention deficit hyperactivity disorder, can be very harmful as they are already taking stimulant medications.[16]
- Patients of ion channelopathies and hypertrophic cardiomyopathy should not take energy drinks because of the risk of hypertension, syncope, arrhythmias, and sudden death due to unwanted stimulant effect of caffeine.[17] In August 2008, a study conducted by the Cardiovascular Research Centre at the Royal Adelaide Hospital in Australia assessed the cardiovascular status of 30 young adults one hour before and after the intake of a popular energy drink and found that it could increase the risk of stroke and heart attack.[1]
- High amounts of caffeine help to counter caloric-restriction–associated fatigue, and suppress appetite, and thus have often been taken by patients of anorexia nervosa. But as these patients have a propensity for

cardiac morbidity/mortality and electrolyte disorders, intake of high-caffeine energy drinks can trigger cardiac dysrhythmias and intracardiac conduction abnormalities.[18.]

- Other high-risk groups include adolescents with obesity, hemodynamic compromise, diabetics and individuals with pre-existing cardiovascular, meta-bolic, hepatorenal, and neurologic disease, those who are taking medications that may be affected by high glycemic load foods, caffeine, and/or other stimulants, and adolescents in rapid growth phase.[12]
- Caffeine also acts as a diuretic; therefore, energy drinks should be avoided during exercise as fluid losses from sweating coupled with diuresis can lead to dehydration.

WHERE WE STAND?

Considering the potential adverse effects, energy drinks have been banned in some countries like Denmark, Uruguay and Turkey. Energy drinks with caffeine more than 320 ppm are banned in Australia.[19] European countries have stipulated that energy drinks with caffeine more than 150 ppm should be labeled as having 'high caffeine content'.

In the first year of the launch of a leading energy drink, there was a tussle between the manufacturers and government agencies on labeling of the product. The central food laboratory continued to label it as carbonated beverage (maximum allowable caffeine content–200 ppm, now lowered to 145 ppm). The manufacturers maintained it as proprietary product (caffeine content–320 ppm), and claimed it to be safe. The maximum limit of caffeine of 200 ppm in carbonated beverages was reduced to maximum level of 145 ppm on recommendations by Central Committee on Food Standards (India) and notified vide notification GSR 431(E) dated 19.06.2009. Food Safety and Standards Authority of India (FSSAI) then constituted an expert group on energy drinks and made certain observations (Box 6.1).[1]

Center for Science and Environment (CSE), a Delhi-based NGO, tested eight brands of energy drinks and showed that caffeine levels were exceeding 145 ppm in 6 of them.[20] FSSAI constituted an expert group, followed by a risk assessment study commissioned by National Institute of Nutrition (NIN), Hyderabad. On the basis of NIN report, FSSAI has now recommended a limit of 320 ppm of caffeine in energy drinks. In June 2012, FSSAI announced the mandatory use of statutory safety warnings and that all energy drinks should be renamed as "caffeinated beverages."

Box 6.1: Food safety and standards authority of India observations on energy drinks

- Caffeine is not an additive but a chemical with addictive property. Caffeine up to 200 ppm is added as a flavoring agent but above 200 ppm it is a functional ingredient. The functionality of caffeine at 320 ppm needs to be ascertained along with justification for fixing a cut-off limit at 320 ppm.
- Energy drink is a beverage which is fortified with vitamins and there is no case for encouraging its consumption. The name 'energy drinks' is a misnomer as it gives the impression that this should be taken to get energy.
- The vegetarian and non-vegetarian symbol should also be given on the label of energy drinks as per the source of ingredients added.
- Standards for energy drinks, both carbonated and non-carbonated need to be laid down to enable better regulation of the product. These may be termed as 'caffeinated drinks'.
- There is a need to limit consumption of energy drinks by a person per day taking into account total caffeine content from all ingredients and items in the diet.
- Alternatively, instead of laying down separate standards for carbonated energy drinks, standards for carbonated beverages per se can be amended to include other ingredients like taurine, glucuronolactone, etc. which are found in energy drinks.
- There is also a need to get the market data of availability of energy drinks in India and analyze samples as a basis for fixation of standards according to Indian requirements.

TABLE 6.2: Caffeine content of common fast moving consumer goods

Products	Caffeine content/250 mL
Tea	60 mg
Coffee	80–120 mg
Carbonated beverages	25–40 mg
Dark chocolate (100 g)	43 mg
Hershey's syrup (2 tbsp/ 39 g)	5 mg

Following this, the energy drinks now boldly write "contains caffeine". Further, they mention clearly "Not recommended for children, pregnant or lactating women and persons sensitive to caffeine. Use not more than 2 cans a day." FSSAI has also proposed that such products be packed in only 250 mL containers. However, consumers need to keep in mind that there are other sources of caffeine intake like coffee, tea, chocolate products, and carbonated drinks. Table 6.2 depicts the caffeine content of commonly consumed beverages. As of now, this caffeine cap of 320 ppm for energy drinks does not take into account the total caffeine content from other beverages. There is no sample study in India to determine the caffeine intake of the population as such. Also the justification for propagating the use of energy drinks for a source of vitamins, minerals, and amino acids is not acceptable as these can be easily obtained from a normal healthy diet.

CONCLUSION

Intake of energy drinks prior to physical activities may be undertaken while keeping their possible deleterious effects in mind. Their use during physical activity is not recommended. Sports drinks (non-caffeinated) are designed to be taken during physical activity and should be preferred. Energy drinks claim to have stimulant effects; these may be pleasant at times. However, intake of these drinks can be harmful. Considering this fact and the growing popularity of these drinks, one should be cautious before and during intake of energy drinks. More awareness needs to be created in the younger generation regarding their appropriate intake. Further research should be done to assess the benefits and ill-effects of various ingredients present in these drinks. Indian Academy of Pediatrics should lead a campaign to educate parents and pediatricians about the risk of caffeinated drinks.

REFERENCES

1. Food Safety and Standards Authority of India. Proposed Regulation of Energy Drinks and Caffeine (revised). Available from: *http://www.fssai.gov.in/portals/0/standards_of_energy_drinks_.pdf.* Accessed February 19, 2014.
2. Schubert MM, Astorino TA, Azevedo JL Jr. The effects of caffeinated "energy shots" on time trial performance. Nutrients. 2013;5:2062–75.
3. Committee on Nutrition and the Council on Sports Medicine and Fitness. Sports drinks and energy drinks for children and adolescents- Are they appropriate? Pediatrics. 2011;127:1182–9.
4. Reissig CJ, Strain EC, Griffiths RR. Caffeinated energy drinks–a growing problem. Drug Alcohol Depend. 2009;99:1–10.
5. Mukherjee A. Burst of Energy: A host of newcomers has entered the energy drinks market. But making an impact will not be easy. Business Today 10 November 2013. Available from: *http://businesstoday.intoday.in/story/challenges-ahead-for-newcomers-in-energy-drinks-market/1/199794.html.* Accessed February 17, 2014.
6. Chatterjee P. New entrants to boost energy drinks market. The Hindu 9 April, 2013. Available from: *http://www.thehindubusinessline.com/companies/new-entrants-to-boost-energy-drinks-market/article4598806.ece.* Accessed February 17, 2014.
7. National Institute of Nutrition. Dietary Guidelines for Indians. A manual. 2nd ed. Hyderabad: National Institute of Nutrition; 2010. p73. Available from: *http://ninindia.org/DietaryguidelinesforIndians-Finaldraft.pdf.* Accessed February 20, 2014.
8. Heckman MA, Weil J, Mejia EG. Caffeine (1, 3, 7-trimethylxanthine) in foods: A comprehensive review on consumption, functionality, safety, and regulatory matters. J Food Sci. 2010;75:R 75–87.
9. Yunusa I, Ahmed IM. Energy drinks: composition and health benefits. Bayero J Pure Applied Sci. 2011;4:186–91.

10. Triebel S, Sproll C, Reusch H, Godelmann R, Lachenmeier DW. Rapid analysis of taurine in energy drinks using amino acid analyzer and Fourier transform infrared (FTIR) spectroscopy as basis for toxicological evaluation. Amino Acids. 2007;33:451–7.

11. Kponee KZ, Siegel M, Jernigan DH. The use of caffeinated alcoholic beverages among underage drinkers: results of a national survey. Addict Behav. 2014;39:253–8.

12. Wolk BJ, Ganetsky M, Babu KM. Toxicity of energy drinks. Curr Opin Pediatr. 2012;24:243–51.

13. Savoca MR, Evans CD, Wilson ME, Harshfield GA, Ludwig DA. The association of caffeinated beverages with blood pressure in adolescents. Arch Pediatr Adolesc Med. 2004;158:473–7.

14. Ressing CJ, Strain EC, Griffiths RR. Caffeinated energy drinks–A growing problem. Drug Alcohol Depend. 2009; 99:1–10.

15. Higgins JP, Tuttle TD, Higgins CL. Energy beverages: content and safety. Mayo Clin Proc. 2010;85:1033–41.

16. Goldman RD. Caffeinated energy drinks in children. Can Fam Physician. 2013;59:947–8.

17. Seifert SM, Schaechter JL, Hershorin ER, Lipshultz SE. Health effects of energy drinks on children, adolescents, and young adults. Pediatrics. 2011; 127:511–28.

18. Campbell B, Wilborn C, La Bounty P, Taylor L, Nelson MT, Greenwood M, et al. International Society of Sports Nutrition Position Stand: Energy Drinks. J Int Soc Sports Nutr. 2013;10:1.

19. Centre for Science and Environment. Food safety and toxins. FSSAI takes energy out of the drinks. Available from: http://www.cseindia.org/content/fssai-takes-energy-out-drinks. Accessed Dec. 25, 2013.

20. Centre for Science and Environment. High on caffeine. Available from: http://www.downtoearth.org.in/content/high-caffeine. Accessed Dec. 25, 2013.

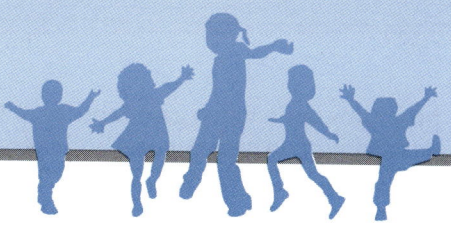

Undesirable Effects of Media on Children: Why Limitation is Necessary?

Aysu Turkmen Karaagac

Teachers, pediatricians and pediatric psychiatrists agree on the fact that sustained intellectual exercise contributes to the brain growth and more sophisticated thinking, and thus brain must be challenged regularly. Communication and analytical thinking abilities of children develop if they regularly converse with their families and/or develop good reading habits. Families may unintentionally contribute to the mental deprivation and limited brain growth of their children by allowing unlimited use of media devices.[1-3]

The social media network sites which have provided children with easy ways of establishing friendships, and satisfy their feelings of belonging and acceptance by others, have become more and more popular especially in developing countries.[4] However, there is no sufficient research/guideline on protecting children's safety in use of media devices in developing countries.[5] The results of the national school violence study in South Africa showed that 80.2% of secondary school learners have a mobile phone, while 54.3% have access to a computer or a tablet computer. About 70% of these children were reported to use social network sites and talk with strangers at least once a week.[5] Research findings in Vietnam have revealed that up to 25% of children in the urban areas and 20% of children

in the rural areas had shared personal information such as their phone number or name of their school with strangers online. It was also reported that 49% of the urban children and 20% of the rural children in Vietnam were subjected to cyberbullying, or were threatened or embarrassed online. Unfortunately, only 1 in 10 of these victims informed a parent or an adult about this abuse.[4,5] Several studies have reported that victims of bullying are 2 to 9 times more likely to consider committing suicide.[3-5] Families should help their children realize the danger of cyberbullying by controlling their computer/tablet computer use.

Watching television (TV) is the first-choice lesiure time activity of the families, especially in the urban areas of developing countries.[6] Burdette, *et al.*[7] reported that children in urban areas spent an avarage of 2.2 hours per day watching TV. Children's exposure to media violence plays an important role in the etiology of violent behaviors.[7,8] TV programs in US show 812 violent acts per hour, a typical American child would have followed 200,000 acts of violence, containing more than 16,000 murders, until the age of 18 years.[8] Furthermore, 15–20% of music videos and many of video games include violence.[8] Children tend to imitate the characters they watch on TV programs or on video games because they can not distinguish between fact and fantasy until 5 years of age. They may accept the violence as an ordinary means to solve problems over the time.[8,9] Therefore, physicians, especially pediatricians, should make parents and teachers media-literate meaning that they should comprehend the risks of exposure to violence, and teach their children how to interpret what they see on TV, in the movies, or in the cartoons.

How does media affect weight in children? Watching television or playing with computer over 2 hours/day might result in obesity in children due to the lack of activity. Studies also suggest that 80% of obese children might become obese in adult life.[9,10] The incidence of childhood obesity–which may lead to hypertension, diabetes mellitus, coronary artery disease, cholecystitis, dyslipidemia, osteoarthritis or sleep apnea in adulthood–has doubled in the last two decades in America in proportion to the increase in children's media use.[11]

Moreover, American Academy of Pediatrics has declared that an average child watches 20,000 or more commercials every year, more than 60% of which promote junk foods related with obesity.[12,13] Costa, *et al.*[14] reported that 13.8% of 1369 commercials screened during 176 hours of TV programming in Brazil were related with foods as sugars, sweets (48.1%) and fats (29.1%). It has been suggested that the content and the timing of commercials should be carefully controlled because children under the age of 8 years are unable to differentiate the advertisements from the regular programs, and commercials have considerable influence on them.[13]

Yousef, *et al.* reported a positive correlation between excessive TV watching (>2 h/d) and aggressive behaviors, attention problems, low self-esteem and internalizing and externalizing problems of children.[15] The use of electronic media devices beginning from the preschool age has been associated with 1.2–2 folds higher rate of emotional disorders like major depression, bipolar disorder or anxiety attacks. In addition, poorer family functioning has been reported with excessive TV watching or computer use.[16]

Obesity and impaired glycemic control due to lack of exercise is one of the major risk factors for cardiovascular diseases.[17] If children's media use is not limited, they neglect regular activities as hiking, running, swimming and riding bicycle.[14] Therefore, it is important to encourage families to monitor their children's media use and to spend more time doing physical activities with their children to improve cardiovascular health in their adulthood.

Children usually sit in unsuitable body postures for a long time in front of TV or computers. Drzal, *et al.*[18] demonstrated that prolonged sitting position resulted in decreased angle of inclination of the thoracolumbar spine, reduced thoracic kyphosis and lumbar lordosis, and pelvic asymmetry in children aged 11 years to 13 years in Poland. Posture education programs should be advocated for school children to avoid such advanced spine abnormalities.

Melatonin is a very important antioxidant that protects nuclear DNA and cell membrane lipids from oxidative damage. It has been strongly suggested that prolonged exposure to magnetic fields might cause hematopoetic system cancers, especially in children, due to melatonin supression.[19]

The most effective way of protecting children from the undesired effects of media is to provide the family control via media literacy education programs. The success of media literacy education of families depends on the power of communication between parents and children. One of the most important steps of this education is to set some rules about limiting the time their children spend watching TV or playing video games. Children's media use should be limited to 1–2 hours/day after they finish their homework and/or sport activities.[20] Parents should watch TV with their children to teach them how to interpret the media messages or content of commercials. Parental supervision during watching cartoons and movies enables the children to distinguish between reality and fantasy. Families should talk with their children about how violent scenes create false excitement, and how problems can be solved non-violently.[19,20] Besides family relationships and willingness, several demographic factors such as age, educational status or income of the parents may affect the results of media literacy applications. Studies have shown that the educated parents can have a better control of children's media use and its content. On the other hand, two-thirds of 8- to 18-year-old children of the families with higher socio-economic status have their own TV sets, computers or video game consoles, which makes family control difficult.[20,21]

In conclusion, harmful effects of un-controlled media use by children is a common problem shared by most of the countries throughout the world. It is impossible to forbid children's media use; however, physicians can promote healthy use through public education. Media organizations should also be trained to be more sensitive about the determination of program contents and timing. Pediatricians should play a key role in raising awareness of media literacy of families as well as encouraging politicians to create effective media-literacy education policies.

REFERENCES

1. Jordan AB, Hersey JC, McDivitt JA, Heitzler CD. Reducing children's television-viewing time: A qualitative study of parents and their children. Pediatrics. 2006;118:1303–10.

2. Yýlmaz G. The effects of media on child health. Turk Arch Pediatr. 2007;42:1–5.

3. Diamond MC. Plasticity of the Brain: Enrichment *vs.* Impoverishment. *In:* Clark C and King K, editors. Television and the Preparation of the Mind for Learning. Washington, DC: US Department of Health and Human services,1992. p. 8–19.

4. Schouten AP, Valkenburg PM, Peter J. Precursors and underlying processes of adolescents online self-disclosure: developing and testing an "Internet-Attribute-Perception" model. Media Psychol. 2007; 10:292–315.

5. Beger G, Sinha A. South African Mobile Generation. Study on South African Young People on Mobiles, UNICEF 2012. Available from: *http://www.unicef.org/southafrica/SAF_resources_MXitstudy.pdf.* Accessed April 1, 2015.

6. Gupta R, Rasania KS, Acharya AS. The influence of television on urban adolescents of Delhi. Indian J Community Med. 2014;39:47–8.

7. Burdette HL, Whitaker RC, Kahn RS, Harvey BJ. Association of maternal obesity and depressive symptoms with television-viewing time in low-income preschool children. Arch Pediatr Adolesc Med. 2003;157:894–9.

8. Beresin EV. The impact of media violence on children and adolescents: opportunities for clinical interventions. American Academy of Child and Adolescent Psychiatry. *https://www.aacap.org/AACAP/Medical_Students_and_Residents/Mentorship_Matters/DevelopMentor/The_Impact_of_Media_Violence_on_Children_and_Adolescents_OpportunitiesforClinical Interventions.aspx.* Accessed April 1, 2014.

9. Bishwalata R, Singh AB, Singh AJ, Devi LU, Singh RK. Over weight and obesity among school children in Munipur, India. Natl Med J India. 2010;23:263–6.

10. Goyal JP, Kumar N, Parmar I, Shah VB, Patel B. Determinants of overweight and obesity in affluent adolescent in Surat city, South Gujarat region, India. Indian J Community Med. 2011;36:296–300.

11. Dietz WH. Overweight in childhood and adolescence. N Engl J Med. 2004;350:855–7.

12. American Academy of Pediatrics, Committee on Communications. Children, Adolescents, and Television (RE0043). Pediatrics. 2001;107:423–6.

13. Canadian Pediatric Society. Healthy active living for children and youth. Pediatric Child Health. 2002;7:339–45.

14. Costa SM, Horta PM, Santos LC. Analysis of television food advertising on children's programming on "free-to-air" broadcast stations in Brazil. Rev Bras Epidemiol. 2013;16:976–83.

15. Yousef S, Eapen V, Zoubeidi T, Mabrouk A. Behavioral correlation with television watching and video game playing among children in the United Arab Emirates. Int J Psychiatry Clin Pract. 2014;18:203–7.

16. Hinkley T, Verbestel V, Ahrens W, Lissner L, Molnar D, Moreno LA, *et al*. Early childhood electronic media use as a predictor of poorer well-being: a prospective cohort study. JAMA Pediatr. 2014;168:485–92.

17. Williams CL, Hayman LL, Daniels SR, Robinson TN, Steinberger J, Paridon S, *et al*. Cardiovascular health in childhood. J Circulation. 2002;106: 143–60.

18. Drzal GJ, Snela S, Rykala J, Podgorska J, Rachwal M. Effects of the sitting position on the body posture of children aged 11 to 13 years. Work. 2014; 6:1–8.

19. Wood B, Rea SM, Plitnick B, Figueiro GM. Light level and duration of exposure determine the impact of self-luminous tablets on melatonin suppression. Applied Ergonomics J. 2013; 44:237–40.

20. DeGaetano G. Raising Media Literate Children. Parent Coaching Institute Articles and Research, 2007. Available from: *http://www.thepci.org/articles/ degaetano_Media Literate Children.html*. Accessed January 20, 2015.

21. Roberts DF, Foehr UG, Rideout V. Generation M. Media in the lives of 8–18 years olds. Menlo Park, Calif.: Keiser Family Foundation Study. 2005: 41–55.

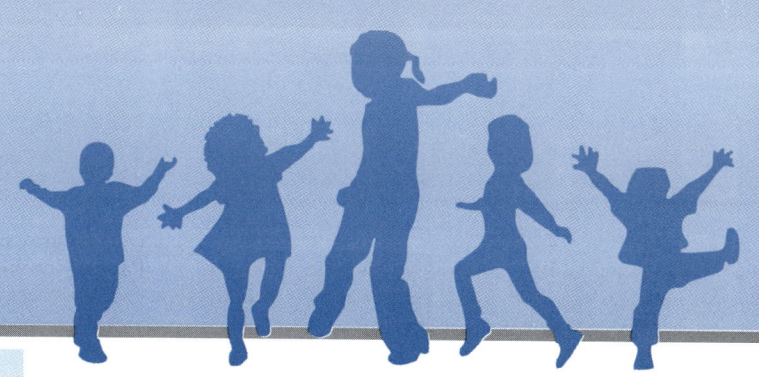

Section

II

A Review of Important Topics

Surfactant Replacement Therapy in Extremely Low Gestational Age Newborns

M Eibisberger, E Resch, B Resch

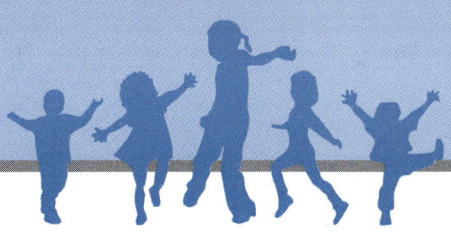

Many trials have been carried out to establish the relative efficacy of various surfactant products in improving clinical outcome in preterm infants with respiratory distress syndrome (RDS). Meta-analyses of trials comparing natural and synthetic surfactants showed a clear reduction in air leaks and suggested improved survival with natural surfactants.[1] In 2000, Ainsworth, *et al.*[2] reported a higher mortality rate in infants receiving a synthetic surfactant compared with the natural surfactant. A Cochrane review of eleven trials demonstrated a significant reduction in the risk of pneumothorax and mortality rate by use of natural surfactant.[3] Both natural surfactant extracts and synthetic surfactant extracts were effective in the treatment and prevention of RDS but natural surfactant treatment was associated with greater early improvement in the requirement for ventilatory support.

Prophylactic surfactant administration to infants judged to be at risk of developing RDS (intubated infants less than 30–32 weeks gestation) demonstrated a decreased incidence of pneumothorax, pulmonary interstitial emphysema and mortality.[4] Results suggested that there would be two less cases of pneumothorax and five less deaths per 100 infants treated with prophylactic surfactant compared

to rescue treatment when surfactant was given within 15 minutes of birth. This regimen was shown to be as effective as treatment before the first breath.[5]

In contrast, no difference between early and late surfactant therapy was observed in a controlled clinical study having a high rate of antenatal steroid treatment in the study population.[6] In most of the earlier trials, the rate of antenatal steroid use was low. The latest Cochrane review of trials comparing early selective treatment of RDS (within the first 2 hours of life) to late selective treatment found evidence of the benefit of early therapy.[7]

RECENT TRIALS

Some recent trials focussed on continuous positive airway pressure (CPAP) treatment and optimal surfactant timing in extremely low gestational age newborns.[8–11] The Continuous Positive Airway Pressure or Intubation at Birth (COIN) trial assigned 610 infants who were born at 25–28 weeks of gestational age to CPAP or intubation and ventilation at 5 minutes after birth.[8] At 28 days, there was a lower risk of death or need for oxygen therapy in the CPAP group than in the intubation group (OR 0.63; 95% CI 0.46 to 0.88; P=0.006). At 36 weeks of gestational age, 33.9% of 307 infants who were assigned to receive CPAP had died or had bronchopulmonary dysplasia (BPD), as compared with 38.9% of 303 infants who were assigned to receive intubation (OR favoring CPAP 0.80; 95% CI, 0.58 to 1.12; P=0.19). There was little difference in overall mortality. In the CPAP group, 46% of infants were intubated during the first 5 days, and the use of surfactant was halved. The incidence of pneumothorax was significantly increased with 9% in the CPAP as compared with 3% in the intubation group (P <0.001), but there were no other serious adverse events. The CPAP group had fewer days of ventilation. Results showed that primary CPAP treatment with surfactant administration, only if ventilation is required, was comparable to intubation and immediate surfactant replacement therapy.

The Surfactant Positive Pressure and Pulse Oximetry Randomized Trial (SUPPORT) by the NICHD Neonatal Research Network included infants between 24 and 27 week of gestational age, who were assigned to intubation and surfactant treatment within 1 hour after birth or to CPAP treatment, including the possibility of surfactant administration if intubation criteria were met.[9] Overall, death or BPD was not significantly different between the study groups. A significantly lower mortality rate was found in infants who were born between 24 and 25 weeks and treated with CPAP compared to the same age group treated with intubation and surfactant therapy (death during hospitalization: 23.9% *vs* 32.1%, P=0.03; death at 36 weeks: 20.0% *vs* 29.3%, P=.01). This study demonstrated that CPAP with subsequent surfactant therapy (if needed) is an equivalent alternative to intubation and primary surfactant treatment. The Breathing Outcomes Study, a prospective secondary study to the SUPPORT trial, assessed respiratory morbidity at 6-month intervals from hospital discharge to 18–22 months corrected age.[10] Treatment with early CPAP rather than intubation/surfactant was associated with less respiratory morbidity defined as wheezing more than twice per week during the worst 2-week period or cough longer than 3 days without a cold.

A multicentre randomized trial by the Vermont Oxford Network DRM study group[11] compared three approaches to the initial respiratory management of preterm neonates born at 26 to 29 weeks of gestational age: prophylactic surfactant followed by a period of mechanical ventilation (prophylactic surfactant); prophylactic surfactant with rapid extubation to bubble nasal CPAP (intubate-surfactant-extubate) or initial management with bubble CPAP and selective surfactant treatment (nCPAP). The primary composite outcome of death or BPD at corrected 36 weeks of gestational age in 648 infants enrolled at 27 centres did not differ between the groups. In the nCPAP group, 48% were managed without intubation and ventilation, and 54% without surfactant treatment. The authors concluded that initial CPAP was a possible and less invasive and probably even less expensive alternative to surfactant prophylaxis.

Prophylactic surfactant followed by nCPAP, and nCPAP with early selective surfactant therapy were compared in the CURPAP trial.[12] Of 208 inborn infants born at 25 to 28 weeks of gestational age, who were not intubated at birth, 105 were randomly assigned to prophylactic surfactant or nCPAP within 30 minutes of birth. Thirty-three (31.4%) infants in the prophylactic surfactant group (n=103), needed mechanical ventilation in the first 5 days of life compared with 34 (33.0%) in the nCPAP group (RR 0.95, 95% CI0.64–1.41; P=0.80). Death and type of survival at 28 days of life and at corrected 36 weeks of gestational age, and incidence of main morbidities of prematurity (secondary outcomes) were similar between groups. A total of 78.1% of infants in the prophylactic surfactant group and 78.6% in the nCPAP group survived in room air at corrected

36 weeks of gestational age.[12] In summary, prophylactic surfactant was not superior to nCPAP and early selective surfactant in decreasing the need for mechanical ventilation and the other morbidities of prematurity in spontaneously breathing very preterm infants on nCPAP.

Taking these results together, primary nCPAP treatment and early surfactant therapy after establishment of respiratory distress syndrome signs seem to be appropriate for clinical practice in extremely low gestational age infants.

The Intubation Surfactant Extubation (INSURE) procedure is discussed as an alternative procedure that may have the potential to combine the positive effects of surfactant and early CPAP.[13] Another mode of surfactant administration, via a thin endotracheal catheter during spontaneous breathing with CPAP, has recently come into clinical use.[14–16] Results of a multicentre German study showed that the application of surfactant to spontaneously breathing preterm infants was feasible, and it reduced the need for subsequent mechanical ventilation.[17] This effect was even more pronounced in the subgroup of infants who were stabilized with CPAP after birth. The intervention group had significantly fewer median days on mechanical ventilation, and a lower need for oxygen therapy at 28 days compared with the standard treatment group. The authors recorded no differences in mortality or serious adverse events between the groups. The main limitations of the new method were the need for expertise, and a risk of trauma.[18] This minimally invasive surfactant therapy (MIST) was also successfully evaluated in eleven preterm infants (25 to 28 weeks of gestational age) in Australia.[19] The subsequent initiated Collaborative Paired Trials Investigating Minimally-Invasive Surfactant Therapy (OPTIMIST) trial is planned to enroll a total of 606 infants from more than 30 centres worldwide, and is expected to be completed by end-2017.[20]

Klebermass, *et al.*[21] used this less invasive surfactant administration (LISA) technique in a prospective cohort of 224 preterm infants (23 to 27 weeks of gestational age), and compared the results with a historical control group.[21] LISA was well tolerated by 94% of all infants, and 68% of infants stayed on CPAP on day 3. The rate of mechanical ventilation was 35% within the first week and 59% during the entire hospital stay. Compared to historical controls, significantly higher survival rates and significantly less intraventricular hemorrhage and cystic periventricular leukomalacia, but higher rates of patent ductus arteriosus and retinopathy of prematurity were documented. Experience with the MIST technique used in 44 preterm infants was recently compared to the INSURE procedure of a historical control group of 31 infants. It resulted neither in any difference regarding the rate of intubation and mechanical ventilation during the first 72 hours, nor secondary respiratory outcomes and relevant morbidities between the groups.[22] Interestingly, significantly more babies in the MIST group (35%) compared to the INSURE group (6.5%) needed a second dose of surfactant.

A meta-narrative review of the efficacy and safety of minimally invasive surfactant administration using a thin catheter, aerosolization, a laryngeal mask airway, and pharyngeal administration in preterm infants with or at risk for respiratory distress syndrome recently reported on 10 studies (6 randomized and 4 observational), including 3081 neonates.[23] None of the studies reported any significant harm with any of the techniques. No statistically significant reduction in BPD but a potential reduction in the need for mechanical ventilation within 72 hours of birth when compared with standard care was observed in eligible studies. The authors concluded that surfactant administration via a thin catheter might be an efficacious and potentially safe method.

GUIDELINES AND RECOMMENDATIONS

Updated guidelines of the European Association of Perinatal Medicine[24] recommend the early use of CPAP of at least 5–6 cm H_2O in spontaneously breathing babies via mask or nasal prongs. Babies with or at high risk of RDS should be given a natural surfactant preparation and prophylaxis (within 15 min of birth) should be given to almost all babies below 26 weeks of gestational age. These guidelines also recommend prophylaxis for all preterm babies with RDS who require intubation for stabilization. Early rescue surfactant is recommended for previously untreated babies if there is evidence of RDS. Immediate (or early) extubation to non-invasive respiratory support following surfactant administration should be considered provided the baby is otherwise stable. Up to three doses of surfactant are recommended if there is ongoing evidence of RDS such as a persistent oxygen requirement and need for mechanical ventilation.

The latest guidelines of the American Academy of Pediatrics Committee on Fetus and Newborn[25] implicate the following for the use of surfactant in case of RDS. Preterm infants born at <30 weeks gestation who need mechanical ventilation because of severe RDS should be given surfactant after initial stabilization. Using CPAP immediately after birth with subsequent selective surfactant administration should be considered as an alternative to routine intubation with prophylactic or early surfactant administration in preterm infants. Rescue surfactant may be considered for infants with hypoxic respiratory failure attributable to secondary surfactant deficiency. Preterm and term neonates who are receiving surfactant should be managed by nursery and transport personnel with the technical and clinical expertise to administer surfactant safely, and unexperienced personnel should wait for the transport team to arrive.

The Committee on Fetus and Newborn recently recommended the early use of CPAP with subsequent selective surfactant administration in extremely preterm infants resulting in lower rates of BPD/death when compared with treatment with prophylactic or early surfactant therapy.[26] Early CPAP is likely to result in a reduction in duration of mechanical ventilation and postnatal corticosteroid therapy. Additionally the Expert committee states the necessity of individualized patient care that is provided in a variety of care-settings, and thus the capabilities of the health care team need to be considered as well. Finally the committee recommends that the use of CPAP immediately after birth with subsequent selective surfactant administration may be considered as an alternative to routine intubation with prophylactic or early surfactant administration in preterm infants, and if it is likely that respiratory support with a ventilator will be needed, early administration of surfactant followed by rapid extubation is preferable to prolonged ventilation.

CONCLUSION

There is a growing body of evidence in recent years suggesting CPAP ventilation being the first choice of ventilatory support in extremely low gestational age newborns, and early rescue surfactant treatment being as effective as prophylactic therapy. The new minimal or less- invasive surfactant administration technique shows some short-term benefits but still cannot be recommended for general use in this vulnerable population of preterm infants. It is highly encouraging to observe all those new studies being in search for the optimal clinical management of RDS in extremely low gestational age newborns. Long-term follow-up studies are needed to formulate recommendations on surfactant therapy in this high-risk population.

REFERENCES

1. Halliday HL. Natural vs. synthetic surfactants in neonatal respiratory distress syndrome. Drugs 1996;51:226–37.

2. Ainsworth SB, Beresford MW, Milligan DWA, Shaw NJ, Fenton AC, Ward P. Pumactant and poractant alfa for treatment of respiratory distress syndrome in neonates born at 25–29 weeks' gestation: A randomised trial. Lancet. 2000;355: 1387–92.

3. Soll RF, Blanco F. Natural surfactant extract versus synthetic surfactant for neonatal respiratory distress syndrome. Cochrane Database Syst Rev 2001:CD000144.

4. Soll RF, Morley CJ. Prophylactic versus selective use of surfactant in preventing morbidity and mortality in preterm infants. Cochrane Database Syst Rev 2001:CD000510.

5. Kendig JW, Ryan RM, Sinkin RA, Maniscalco WM, Notter RH, Guillet C, et al. Comparison of two strategies for surfactant prophylaxis in very premature infants: a multicenter randomized trial. Pediatrics 1998;101:1006–12.

6. Gortner L, Wauer RR, Hammer H, Stock GJ, Heitmann F, Reiter HL, et al. Early versus late surfactant treatment in preterm infants of 27 to 32 weeks' gestational age: A multicenter controlled clinical trial. Pediatrics 1998;102:1153–60.

7. Bahadue FL, Soll R. Early versus delayed selective surfactant treatment for neonatal respiratory distress syndrome. Cochrane Database Syst Rev 2012:CD001456.

8. Morley CJ, David PG, Doyle LW, Brion LP, Hascoet JM, Carlin JB; COIN Trial Investigators. Nasal CPAP or intubation at birth for very preterm infants. N Engl J Med 2008;358:700–8.

9. SUPPORT Study Group of the Eunice Kennedy Shriver NICHD Neonatal Research Network, Finer NN, Carlo WA, Walsh MC, Rich W, Gantz MG, Laptook AR, et al. Early CPAP versus surfactant in extremely preterm infants. N Engl J Med 2010;362:1970–9.

10. Stevens TP, Finer NN, Carlo WA, Szilagyi PG, Phelps DL, Walsh MC, et al., SUPPORT Study Group of the Eunice Kennedy Shriver National Institute of Child Health and Human Development Neonatal Research Network. Respiratory outcomes of the surfactant positive pressure and oximetry randomized trial (SUPPORT). J Pediatr 2014;165:240–9.

11. Dunn MS, Kaempf J, de Klerk A, de Klerk R, Reilly M, Howard D, et al. Vermont Oxford Network DRM Study Group. Randomized trial comparing 3 approaches to the initial respiratory management of preterm neonates. Pediatrics. 2011;128:e1069–76.

12. Sandri F, Plavka R, Ancora G, Simeoni U, Stranak Z, Martinelli S, et al. CURPAP Study Group. Prophylactic or early selective surfactant combined with nCPAP in very preterm infants. Pediatrics. 2010;125:e1402–9.

13. Verder H, Robertson B, Greisen G, Ebbesen F, Albertsen P, Lundstrøm K, et al. Surfactant therapy and nasal continuous positive airway pressure for newborns with respiratory distress syndrome. Danish-Swedish Multicenter Study Group. N Engl J Med 1994;331:1051–5.

14. Kribs A, Pillekamp F, Hünseler C, Vierzig A, Roth B. Early administration of surfactant in spontaneous breathing with nCPAP: Feasibility and outcome in extremely premature infants (postmenstrual age ≤27 weeks). Paediatr Anaesth 2007;17:364–9.

15. Kribs A, Vierzig A, Hünseler C, Eifinger F, Welzing L, Stützer H, et al. Early surfactant in spontaneously breathing with nCPAP in ELBW infants—a single centre four year experience. Acta Paediatr 2008;97:293–8.

16. Kribs A, Härtel C, Kattner E, Vochem M, Küster H, Möller J, et al. Surfactant without intubation in preterm infants with respiratory distress: First multi-center data. Klin Padiatr 2010;222:13–7.

17. Göpel W, Kribs A, Ziegler A, Laux R, Hoehn T, Wieg C, et al. German Neonatal Network. Avoidance of mechanical ventilation by surfactant treatment of spontaneously breathing preterm infants (AMV): an open-label, randomised, controlled trial. Lancet 2011;378:1627–34.

18. Kribs A. How best to administer surfactant to VLBW infants? Arch Dis Child Fetal Neonatal Ed 2011;96:F238-40.

19. Dargaville PA, Aiyappan A, Cornelius A, Williams C, De Paoli AG. Preliminary evaluation of a new technique of minimally invasive surfactant therapy. Arch Dis Child Fetal Neonatal Ed 2011;96:F243-8.

20. Dargaville PA, Kamlin CO, De Paoli AG, Carlin JB, Orsini F, Soll RF, et al. The OPTIMIST-A trial: evaluation of minimally-invasive surfactant therapy in preterm infants 25–28 weeks gestation. BMC Pediatr 2014;14:213.

21. Klebermass-Schrehof K, Wald M, Schwindt J, Grill A, Prusa AR, Haiden N, *et al.* Less invasive surfactant administration in extremely preterm infants: impact on mortality and morbidity. Neonatology 2013;103:252–8.

22. Aguar M, Cernada M, Brugada M, Gimeno A, Gutierrez A, Vento M. Minimally invasive surfactant therapy with a gastric tube is as effective as the intubation, surfactant, and extubation technique in preterm babies. Acta Paediatr 2014;103: e229–33.

23. More K, Sakhuja P, Shah PS. Minimally invasive surfactant administration in preterm infants: A meta-narrative review. JAMA Pediatr 2014;168: 901–8.

24. Sweet DG, Carnielli V, Greisen G, Hallman M, Ozek E, Plavka R, *et al.* European Association of Perinatal Medicine. European consensus guidelines on the management of neonatal respiratory distress syndrome in preterm infants–2010 update. Neonatology 2010;97:402–17.

25. Polin RA, Carlo WA. Committee on Fetus and Newborn; American Academy of Pediatrics. Surfactant replacement therapy for preterm and term neonates with respiratory distress. Pediatrics 2014;133:156–63.

26. Committee on Fetus and Newborn; American Academy of Pediatrics. Respiratory support in preterm infants at birth. Pediatrics 2014;133: 171–4.

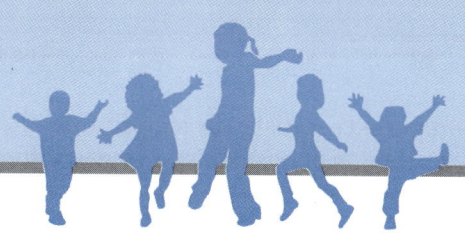

Surfactant Replacement Therapy Beyond Respiratory Distress Syndrome

Bonny Jasani, Nandkishor Kabra, Ruchi Nanavati

Surfactant replacement therapy is an established effective and safe therapy for immaturity-related surfactant deficiency.[1]

Meta-analysis of randomized controlled trials (RCTs) has confirmed that natural surfactant administration in preterm infants with RDS reduces mortality, decreases the incidence of pulmonary air leak (pneumothorax and pulmonary interstitial emphysema), and lowers the risk of bronchopulmonary dysplasia (BPD) or death at 28 days of age.[2]

Although RDS is characterized by the absence or reduction of surfactant, there are other neonatal lung disorders in which inadequate functional surfactant—either by inactivation or inhibition of synthesis may be a prominent element of the pathophysiology either by inactivation or inhibition of synthesis. These include meconium aspiration syndrome (MAS), pulmonary hemorrhage, pneumonia, congenital diaphragmatic hernia and BPD. The objective of this review is to critically evaluate the role of surfactant replacement therapy in neonatal respiratory conditions other than RDS.

MECONIUM ASPIRATION SYNDROME

The pathophysiology of meconium aspiration syndrome (MAS) is complex and multi-factorial. Constituents of meconium, especially bile salts, can inactivate surfactant. Inflammatory mediators, such as cytokines and eicosanoids, can also inhibit surfactant, as can the protein that leaks into the alveolar spaces.[3] Reduced pulmonary blood flow may cause pulmonary ischemia, with damage to the type II cells and reduced surfactant production. Airway obstruction may cause increased resistance and surfactant deficiency. Parenchymal lung changes may require high ventilator support and substantial supplemental oxygen, contributing to lung injury. Thus, surfactant replacement to break this vicious cycle is an attractive option. Two approaches have been attempted: surfactant replacement and surfactant lavage.

Surfactant Replacement

Evidence

In a meta-analysis of four trials (n=326),[4] surfactant replacement by bolus or slow infusion in infants with severe MAS had no statistically significant effect on mortality [typical risk ratio (RR) 0.98, 95% CI 0.41 to 2.39]. The risk of requiring extracorporeal membrane oxygenation (ECMO) was significantly reduced in a meta-analysis of two trials (n=208); [typical RR 0.64, 95% CI 0.46 to 0.9]. Findlay, *et al.*[5] in a trial of 40 term neonates, reported a statistically significant reduction in the length of hospital stay (mean difference -8 days, 95% CI–14 to –3 days). There was no statistically significant reduction in duration of assisted ventilation, duration of supplemental oxygen, air leaks, chronic lung disease, need for oxygen at discharge or intraventricular hemorrhage. Another meta-analysis incorporated eight RCTs of surfactant for MAS with a total of 512 patients.[6] It reported that surfactant significantly treatment reduced oxygenation index, increased arterial oxygen/alveolar oxygen ratio, shortened hospitalization days and decreased mortality rate. There was no statistical difference in the durations of mechanical ventilation and oxygen therapy, and the incidences of air leaks, pulmonary hemorrhage and intracranial hemorrhage between the two groups.

Surfactant Lavage

An alternative approach to treatment of MAS is the technique of lung lavage. This takes advantage of the detergent-like property of pulmonary surfactant, in which meconium might be solubilized and literally "washed" from the lung. Thus, in addition to replenishing the lung with functional surfactant, lavage might theoretically remove particulate meconium and prevent some of the pathophysiology attributed to obstruction and toxicity.[7] Surfactant lavage has been performed in several animal and human studies, with an optimal total lavage fluid volume of 15 to 30 mL/kg.[8–12] The surfactant was diluted in these studies in physiological saline to obtain a final phospholipid concentration of 5 mg/mL.[13]

Evidence

In a recent meta-analysis of surfactant lavage, lung lavage with diluted surfactant was shown to be beneficial to infants with MAS in terms of reduction in composite outcome of death or use of ECMO (RR 0.33, 95% CI 0.11 to 0.96; n=88).[14] Additional controlled clinical trials of

lavage therapy should be conducted to confirm this effect, to refine the method of lavage, and to compare lavage with other approaches including surfactant bolus therapy.[14] In a study of newborn lambs with respiratory failure and pulmonary hypertension induced by MAS, gas exchange and lung compliance were improved by lung lavage with dilute surfactant but not by bolus treatment.[15] Till further robust evidence is available, lung lavage with surfactant in MAS should be considered as an experimental therapy. In infants with MAS, if ECMO is not available, surfactant administration may reduce the severity of respiratory illness, mortality and decrease the number of infants with progressive respiratory failure requiring support with ECMO.

Recent Developments

Henn, et al.[16] assessed the effect of surfactant administration in 21 newborn pigs, preceded or not by bronchoalveolar lavage (BAL) with dilute surfactant, on pulmonary function in experimental severe MAS. BAL with dilute surfactant, followed by an additional dose of surfactant, produced significant improvements in arterial blood gases and pulmonary mechanics as compared with a single dose of surfactant.

A synthetic surfactant (CHF5633), containing SP-B and SP-C analogs, was tested in 26 newborn pigs for resistance to meconium inactivation in comparison to poractant alfa.

Surfactant was inactivated in both groups 6 hours after meconium instillation, but CHF5633 was more resistant than poractant alfa in terms of lipid peroxidation. This study indicates that CHF5633 may be as efficient as poractant alfa in experimental MAS.[17]

In a recent study by Mikolka, et al.[18] budesonide was added into surfactant preparation curosurf to enhance efficacy of the surfactant therapy in experimental model of MAS. Combined therapy improved gas exchange, and showed a longer-lasting effect than surfactant-only therapy. In conclusion, budesonide additionally improved the effects of exogenous surfactant in experimental MAS.

PNEUMONIA

Surfactant inactivation may be associated with pneumonia.[19,20] Facco, et al.[21] studied kinetics of surfactant's major component, disaturated-phosphatidylcholine (DSPC), in neonatal pneumonia and concluded that DSPC half-life and pool size were markedly impaired in neonatal pneumonia, and that they inversely correlated with the degree of respiratory failure. In a small randomized trial of surfactant rescue therapy, the subgroup of infants with sepsis showed improved oxygenation and a reduced need for ECMO compared with a similar group of control infants.[19] Newborn infants with pneumonia or sepsis receiving rescue surfactant also demonstrated improved gas exchange compared with infants without surfactant treatment.[20]

PULMONARY HEMORRHAGE

Experimental data suggest that the molecular components involved in pulmonary hemorrhage can biophysically inactivate endogenous lung surfactant, and exogenous surfactant replacement may be capable of reversing this process even in the continued presence of inhibitor molecules.[22,23]

Evidence

In two clinical studies, the mean oxygenation index improved in preterm and term infants who received surfactant following clinically significant pulmonary hemorrhage, with no clinical deterioration in any patient.[24,25] Case reports have also described the successful use of surfactant treatment after idiopathic[26] or iatrogenic[27] pulmonary hemorrhage. However, a recent systematic review[28] found no randomized or quasi-randomized trials evaluating the effects of surfactant in pulmonary hemorrhage in neonates, suggesting the need for such trials.

Recent Developments

A recent study evaluated the impact of surfactant upon in vitro clot formation in order to assess the role of surfactant in the pathogenesis of pulmonary hemorrhage. The presence of surfactant impairs coagulation in vitro hence conferring greater risk of pulmonary haemorrhage in extremely preterm infants.[29] Bozdağ, et al.[30] in an RCT compared efficacy of two natural surfactants (poractant alfa and beractant) for pulmonary hemorrhage in 42 very low-birth-weight (VLBW) infants. They concluded that both natural surfactants improved oxygenation, and the type of surfactant did not seem to have any effect on BPD and mortality rates in these patients.

CONGENITAL DIAPHRAGMATIC HERNIA (CDH)

Pulmonary hypoplasia and pulmonary hypertension are the hallmarks of CDH, but morphologic and biochemical immaturity of the lung have also been noted, and exogenous surfactant as adjuvant treatment for the severe respiratory distress associated with this disease is an attractive concept. Data from human studies in CDH are conflicting. In human fetuses with CDH, amniotic fluid lecithin to sphingomyelin (L/S) ratios and phosphatidylglycerol (PG) levels have been inconsistent; some investigators have found normal values and others document values suggestive of lung immaturity.[31–35] Moreover, surfactant phosphatidylcholine synthesis and pool size do not appear to be altered by CDH, although turnover of phosphatidylcholine is faster in CDH, possibly due to increased catabolism and/or recycling.[36] Of the few studies that have examined surfactant proteins (SP) expression in CDH, data are available only for SP-A. The concentration of SP-A in tracheal aspirates of infants with CDH has been shown to be either unchanged[37] or reduced[38] by CDH.

Evidence

There have been no multicenter randomized trials of surfactant for respiratory failure due to CDH. In two retrospective analyses of patients in the CDH Study Group, surfactant treatment did not improve outcomes,[39] and was associated with increased ECMO use, a higher incidence of chronic lung disease, and lower survival.[40] In preterm infants with CDH, the usage of surfactant was associated with a lower survival rate.[41]

Recent Developments

Janssen, et al.[42] studied endogenous surfactant metabolism in the most severe CDH patients who required ECMO. These patients have a decreased surfactant phosphatidylcholine synthesis that may be part of the pathogenesis of severe pulmonary insufficiency and has a negative impact on weaning from ECMO. Cogo, et al.[43] measured DSPC and SP-B concentration in tracheal aspirates and their synthesis rate in infants with CDH compared to infants without lung disease. Infants with CDH had a lower rate of synthesis of SP-B and less SP-B in tracheal aspirates. In these infants, partial SP-B deficiency could contribute to the severity of respiratory failure and its correction might represent a therapeutic goal.[43]

BRONCHOPULMONARY DYSPLASIA (BPD)

BPD describes the end product of a multitude of injuries and exposures to the preterm lung occurring prenatally, perinatally, and post-natally. The etiology of BPD is multifactorial, and involves derangements in multiple aspects of lung function (for example, sur-factant production), repair from injury (for example, elastin deposition), and growth and development (for example, alveologenesis). These derangements of normal development are likely mediated, in part, by chronic inflam-mation that develops in the immature lung exposed to repetitive ventilator stretch with oxygen-enriched gas, often complicated by infection.[44] Surfactant dysfunction (defined as elevation in the values of minimum surface tension *in vitro*) occurs in a high proportion (43–76%) of preterm infants who remain

intubated and ventilated at 1–2 weeks of age.[45-47] Infants are twice as likely to develop surfactant dysfunction during episodes of respiratory deterioration or infection, and higher minimum surface tension is directly correlated with an index of lung disease severity.[45,46] In these ventilated preterm infants, elevated minimum surface tension as measured in tracheal aspirates was associated with altered lipid composition, lower total protein in the surfactant fraction, and markedly lower content of surfactant proteins B and C. SP-B content had the strongest correlation with surface tension and was inversely related.[45] Similar findings relating SP-B content to surfactant dysfunction have been described in acute lung injury, thereby supporting the validity of using SP-B content as an indicator of surfactant function.[48] Heavy isotope labeling studies of intubated infants with BPD have demonstrated altered surfactant phospholipid pools and reduced recycling of alveolar surfactant phos-pholipids.[49,50]

Evidence

There is limited data evaluating late surfactant therapy for premature infants who require continuing ventilatory support beyond one week of life. Pandit, et al.[51] found that FiO$_2$ decreased significantly at 24 to 72 hours after a single dose of surfactant to ten premature infants. Bissinger, et al.[52] also demonstrated a transient improvement in oxygenation of premature infants >7 days after treatment with two doses of surfactant. Katz and Klein,[53] in a retrospective cohort study of 25 premature infants, found that late surfactant treatment was well tolerated, and that 70% of those treated had a short-term improvement in respiratory status. Laughon, et al.[54] in a multi-center pilot study administered surfactant to 136 intubated infants on days 3 to 10 of life, and reported a trend toward improved survival without BPD. Merill, et al.[47] in an open label pilot study of 87 very low birthweight infants reported a nonsignificant increase in the proportion of survivors without BPD when the number of late doses was increased.

Recent Developments

Keller, *et al.*[55] conducted a study to assess the safety and efficacy of late administration of SP-B containing surfactant (calfactant) in combination with prolonged inhaled nitric oxide (iNO) in infants ≤1,000 g birth weight. They randomized 85 preterm infants ventilated at 7–14 d after birth to receive late administration of surfactant (up to 5 doses) plus prolonged iNO or iNO alone. Late administration of surfactant had minimal acute adverse effects. Clinical status as well as surfactant recovery and SP-B content in tracheal aspirate were transiently improved as compared to the controls; these effects waned after 1 day. They concluded that late therapy with surfactant in combination with iNO is safe and transiently increases surfactant SP-B content, possibly leading to improved short- and long-term respiratory outcomes.[55]

An ongoing trial multi-center, blinded, randomized controlled clinical trial (NCT01022580) aims to evaluate the effects of booster doses of exogenous surfactant in addition to iNO on the outcome of survival without BPD at post-menstrual age of 36 weeks in extremely low gestational age infants.

CONCLUSION

Evidence demonstrating the utility of surfactant replacement therapy across the varied spectrum of neonatal respiratory disorders other than RDS exists, but there still remains a paucity of high-quality RCTs to recommend routine incorporation into clinical practice. Considering the evidence in support of surfactant replacement therapry as an effective management strategy in infants with MAS, large multicentric trials comparing bolus route and lung lavage route should be conducted. The outcomes should include short- and long-term clinical outcomes and any adverse effects.

In addition, future studies should focus on carefully designed RCTs of surfactant replacement therapy in term or late preterm infants with proven bacterial pneumonia. In addition, experimental studies exploring the pharmacokinetics, optimal dose and dosing interval, concentration, method of delivery and duration of treatment regimen in each of these conditions are needed to further optimize neonatal outcomes.

REFERENCES

1. Engle WA. American Academy of Pediatrics Committee on Fetus and Newborn. Surfactant replacement therapy for respiratory distress in the preterm and term neonate. Pediatrics 2008; 121:419–32.
2. Seger N, Soll R. Animal derived surfactant extract for treatment of respiratory distress syndrome. Cochrane Database Syst Rev 2009;2:CD007836.
3. Dargaville PA, South M, McDougall PN. Surfactant and surfactant inhibitor in meconium aspiration syndrome. J Pediatr 2001;138:113–5.
4. El Shahed AI, Dargaville P, Ohlsson A, Soll RF. Surfactant for meconium aspiration syndrome in term and late preterm infants. Cochrane Database Syst Rev 2014;12:CD002054.
5. Findlay RD, Taeusch HW, Walther FJ. Surfactant replacement therapy for meconium aspiration syndrome. Pediatrics. 1996;97:48–52.
6. Luo FF, Yang DY, Chen P, Hua ZY. Efficacy of pulmonary surfactant therapy in neonates with meconium aspiration syndrome: a meta-analysis. Zhongguo Dang Dai Er Ke Za Zhi 2012;14:413–7.
7. Donn SM, Dalton J. Surfactant replacement therapy in the neonate: beyond respiratory distress syndrome. Respir Care 2009;54:1203–8.
8. Dargaville PA, Copnell B, Mills JF, Haron I, Lee JK, Tingay DG, *et al.* Randomized controlled trial of lung lavage with dilute surfactant for meconium aspiration syndrome. J Pediatr 2011;158:383–9.
9. Wiswell TE, Knight GR, Finer NN, Donn SM, Desai H, Walsh WF, *et al.* A multicenter, randomized controlled trial comparing Surfaxin (Lucinactant) lavage with standard care for treatment of meconium aspiration syndrome. Pediatrics 2002;109:1081–7.
10. Dargaville PA, Mills JF, Headley BM, Chan Y, Coleman L, Loughnan PM, *et al.* Therapeutic lung

lavage in the piglet model of meconium aspiration syndrome. Am J Respir Crit Care Med 2003;168:456–463.

11. Lopez E, Gascoin G, Flamant C, Merhi M, Tourneux P, Baud O; French Young Neonatologist Club. Exogenous surfactant therapy in 2013: what is next? Who, when and how should we treat newborn infants in the future? BMC Pediatr 2013;13:165.

12. Lista G, Bianchi S, Castoldi F, Fontana P, Cavigioli F. Bronchoalveolar lavage with diluted porcine surfactant in mechanically ventilated term infants with meconium aspiration syndrome. Clin Drug Investig 2006;26:13–9.

13. Dargaville PA, Mills JF, Copnell B, Loughnan PM, McDougall PN, Morley CJ. Therapeutic lung lavage in meconium aspiration syndrome: A preliminary report. J Paediatr Child Health 2007;43:539–45.

14. Hahn S, Choi HJ, Soll R, Dargaville PA. Lung lavage for meconium aspiration syndrome in newborn infants. Cochrane Database Syst Rev 2013;4:CD003486.

15. Rey-Santano C, Alvarez-Diaz FJ, Mielgo V, Murgia X, Lafuente H, Ruiz-Del-Yerro E, et al. Bronchoalveolar lavage versus bolus administration of lucinactant, a synthetic surfactant in meconium aspiration in newborn lambs. Pediatr Pulmonol 2011;46:991–9.

16. Henn R, Fiori RM, Fiori HH, Pereira MR, Colvero MO, Ramos Garcia PC, et al. Surfactant with and without bronchoalveolar lavage in an experimental model of meconium aspiration syndrome. J Perinat Med 2015 Feb 20 [Epub ahead of print].

17. Salvesen B, Curstedt T, Mollnes TE, Saugstad OD. Effects of natural versus synthetic surfactant with SP-B and SP-C analogs in a porcine model of meconium aspiration syndrome. Neonatology 2014;105:128–35.

18. Mikolka P, Mokrá D, Kopincová J, Toměíková-Mikušiaková L, Calkovská A. Budesonide added to modified porcine surfactant Curosurf may additionally improve the lung functions in meconium aspiration syndrome. Physiol Res 2013;62:S191–200.

19. Tan K, Lai NM, Sharma A. Surfactant for bacterial pneumonia in late preterm and term infants. Cochrane Database Syst Rev 2012;2:CD008155.

20. Vento GM, Tana M, Tirone C, Aurilia C, Lio A, Perelli S, et al. Effectiveness of treatment with surfactant in premature infants with respiratory failure and pulmonary infection. Acta Biomed 2012;83:33–6.

21. Facco M, Nespeca M, Simonato M, Isak I, Verlato G, Ciambra G, et al. In vivo effect of pneumonia on surfactant disaturated-phosphatidylcholine kinetics in newborn infants. PLoS One 2014;9: e93612.

22. Holm BA, Notter RH. Effects of hemoglobin and cell membrane lipids on pulmonary surfactant activity. J Appl Physiol 1987;63:1434–42.

23. Wang Z, Notter RH. Additivity of protein and nonprotein inhibitors of lung surfactant activity. Am J Respir Crit Care Med 1998;158:28–35.

24. Pandit PB, Dunn MS, Colucci EA. Surfactant therapy in neonates with respiratory deterioration due to pulmonary hemorrhage. Pediatrics 1995;95:32–36.

25. Amizuka T, Shimizu H, Niida Y, Ogawa Y. Surfactant therapy in neonates with respiratory failure due to haemorrhagic pulmonary oedema. Eur J Pediatr 2003;162:697–702.

26. Neumayr TM, Watson AM, Wylam ME, Ouellette Y. Surfactant treatment of an infant with acute idiopathic pulmonary hemorrhage. Pediatr Crit Care Med 2008;9:e4–e6.

27. Haas NA, Kulasekaran K, Camphausen CK. Successful use of surfactant to treat severe intrapulmonary hemorrhage after iatrogenic lung injury–a case report. Pediatr Crit Care Med 2006; 7:583–5.

28. Aziz A, Ohlsson A. Surfactant for pulmonary haemorrhage in neonates. Cochrane Database Syst Rev 2012;7:CD005254.

29. Strauss T, Rozenzweig N, Rosenberg N, Shenkman B, Livnat T, Morag I, et al. Surfactant impairs coagulation in-vitro: A risk factor for pulmonary hemorrhage? Thromb Res 2013;132: 599–603.

30. Bozdað Þ, Dilli D, Gökmen T, Dilmen U. Comparison of two natural surfactants for pulmonary hemorrhage in very low-birth-weight infants: A randomized controlled trial. Am J Perinatol 2015;32:211–8.

31. Sullivan KM, Hawgood S, Flake AW, Harrison MR, Adzick NS. Amniotic fluid phospholipid analysis in the fetus with congenital diaphragmatic hernia. J Pediatr Surg 1994;29:1020–3.

32. Moya FR, Thomas VL, Romaguera J, Mysore MR, Maberry M, Bernard A, et al. Fetal lung maturation in congenital diaphragmatic hernia. Am J Obstet Gynecol 1995;173:1401–5.

33. Hisanaga S, Shimokawa H, Kashiwabara Y, Maesato S, Nakano H. Unexpectedly low lecithin/sphingomyelin ratio associated with fetal diaphragmatic hernia. Am J Obstet Gynecol 1984;149:905–6.

34. Wilcox DT, Glick PL, Karamanoukian HL, Azizhan RG, Holm BA. Pathophysiology of congenital diaphragmatic hernia, XII: amniotic fluid lecithin/sphingomyelin ratio and phosphatidylglycerol concentrations do not predict surfactant status in congenital diaphragmatic hernia. J Pediatr Surg 1995;30:410–2.

35. Ijsselstijn H, Zimmermann LJ, Bunt JE, de Jongste JC, Tibboel D. Prospective evaluation of surfactant composition in bronchoalveolar lavage fluid of infants with congenital diaphragmatic hernia and of age-matched controls. Crit Care Med 1998;26:573–80.

36. Cogo PE, Zimmermann LJ, Verlato G, Midrio P, Gucciardi A. A dual isotope tracer method for the measurement of surfactant disaturated phosphatidylcholine net synthesis in infants with congenital diaphragmatic hernia. Pediatr Res 2004;56:184–90.

37. Lotze A, Knight GR, Anderson KD, Hull WM, Whitsett JA. Surfactant (beractant) therapy for infants with congenital diaphragmatic hernia on ECMO: Evidence of persistent surfactant deficiency. J Pediatr Surg 1994;29:407–12.

38. Cogo PE, Zimmermann LJ, Rosso F, Tormena F, Gamba P. Surfactant synthesis and kinetics in infants with congenital diaphragmatic hernia. Am J Respir Crit Care Med 2002;166:154–8.

39. Colby CE, Lally KP, Hintz SR, Lally PA, Tibboel D, Moya FR, et al. Surfactant replacement therapy on ECMO does not improve outcome in neonates with congenital diaphragmatic hernia. J Pediatr Surg 2004;39:1632–7.

40. Van Meurs K. Is surfactant therapy beneficial in the treatment of the term newborn infant with congenital diaphragmatic hernia? J Pediatr. 2004; 145:312–6.

41. Lally KP, Lally PA, Langham MR, Hirschl R, Moya FR, Tibboel D. Surfactant does not improve survival rate in preterm infants with congenital diaphragmatic hernia. J Pediatr Surg 2004;39: 829–33.

42. Janssen DJ, Zimmermann LJ, Cogo P, Hamvas A, Bohlin K, Luijendijk IH, et al. Decreased surfactant phosphatidylcholine synthesis in neonates with congenital diaphragmatic hernia during extracorporeal membrane oxygenation. Intensive Care Med 2009;35:1754–60.

43. Cogo PE, Simonato M, Danhaive O, Verlato G, Cobellis G, Savignoni F, et al. Impaired surfactant protein B synthesis in infants with congenital diaphragmatic hernia. Eur Respir J 2013;41: 677–82.

44. Bose CL, Dammann CE, Laughon MM. Bronchopulmonary dysplasia and inflammatory biomarkers in the premature neonate. Arch Dis Child Fetal Neonatal Ed 2008;93:F455–F61.

45. Merrill JD, Ballard RA, Cnaan A, Hibbs AM, Godinez RI, Godinez MH, et al. Dysfunction of pulmonary surfactant in chronically ventilated premature infants. Pediatr Res 2004;56:1–9.

46. Ballard PL, Merrill JD, Truog WE, Godinez RI, Godinez MH, McDevitt TM, et al. Surfactant function and composition in premature infants treated with inhaled nitric oxide. Pediatrics 2007;120:346–53.

47. Merrill JD, Ballard PL, Courtney SE, Durand DJ, Hamvas A, Hibbs AM, et al. Pilot trial of late booster doses of surfactant for ventilated premature infants. J Perinatol 2011;31:599–606.

48. Günther A, Schmidt R, Harodt J, Schmehl T, Walmrath D, Ruppert C, et al. Bronchoscopic administration of bovine natural surfactant in ARDS and septic shock: impact on biophysical and biochemical surfactant properties. Eur Respir J 2002;19:797–804.

49. Cogo PE, Toffolo GM, Gucciardi A, Benetazzo A, Cobelli C, Carnielli VP. Surfactant disaturated phosphati-dylcholine kinetics in infants with bronchopulmonary dysplasia measured with stable isotopes and a two-compartment model. J Appl Physiol 2005;99:323–9.

50. Spence KL, Zozobrado JC, Patterson BW, Hamvas A. Substrate utilization and kinetics of surfactant metabolism in evolving bronchopulmonary dysplasia. J Pediatr 2005;147:480–5.

51. Pandit PB, Dunn MS, Kelly EN, Perlman M. Surfactant replacement in neonates with early chronic lung disease. Pediatrics 1995;95:851–4.

52. Bissinger R, Carlson C, Hulsey T, Eicher D. Secondary surfactant deficiency in neonates. J Perinatol 2004;24:663–6.

53. Katz LA, Klein JM. Repeat surfactant therapy for postsurfactant slump. J Perinatol 2006;26:414–22.

54. Laughon M, Bose C, Moya F, Aschner J, Donn SM, Morabito C, et al. A pilot randomized, controlled trial of later treatment with a peptide-containing, synthetic surfactant for the prevention of bronchopulmonary dysplasia. Pediatrics. 2009;123: 89–96.

55. Keller RL, Merrill JD, Black DM, Steinhorn RH, Eichenwald EC, Durand DJ, et al. Late administration of surfactant replacement therapy increases surfactant protein-B content: a randomized pilot study. Pediatr Res 2012;72:613–9.

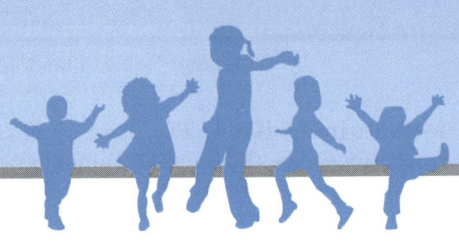

Continuous Positive Airway Pressure in Preterms Neonates

Neeraj Gupta, Shiv Sajan Saini, Srinivas Murki, Praveen Kumar, Ashok Deorari

Continuous Positive Airway Pressure (CPAP) is a well-established mode of respiratory support in preterm newborns. Advancement in technology, increasing survival of extremely preterm newborns and better understanding of various respiratory diseases led to new evidence in this field over last decade. It is important to update ourselves on the recent changes in the practice of CPAP and its implications for resource-limited settings.

We reviewed evidence for the clinical use of CPAP as a primary treatment for respiratory distress syndrome (RDS), delivery room CPAP, CPAP generator, heated humidified high flow nasal cannula (HHHFNC) and CPAP interface in neonates.

EVIDENCE ON CLINICAL USE

Primary Treatment of RDS

CPAP vs no CPAP (Hood oxygen): Meta-analysis evaluating CPAP against head box oxygen showed that CPAP use reduced the overall rate of mortality [RR 0.52 (95% CI 0.32, 0.87)] and the rate of the combined outcome of death or assisted ventilation [RR 0.70 (95% CI 0.55, 0.88)]. However, there was increased risk of pneumothorax [RR 2.64 (95% CI 1.39, 5.04); NNH 17 (17, 25)].[1] Use of CPAP has also shown to decrease the need for up-transfers to

higher centers.[2] The introduction of CPAP in a level II special newborn care unit significantly reduced the need for up-transfers as compared to pre-CPAP epoch, especially in very low birth weight (VLBW) and preterm infants.[3]

Early vs late CPAP: The application of CPAP early in the course of the disease before alveolar collapse occurs may work better than late CPAP by reducing lung damage and promoting lung function and surfactant pool. In the systematic review that compared early CPAP (starting CPAP at the time of randomization) *vs* late CPAP (initiating late in the course of disease when FiO_2 requirement is >0.60), early CPAP was associated with a significant reduction in subsequent use of mechanical ventilation [RR 0.55, (95% CI 0.32, 0.96); NNT 6]. But early CPAP had no effect on overall mortality, bronchopulmonary dysplasia (BPD) or pneumothorax.[4]

Delivery room/very early CPAP: The conventional approach of managing extreme premature infants was intubation, surfactant administration and mechanical ventilation. Gradually it was realized that both CPAP and surfactant lead to the same final goal of establishing functional residual capacity. Recently CPAP has been used to stabilize neonates immediately after resuscitation in the delivery room. Three high-quality randomized controlled trials compared delivery room CPAP (DR CPAP or prophylactic CPAP) with conventional approach[5-7] (Table 10.1). When used early in the delivery room in extreme preterm infants (gestation <28 weeks), either prophylactic[6,7] or early rescue,[5] CPAP

TABLE 10.1: Studies comparing delivery room CPAP or prophylactic CPAP with conventional approach

Author	Study design and population	Comparison	Results
Morley, et al. 2008 (COIN trial)	Multicentric RCT (N=610); 25–28+6 weeks who were spontaneously breathing in delivery room with mild to moderate respiratory distress.	Delivery room CPAP (DR CPAP) vs Conventional approach*	a. No difference in composite outcome of BPD or death at 36 weeks of post conceptional age (PCA) [OR 0.80 (95% CI 0.58–1.12)] b. DR CPAP group spent less time on mechanical ventilation (MV), surfactant need was almost half and required less postnatal steroids for BPD (P <0.05) c. Incidence of pneumothorax was high in DR CPAP group 9.1% vs 3.0%) compared to conventional group (P < 0.05)
Finer, et al. 2010 (SUPPORT trial)	Multicentric RCT (randomized before delivery) N=1316; 24–27+6 weeks All neonates independent of respiratory status	Prophylactic CPAP vs Conventional approach*	a. No difference in the composite outcome of BPD or death at 36 weeks of PCA [OR 0.95 (95% CI 0.85–1.05)] b. Need of surfactant, intubation and MV, duration of MV and use of postnatal steroid for BPD was less in prophylactic CPAP group compared to conventional group (P <0.05) c. No statistically significant difference in air leaks
Dunn, et al. 2011 (VON DRM trial)	Multicentric RCT(randomized before delivery) N=648; 26–29+6 weeks. All neonates independent of respiratory status	Prophylactic CPAP (nCPAP) vs prophylactic surfactant followed by mechanical ventilation [prophylactic surfactant (PS)] = conventional approach*) vs prophylactic surfactant with rapid extubation to CPAP [intubate-surfactant-extubate (ISX)]	a. No difference in composite outcome of BPD or death in PS group at 36 weeks of post conceptional age compared to nCPAP group [OR 0.83 (95% CI 0.64–1.09)] or ISX group [OR 0.78 (95% CI 0.59– 1.03)] b. In nCPAP group 48% were managed without intubation and ventilation, and 54% without surfactant treatment

*Conventional approach: Intubation, prophylactic surfactant followed by mechanical ventilation

was associated with almost 50% reduction in need for intubation mechanical ventilation, and surfactant usage in comparison to 'mechanical ventilation with or without surfactant'. The risk of death or BPD at 36 weeks was comparable between the two-treatment approaches in these trials. Thus it is clear that initial stabilization on CPAP and provision of rescue surfactant should be the preferred approach among preterm neonates ≤28 weeks of gestation.

CPAP and surfactant (InSurE strategy): CPAP and surfactant work together towards establishing and maintaining functional residual capacity in RDS. Verder, *et al.*[9] described a technique, InSurE (Intubation, surfactant, extubation), of administering surfactant to symptomatic preterm neonates who were stabilized on CPAP. Meta-analysis of six trials comparing early surfactant administration with brief mechanical ventilation (1 hour) followed by extubation *vs* later selective surfactant and continued mechanical ventilation in neonates with RDS reported that earlier strategy is associated with a significant reduction in need of mechanical ventilation (RR 0.67, 95% CI 0.57–0.79) and BPD (RR 0.51, 95% CI 0.26–0.99), but the relative contribution of early surfactant in decreasing the incidence of BPD remains speculative.[9]

Verder, *et al.*[10] and Reininger, *et al.*[11] showed that CPAP along with surfactant (by InSurE) as compared to CPAP alone in symptomatic preterm neonates with RD decreases the need of mechanical ventilation. The CURPAP trial[12] and the VON DRM trial[7] reported that prophylactic surfactant was not superior to nasal CPAP and early rescue surfactant in decreasing the need for mechanical ventilation in the first few days of life. Moreover, there was no difference in death or BPD at 36 weeks' postmenstrual age. A recent Cochrane systematic review (that included the SUPPORT and VON DRM trials) of prophylactic *vs* selective use of surfactant concluded that the benefits of prophylactic surfactant in terms of decreased air leaks and decrease mortality no longer holds true in contrast to the results of previous meta-analysis, which included studies when prophylactic or DR CPAP application was not practiced and the rate of coverage of antenatal steroids was low.[13] Moreover, a meta-analysis of these two studies alone demonstrated a compelling trend toward an increase in the risk of neonatal mortality or BPD associated with the use prophylactic surfactant when compared with early stabilization on CPAP with selective use of surfactant (typical RR 1.12, 95% CI 1.02, 1.24).[13] The same has been highlighted in the recent recommendations from American Academy of Pediatrics regarding the use of prophylactic surfactant in neonates <30 weeks gestation. There was a trend towards increased risk of BPD (RR 1.13, 95% CI 1.00–1.28) and death or BPD (RR 1.13; 95% CI 1.02–1.25) with use of prophylactic surfactant in infants born at <30 weeks gestation as compared to infants who were routinely applied CPAP in the delivery room.[14]

Two trials studied the ideal timing of rescue surfactant administration in moderately preterm infants (27 to 33 weeks of gestation) supported with CPAP within the first 1–2 hours of life. In both these trials for infants with RDS on CPAP, early addition of surfactant in comparison to CPAP alone was associated with lesser need for subsequent mechanical ventilation (Table 10.2).[15,16]

Overall, the current evidence supports CPAP as an acceptable safer alternative to endotracheal intubation in the delivery room, and to early rescue surfactant (InSurE) for preterm infants with RDS. However, it is important to note that all these recent trials (COIN, SUPPORT, VON DRM and CURPAP) have been done in extremely preterm neonates (<28 weeks) where the use of antenatal steroid coverage was very high (>90%).

Post-Extubation

Atelectasis and apnea often follow extubation in preterm neonates and nasal CPAP

TABLE 10.2: Macronutrient content and cost (per 100 g) of organic and conventional food items

Author	Study design and population	Comparison	Results
Rojas, et al. 2009	Multicentric RCT (N=279); 27–31^{+6} weeks who were spontaneously breathing in delivery room with evidence of respiratory distress and were on supplemental oxygen within first hour of life (15 min to 60 min)	Very early rescue surfactant by InSurE* followed by CPAP vs CPAP alone	a. Need for mechanical ventilation was significantly less in early rescue surfactant group (26% vs 39%); [RR 0.69 (95% CI 0.49-0.97)] b. Incidence of pneumothorax was less in early rescue surfactant group (2% vs 9%); [RR 0.25 (0.07-0.85) c. Trend toward less BPD in early rescue surfactant group (49% vs 59%) [RR 0.84 (95% CI 0.66–1.05)]
Kandraju, et al. 2013	RCT (N=153); 28–33^{+6} weeks All symptomatic neonates with RDS within first 2 hours of life	Early rescue surfactant by InSurE* followed by CPAP vs CPAP alone initially with late (FiO$_2$ > 0.50) selective surfactant	a. Need for mechanical ventilation was significantly less in early rescue surfactant group (16.2% vs 31.6%); [RR 0.41 (95% CI 0.19–0.91)] b. No significant difference in incidence of pneumothorax and BPD

*InSurE—Intubation, surfactant, extubation

is used in an attempt to reduce the need for re-ventilation. A meta-analysis of nine trials showed that neonates extubated to CPAP as compared to head box oxygen had less incidence of respiratory failure (apnea, respiratory acidosis and increased oxygen requirements).[17]

Apnea of Prematurity

There is widespread use of CPAP along with methylxanthines in treatment of apnea of prematurity. However, there is no RCT which used current CPAP interface to support this practice. Moreover, ethically it may not be possible to compare CPAP with 'no treatment group' to treat apnea of prematurity.

Other Applications

CPAP may be useful in other conditions that result in alveolar collapse or airway narrowing. It relieves the signs of cardiac failure due to patent ductus arteriosus. Similarly, it is often used in the management of pneumonia, transient tachypnea of newborn, postoperative respiratory management, pulmonary edema and pulmonary hemorrhage. In meconium aspiration syndromes (MAS), application of CPAP can be beneficial by resolving the atelectatic alveoli due to alveolar injury and secondary surfactant deficiency.[18] In an observational study of 66 neonates with MAS, in whom CPAP was started at a mean age of 5.3 hours, Murki, et al.[19] showed that 75% could be managed successfully with CPAP alone, especially if they were inborn. Incidence of pneumothorax in this study was 2.6%.[19] There is no head-to-head comparison of CPAP with mechanical ventilation in MAS. CPAP has been used for the management of laryngo/tracheo/bronchomalacia as positive pressure distends the large airways as well, and overcome their tendency to collapse, especially during expiration.

Appropriate Pressure for CPAP

There is paucity of data regarding the ideal range of CPAP pressures in neonates.[20] In a recent RCT, neonates (n=93) of 23–30 weeks gestation with residual lung disease (needing $FiO_2 > 0.25$) who were being extubated for the first time were randomized to receive low (4–6 cm) or high (7–9 cm) CPAP pressure.[21] The rates of extubation failure and re-intubation within 96 hours of extubation were significantly lower in the high CPAP pressure group. This was mainly due to strikingly lower failure rates in 500–750 g birth weight group.[21]

Weaning

A questionnaire survey done in 58 units in England revealed that 36 (66%) of the units used to wean by 'time off', 2 (4%) by weaning pressure, and in remaining 30%, there was no set method.[22] A randomized trial comparing the strategy of weaning pressure with one of increasing time off-CPAP showed a significant shorter duration of weaning with the 'pressure' strategy (1.5 days in pressure group vs 9 days in 'time off'; P 0.001).[23] A Cochrane review of three RCTs concluded that neonates in whom CPAP pressure was weaned to a pre-defined level, and then CPAP was stopped completely have less total time on CPAP and shorter durations of oxygen therapy and hospital stay compared with those in whom CPAP was removed for a pre-determined number of hours each day.[24] The overall evidence (Table 10.3)[25–27] favors abrupt stoppage of CPAP after achieving the stability criteria without any exposure to nasal cannula. The point at which to attempt abrupt stoppage of CPAP needs to be established in future trials.

TABLE 10.3: Recent trials of CPAP weaning

Author	Study design and population	Comparison	Results
Abdel-Hady, et al. 2011	RCT (N=60); ≥28 weeks who were clinically stable on NCPAP of 5 cmH₂O with $FiO_2 < 0.30$ for at least 24 h	No nasal cannula (No-NC) group: Infants kept on NCPAP until they were on $FiO_2 = 0.21$ for 24 h, and then were weaned off NCPAP completely without any exposure to NC vs Nasal cannula (NC) group: Infants weaned off NCPAP when FiO_2 was ≤0.30 to NC (2 L/min of oxygen) followed by gradual weaning from oxygen	a. No-NC group had fewer days on oxygen and shorter duration of respiratory support b. No difference regarding success of weaning from NCPAP
Todd, et al. 2012	Multicentric RCT (N=177); < 30 weeks who were clinically stabile on CPAP 4–6 cm with $FiO_2 < 25\%$ for at least 12 h	M1: Taken 'OFF' CPAP with with the view to stay 'OFF' vs M2: Cycled on and off CPAP with incremental time 'OFF' vs M3: As with M2, cycled on and off CPAP but during 'OFF' periods were supported by nasal cannula at a flow of 0.5 L/min	Method 1 significantly shortened CPAP weaning time, CPAP duration, oxygen duration, BPD and length of admission
O'Donnell, et al. 2013	2-center RCT (N=78); VLBW infants who were stable on CPAP of 3–5 cm H₂O with $FiO_2 = 0.21$ for 24 h	Nasal prong group: Treated with low-flow (1.0 L/min) nasal prongs with room air vs Spontaneous breathing in room air	No significant difference in failure rate of weaning from CPAP [41% in nasal prong group vs 31% in spontaneous breathing group (P=0.48)].

IDEAL CPAP DEVICE

CPAP Pressure Generator (Table 10.4)[28–33]

Bubble CPAP has the advantage over ventilator CPAP in producing pressure oscillations superimposed over the pressure fluctuations, as a result of spontaneous breathing. The noisy pressure waveform superimposed over pressure fluctuations (stochastic resonance effect) promotes lung recruitment resulting in better oxygenation.[29] Moreover, additional benefits accrue with bubble CPAP due to higher delivered pressure as compared to set pressure because of its flow-dependent nature. In spite of theoretical advantage of variable flow CPAP devices, data supporting its clinical superiority across all the settings are scarce (Table 10.5).[34–38] In a recent RCT comparing Benveniste valve (Jet CPAP) with bubble CPAP in neonates with RDS, there was no difference in the failure rate, mortality or any other morbidity between the two groups. The prong displacements were more common with Benveniste valve (Jet CPAP) as compared to bubble CPAP. However, the pain scores in neonates were lesser with Benveniste valve.[49]

Though, there is some evidence for the superiority of IFD and bubble CPAP over ventilator CPAP but the differences in study design, indications, short study epochs and insufficient relevant clinical outcomes necessitate the need for further studies on this issue.

Heated Humidified High-flow Nasal Cannula (HHFNC)

Simple nasal cannulas with an outer diameter of 3 mm and flows up to 2 L/min, have been reported to deliver CPAP. In humidified high-flow nasal cannula (HHFNC), warm and humidified respiratory gases are delivered at flow rates between 2 to 8 L/min. A systematic review of 19 studies concluded that HHHFNC may be as effective as nasal NCPAP in improving respiratory parameters, but its efficacy and safety in preterm neonates need

TABLE 10.4: Studies comparing bubble CPAP and ventilator CPAP

Author	Study design and population	Results
Lee, *et al.* 1998	Randomized crossover design N=10; 750–2000 g, preterm neonates ready for extubation	39% reduction in infant's lung volume and 7% reduction in respiratory rate but no difference in blood gas parameters in infants on bubble CPAP
Pillow, *et al.* 2007	Experimental (lamb model) N=34; preterm lambs treated with CPAP for 3 h	Bubble CPAP associated with a higher pH, PaO_2, oxygen uptake, and a decreased alveolar protein and ventilation in-homogeneity
Tagare, *et al.* 2010	RCT (pilot study) N=30; Preterm (<37 wk) neonates with respiratory distress and oxygen requirement >30% in first 6 h of life	Success rate and dislodgement rate were comparable
Courtney, *et al.* 2011	Randomized with crossover design N=18; neonates <1500 g and <28 d old and on NCPAP for mild respiratory distress	No significant difference in work of breathing, tidal volume, respiratory rate, heart rate, breathing asynchrony but transcutaneous oxygen was higher with Bubble CPAP
Yadav, *et al.* 2012	RCT (pilot study) N=32; neonates ≥32 wk and <1500 g	Bubble CPAP associated with 50% reduction in the extubation failure rate though difference was not statistically significant
Tagare, *et al.* 2013	RCT N=114; preterm neonates with Silverman-Anderson score >4 and oxygen requirement >30% within first 6 hours of life	Bubble CPAP has higher success rate than ventilator CPAP (82.5% *vs* 63.2%)

TABLE 10.5: Studies comparing various types of constant-flow with variable-flow pressure generators

Author	Study design and population	Comparison	Results
Moa, et al. 1988	Experimental *in vitro* study Lung model simulated breathing pattern of a newborn	Variable flow NCPAP *vs* Continuous flow NCPAP	Pressure variations in airway and external workload were less with variable flow CPAP device
Klausnr, et al. 1996	Experimental *in vitro* study Breathing apparatus simulating breathing pattern of a VLBW newborn	Variable flow NCPAP *vs* Continuous flow NCPAP	Imposed work of breathing and variations in airway pressure was less with variable flow NCPAP device
Ahluwalia, et al. 1998	Crossover study (N=20); Infant of 24–34 wk on CPAP with FiO_2 of 0.3.	Infant Flow Driver (IFD) *vs* Single prong ventilator NCPAP	No significant difference in respiratory rate, heart rate, blood pressure and comfort score
Courtney, et al. 2001	Crossover study (N=32); birth weight 1081 ±316 g, 29 ± 2 wk receiving NCPAP for apnea or mild respiratory distress enrolled at age of 13 ±12 d	IFD *vs* Ventilator NCPAP *via* CPAP prongs *vs* Ventilator NCPAP via modified nasal cannula	Compared with two continuous flow devices, the variable flow nasal CPAP device leads to greater lung recruitment
Pandit, et al. 2001	Crossover trial (N=24); <1800 g receiving constant-flow NCPAP for apnea or mild respiratory distress	Infant flow system NCPAP *vs* Ventilator NCPAP	Work of breathing lower with variable flow (13 to 29%) as compared to ventilator CPAP
Mazella, et al. 2001	RCT (N=36); RDS in <36 wk infants and <12 h old	IFD *vs* Nasopharyngeal bubble CPAP	Oxygen requirement and respiratory rate decreased by 4 h. Probability of remaining supplementary oxygen free over the first 48 h of treatment significantly higher in patients treated with the IFD.
Liptsen, et al. 2005	RCT (N=18); <1500 g birth weight, <28 d of age, requiring NCPAP for mild respiratory distress	IFD *vs* Bubble NCPAP	Resistive work of breathing, respiratory rate and phase angle (time lag between chest and abdominal movement) were all greater with bubble CPAP as compared to IFD
Boumecid, et al. 2007	Crossover study (N=13); 26–32 wk. All were evaluatedon each device applied for 30 min in random order	Variable-flow NCPAP *vs* Continuous flow NCPAP *vs* Nasal cannula	Variable-flow NCPAP increases tidal volume and improves thoraco-abdominal synchrony. Increased tidal volume is probably due to increased contribution of the rib cage.
Pantalitschka, et al. 2009	Crossover trial (N=16); 31 wk; all infants having apnea of prematurity were allocated to four different modes of respiratory support for 6 h each	NIPPV via a conventional ventilator *vs* NIPPV *via* a variable flow device *vs* NCPAP *via* a variable flow device *vs* NCPAP *via* a constant flow underwater bubble system	The median event rate [cumulative event rate of bradycardias ($\leq$80 beats per min) and desaturation events ($\leq$80% arterial oxygen saturation] was significantly less with variable flow CPAP as compared to bubble CPAP (2.8 *vs* 5.4 per hr)
Yaqui, et al. 2011	RCT (N=40); > 1500 g (mean birth weight 2500 g) with FiO_2 > 30% within first 24 h after	Variable flow CPAP *vs* Bubble CPAP	Bubble CPAP showed the same benefits (CPAP failure rate, total CPAP duration, total oxygen

NIPPV: Non-invasive positive pressure ventilation

Contd...

TABLE 10.5: Studies comparing various types of constant-flow with variable-flow pressure generators *(Contd...)*

Author	Study design and population	Comparison	Results
	birth (70% of subjects had TTNB)		duration) as variable flow CPAP in newborns with birth weight ≥1500 g and moderate respiratory distress
Bober, et al. 2012	Multicentric RCT (N=276); infants with birth weight 750–1500 g and ≤32 wk were divided into 'weaning group' (infants that met criteria for intubation and surfactant) and 'elective group' (infants that did not meet intubation criteria but required respiratory support within 6 h of delivery) and then were randomly assigned intervention	Infant flow CPAP vs Ventilator CPAP	Treatment failure (defined as the need for reintubation and mechanical ventilation within 3 days of initial extubation in the 'weaning group' and need for intubation in the first 3 days after first weaning from NCPAP in the 'elective group') was not statistically different between the two groups
Kirchner, et al. 2012	Experimental in vitro study Noise production was measured in a closed incubator at 2 mm lateral distance from the end of the nasal prongs in an experimental model	Variable flow CPAP generator (Infant flow and Medijet) vs Constant flow CPAP generator (Bubble CPAP and Baby flow ventilator CPAP)	Values measured at a continuous constant flow rate of 8 L/min averaged 83 dB for the Infant Flow, 72 dB for the MediJet, 62 dB for the Bubble CPAP and 55 dB for the Baby Flow. Constant flow work more quietly than variable flow CPAP generators

In post extubation setting

Author	Study design and population	Comparison	Results
Roukema et al. 1999	Crossover trial; N=93; <1250 g; Used as post extubation respiratory support to decrease extubation failure	Infant flow NCPAP vs Nasopharyngeal CPAP	Less extubation failure with IFD CPAP
Sun, et al.1999	RCT (N=73); <1250 g had RDS and were mechanically ventilated	Flow driver CPAP vs Conventional NCPAP	Extubation failure rate was higher in conventional NCPAP on day 1 and within 7 d of extubation
Kavvadia, et al. 2000	RCT (N=36); 25–35 wk 12 infants in each group after extubation were put on IFD or single nasal prong NCPAP or no CPAP	IFD vs Single nasal prong NCPAP vs No CPAP	IFD had no short term advantage over single nasal prong NCPAP when used after extubation
Stefanescu, et al. 2003	RCT N=162; <1000 g Used as post extubation respiratory support to decrease extubation failure	Infant flow NCPAP vs Ventilator NCPAP	IFD CPAP as effective as ventilator CPAP in preventing extubation failure
Huckstadt, et al. 2003	Randomized cross over trial (N=20), 26–40 wk; 640–4110 g; Being mechanically ventilated for TTNB, RDS, sepsis	Infant flow CPAP vs Ventilator CPAP	No significant increase in the inspiratory flow and tidal volume and less fluctuations in CPAP pressures during breathing cycle with Infant flow system
Gupta, et al. 2009	RCT (N=140), 24–29 wk; 600–1500 g had RDS and were mechanically ventilated	Bubble CPAP vs IFD	Bubble CPAP as effective as IFD CPAP, associated with a significantly higher rate of successful extubation in infants ventilator for <14 d, and a significantly reduced duration of CPAP support

further research.[50] A recent multicentric RCT in 432 neonate (28 to 42 weeks) comparing HHHFNC with CPAP device for planned nasal CPAP support, as either primary therapy or in post-extubation setting did not find any difference in early failure (10.8% *vs* 8.2%) or subsequent need for any intubation (15.1% *vs* 11.4%). HHHFNC neonates remained on the study mode significantly longer than nasal CPAP neonates (median: 4 *vs* 2 days, P<0.01), but there were no differences for days on supplemental oxygen, and BPD.[51] Another RCT on 132 neonates (<32 weeks gestation) in post-extubation setting did not find any difference in extubation failure rate (22% in HHHFNC *vs* 34% in NCPAP) within 7 days after extubation. However, the nasal trauma score was significantly less in HHHFNC group (3.1 *vs* 11.8; P<0.001) as compared to NCPAP group.[52] A randomized crossover trial found similar patient comfort score in preterm infants (n=20, <34 weeks gestation) who were treated with HHHFNC or NCPAP due to mild respiratory illness. However, parents preferred HHHFNC because of better child satisfaction, interaction and possibility to take part in care.[53] In a recent multicentric non-inferiority RCT done among neonates <32 weeks gestation (n = 303) in post-extubation setting, the use of HHHFNC was not inferior to NCPAP. The treatment failure within seven days after extubation occurred in 34.2% in HHHFNC group as compared to 25.8% in NCPAP group.[54] However, like previous trials, neonates in HHHFNC group had a significantly lower incidence of nasal trauma than those in the NCPAP group (39.5% *vs* 54.3%, P= 0.01). Thus, HHHFNC may have a potential role as an alternative to CPAP in post-extubation setting due to its ease of application and less nasal trauma.

Patient Interface

The most common interfaces used for CPAP are nasal prongs and nasal masks. Nasal prongs can be short (6–15 mm) or long (40–90 mm), and single or binasal. The long nasal prong which is actually a nasopharyngeal prong has the disadvantages of a high resistance, more prone to kinking and blockage by secretions, and difficulty in monitoring local side effects. The short binasal prongs include Argyle, Hudson, Medicorp, F and P, prongs and IFD prongs. Short binasal prongs have the least resistance to flow and are more effective at preventing re-intubation than single nasal or nasopharyngeal prongs [RR 0.59; 95% CI: 0.41, 0.85] in preterm neonates.[55] In patients with RDS, short binasal prongs were found to be superior to nasopharyngeal prongs in terms of lower oxygen requirement and less respiratory rate in first 48 hours.[56] Information about short binasal prongs is limited. A study comparing Hudson with Argyl prongs in preterm neonates, receiving nasal CPAP as initial ventilatory assistance or for weaning from a ventilator, concluded that Argyle prong is more difficult to be retained in the nostrils of active patients and nasal hyperemia occurs more frequently with its use.[57]

In another RCT among VLBW neonates, comparing nasal prongs with nasal mask, no significant difference was noted in the incidence of nasal injury.[58] A randomized trial in neonates <31 weeks gestation comparing nasal mask with binasal prongs showed less intubation rate within 72 hours for the treatment of RDS or in post-extubation setting with nasal mask (28% *vs* 52%; P=0.007).[59] In a recent RCT from India, Chandrasekaran, *et al*.[60] reported a 6% reduction in the oxygen requirement at 2 hours of CPAP initiation with nasal mask as compared to nasal prongs. Moreover, infants on nasal mask had no nasal injury (31.3% *vs* 0%; P<0.01). On post-hoc analysis, the need for surfactant after starting CPAP was markedly lesser (95% CI 33%-89%, P<0.01).[60] More evidence is required before nasal masks can replace short binasal prongs.

'RAM cannula' is a binasal prong like the oxygen prongs but with a diameter much wider than the conventional oxygen prongs. It is easy to apply and retains the benefit of a circuit with inspiratory and expiratory limbs to provide non-invasive ventilation. Preliminary data is promising but more evidence is required to support its use.[61] Nzegwu, et al.[62] in a recent prospective observational study showed that RAM cannula was well tolerated in neonates. The overall success rate in weaning off the RAM cannula was 66% in newborns who were on CPAP with FiO_2 $\leq$0.35.[62]

Recent Advances

Bilevel nasal CPAP, popularly known as BiPAP/SiPAP is a newer mode of non-invasive respiratory support similar to CPAP where two levels of CPAP (Phigh and Plow) are given at preset time intervals [Thigh (time the CPAP pressures are high) and Tlow (time the CPAP pressures are low)]. A study evaluating BiPAP after InSurE failure to prevent the need for mechanical ventilation among VLBW neonates (n=60) found that the need of mechanical ventilation was 27% in the historical controls as compared to 0% in the BiPAP group.[63] A RCT by Lista, et al.[64] comparing BIPAP with CPAP among neonates with RDS between 28–34 weeks of gestation (n=40) found similar cytokine levels in serum on day 1 and 7 of life. However, neonates in CPAP group required longer respiratory support and oxygen therapy, and were discharged later.[64] Another RCT comparing CPAP with BiPAP in the post-extubation setting among neonates (n=136) with birth weight $\leq$1250 g did not find any difference in the incidence of sustained extubation for next 7 days after extubation.[65] Thus, preliminary data is encouraging but more evidence is required in this direction.

Another recent innovation is Sea-PAP, a modification of bubble CPAP, where a segment of the expiratory tube immersed in water has been bent at an angle of 135°.[66] The rationale is to increase the amplitude of the oscillations which are superimposed on the pressure fluctuations, which may result in better recruitment of alveoli and better gas exchange. Preliminary data in animal studies are promising but the device requires clinical evaluation.[67]

LONG TERM OUTCOMES OF CPAP

In a retrospective analysis, Thomas, et al.[68] compared the ventilator support strategy (CPAP vs mechanical ventilation) at 24 h of age to predict neurodevelopmental outcomes. After adjusting for illness severity, those on CPAP at 24 hours of life had better Bayley Scores of Infant Development at 18–22 months of corrected age apart from lower BPD and lower mortality.[68] In the SUPPORT trial, there was no statistically significant difference in the composite outcome of death or neurodevelopmental impairment at 18–22 months of corrected age in early CPAP group as compared to mechanical ventilation and surfactant group.[69] Further studies are required to evaluate long-term impact of CPAP on various development and respiratory outcomes.

IMPLICATIONS AND APPLICABILITY

Assuming the incidence of RDS to be 1.2% among live-births, nearly 1,86,000 infants each year are affected with RDS in India.[70] With a reported mortality of 57% to 89% among infants with RDS, nearly 100,000 infants each year are estimated to die due to RDS.[71] Mechanical ventilation and CPAP are the mainstay in the management of RDS. Even the low-cost indigenously designed CPAP systems have been shown to be effective in reducing the mortality and up-transfers among term and preterm neonates with respiratory distress in low- and middle-income countries.[72–74]

A recent systematic review[75] examining the efficacy and safety of bubble CPAP in neonates with respiratory distress in low- and middle-income countries found that the initial use of bubble CPAP compared with oxygen therapy reduced the need for mechanical ventilation by 30–50%. Although the mortality and the complication rates between the bubble CPAP and ventilator CPAP were similar, the CPAP failure rate was lower in the bubble

CPAP group as compared to ventilator CPAP (3 RCTs, OR 0.32, 95% CI 0.16, 0.67; P<0.003). Better outcomes were seen in neonates with birth weight >1000 g than neonates <1000 g, and in those with mild to moderate respiratory distress compared to neonates with more severe disease. Moreover, bubble CPAP can be effectively and safely applied by nurses and other health workers after their initial training in these settings, and thus may improve neonatal survival and quality of neonatal care.[75]

Most places except few referral neonatal units, teaching hospitals and medical colleges cannot provide invasive ventilation in developing countries. Therefore, CPAP appears to be the best option to manage infant with RDS and to prevent up-transfers to already over-burdened Level III/tertiary care centers. It also reduces cost of care by reducing the need for mechanical ventilation and surfactant.[76] Early use of CPAP will be a simple and cost effective intervention in resource-limited settings.

With the substantial increase in the CPAP use over last decade, future seems promising. However, dependence on imported CPAP devices, lack of an ideal interface, non-availability of round-the-clock air/oxygen supply, surfactant and backup ventilation, lack of awareness and expertise among doctors and inadequately trained nursing staff are the major challenges. This situation is further compounded by overcrowded delivery rooms and lack of NICU beds. Good antenatal care, timely referral, and optimum delivery and newborn care practices should be equally addressed to get maximum benefits from CPAP.

Our initial focus should be primarily on infants with gestation >28 weeks to make a larger impact. However, as survival of extremely low birth weight neonates has improved, tertiary care centers should focus on very early CPAP in the delivery room. The concerns of associated morbidities and long-term sequelae should be addressed with simultaneous improvements in effective resuscitation, asepsis, breast milk feeding, aggressive nutrition, intensive monitoring, and screening for complications.

CPAP is a big boon for resource-limited countries, provided it is started early and used judiciously along with holistic care and proper follow-up services.

REFERENCES

1. Ho JJ, Subramaniam P, Henderson-Smart DJ, Davis PG. Continuous distending pressure for respiratory distress syndrome in preterm infants. Cochrane Database Syst Rev 2002;2:CD002271.
2. Buckmaster AG, Arnolda GR, Wright IM, Henderson-Smart DJ. CPAP use in babies with respiratory distress in Australian special care nurseries. J Paediatr Child Health 2007;43:376–82.
3. Kiran S, Murki S, Pratap OT, Kandraju H, Reddy A. Nasal continuous positive airway pressure therapy in a non-tertiary neonatal unit: Reduced need for up-transfers. Indian J Pediatr 2014 Jun 21 [Epub ahead of print].
4. Ho JJ, Henderson-Smart DJ, Davis PG. Early versus delayed initiation of continuous distending pressure for respiratory distress syndrome in preterm infants. Cochrane Database Syst Rev 2002;2:CD002975.
5. Morley CJ, Davis PG, Doyle LW, Brion LP, Hascoet JM, Carlin JB; COIN Trial Investigators. Nasal CPAP or intubation at birth for very preterm infants. N Engl J Med 2008;358:700–8.
6. SUPPORT Study Group of the Eunice Kennedy Shriver NICHD Neonatal Research Network, Finer NN, Carlo WA, Walsh MC, Rich W, Gantz MG, Laptook AR, et al. Early CPAP versus surfactant in extremely preterm infants. N Engl J Med 2010;362:1970–9.
7. Dunn MS, Kaempf J, de Klerk A, de Klerk R, Reilly M, Howard D; Vermont Oxford Network DRM Study Group. Randomized trial comparing 3 approaches to the initial respiratory management of preterm neonates. Pediatrics. 2011;128:1069–76.
8. Verder H, Agertoft L, Albertsen P, Christensen NC, Curstedt T, Ebbesen F, et al. Surfactant treatment of newborn infants with respiratory distress syndrome primarily treated with nasal continuous positive air pressure. A pilot study. Ugeskr Laeger 1992;154:2136–9.
9. Stevens TP, Harrington EW, Blennow M, Soll RF. Early surfactant administration with brief ventilation vs selective surfactant and continued

mechanical ventilation for preterm infants with or at risk for respiratory distress syndrome. Cochrane Database Syst Rev 2007;4:CD003063.

10. Verder H, Robertson B, Greisen G, Ebbesen F, Albertsen P, Lundstrom K, et al. Surfactant therapy and nasal continuous positive airway pressure for newborns with respiratory distress syndrome. Danish-Swedish Multicenter Study Group. N Engl J Med 1994;331:1051–5.

11. Reininger A, Khalak R, Kendig JW, Ryan RM, Stevens TP, Reubens L, et al. Surfactant adminis-tration by transient intubation in infants 29 to 35 weeks' gestation with respiratory distress syn-drome decreases the likelihood of later mecha-nical ventilation: A randomized controlled trial. J Perinatol 2005;25:703–8.

12. Sandri F, Plavka R, Ancora G, Simeoni U, Stranak Z, Martinelli S, et al. CURPAP Study Group. Prophylactic or early selective surfactant com-bined with nCPAP in very preterm infants. Pediatrics 2010;125:1402-9.

13. Rojas-Reyes MX, Morley CJ, Soll R. Prophylactic versus selective use of surfactant in preventing morbidity and mortality in preterm infants. Cochrane Database Syst Rev 2012;3:CD000510.

14. Polin RA, Carlo WA. Committee on Fetus and Newborn; American Academy of Pediatrics. Sur-factant replacement therapy for preterm and term neonates with respiratory distress. Pediatrics 2014;133:156–63.

15. Rojas MA, Lozano JM, Rojas MX, Laughon M, Bose CL, Rondon MA, et al; Colombian Neonatal Research Network. Very early surfactant without mandatory ventilation in premature infants treated with early continuous positive airway pressure: a randomized, controlled trial. Pediatrics 2009;123:137–42.

16. Kandraju H, Murki S, Subramanian S, Gaddam P, Deorari A, Kumar P. Early routine versus late selective surfactant in preterm neonates with respiratory distress syndrome on nasal conti-nuous positive airway pressure: A randomized controlled trial. Neonatology 2013;103:148–54.

17. Davis PG, Henderson-Smart DJ. Nasal conti-nuous positive airways pressure immediately after extubation for preventing morbidity in preterm infants. Cochrane Database Syst Rev 2003;2:CD000143.

18. Goldsmith JP. Continuous positive airway pres-sure and conventional mechanical ventilation in the treatment of meconium aspiration syndrome. J Perinatol 2008;28: S49–55.

19. Priya B, Murki S. CPAP for Meconium Aspiration Syndrome: Predictors of Failure. In: Thakre R, Pejaver RK. editors. Proceedings of VI Annual Convention of Neonatology Chapter of Indian Academy of Pediatrics: IAP Neocon 2013 Abstracts. Ahmedabad, India: IAP Neonatal Chapter India; 2013;12.

20. Davis PG, Morley CJ. Non-invasive respiratory support: An alternative to mechanical ventilation in preterm infants. In: Bancalari E (ed). The Newborn Lung. Neonatology questions and new controversies. 1st edn. Philadelphia: Saunders 2008;361–76.

21. Buzzella B, Claure N, D'Ugard C, Bancalari E. A randomized controlled trial of two nasal conti-nuous positive airway pressure levels after extubation in preterm infants. J Pediatr 2014;164: 46–51.

22. Bowe L, Clarke P. Current use of nasal conti-nuous positive airways pressure in neonates. Arch Dis Child Fetal Neonatal Ed 2005;90:F92–3.

23. Singh SD, Robinson MJ, Clarke P, Bowe L, Smith J, Glover K, et al. Nasal CPAP weaning of VLBW infants: Is decreasing CPAP pressure or increasing time off the better strategy? Results of a randomized controlled trial. Early Hum Dev 2007;83:125–37.

24. Jardine LA, Inglis GD, Davies MW. Strategies for the withdrawal of nasal continuous positive airway pressure (NCPAP) in preterm infants. Cochrane Database Syst Rev 2011;2:CD006979.

25. Abdel-Hady H, Shouman B, Aly H. Early wean-ing from CPAP to high flow nasal cannula in preterm infants is associated with prolonged oxygen requirement: A randomized controlled trial. Early Hum Dev 2011;87:205–8.

26. Todd DA, Wright A, Broom M, Chauhan M, Meskell S, Cameron C et al. Methods of weaning preterm babies <30 weeks gestation off CPAP: A multicentre randomised controlled trial. Arch Dis Child Fetal Neonatal Ed 2012;97:F236–40.

27. O'Donnell SM, Curry SJ, Buggy NA, Moynihan MM, Sebkova S, Janota J, et al. The NOFLO trial: Low-flow nasal prongs therapy in weaning nasal continuous positive airway pressure in preterm infants. J Pediatr 2013;163:79–83.

28. Lee KS, Dunn MS, Fenwick M, Shennan AT. A comparison of underwater bubble continuous positive airway pressure with ventilator-derived continuous positive airway pressure in pre-mature neonates ready for extubation. Biol Neonate 1998;73:69–75.

29. Pillow JJ, Hillman N, Moss TJ, Polglase G, Bold G, Beaumont C, et al. Bubble continuous positive airway pressure enhances lung volume and gas exchange in preterm lambs. Am J Respir Crit Care Med 2007;176:63–9.

30. Tagare A, Kadam S, Vaidya U, Pandit A, Patole S. A pilot study of comparison of BCPAP vs VCPAP in preterm infants with early onset respiratory distress. J Trop Pediatr 2010;56:191–4.

31. Courtney SE, Pyon KH, Saslow JG, Arnold GK, Pandit PB, Habib RH. Lung recruitment and breathing pattern during variable versus continuous flow nasal continuous positive airway pressure in premature infants: an evaluation of three devices. Pediatrics 2001;107:304–8.

32. Yadav S, Thukral A, Sankar MJ, Sreenivas V, Deorari AK, Paul VK, et al. Bubble vs conventional continuous positive airway pressure for prevention of extubation failure in preterm very low birth weight infants: A pilot study. Indian J Pediatr 2012;79:1163–68.

33. Tagare A, Kadam S, Vaidya U, Pandit A, Patole S. Bubble CPAP versus ventilator CPAP in preterm neonates with early onset respiratory distress–A randomized controlled trial. J Trop Pediatr. 2013; 59:113–9.

34. Moa G, Nilsson K, Zetterström H, Jonsson LO. A new device for administration of nasal continuous positive airway pressure in the newborn: an experimental study. Crit Care Med 1988;16: 1238–42.

35. Klausner JF, Lee AY, Hutchison AA. Decreased imposed work with a new nasal continuous positive airway pressure device. Pediatr Pulmonol. 1996;22:188–94.

36. Ahluwalia JS, White DK, Morley CJ. Infant flow driver or single prong nasal continuous positive airway pressure: short-term physiological effects. Acta Paediatr 1998;87:325–7.

37. Courtney SE, Pyon KH, Saslow JG, Arnold GK, Pandit PB, Habib RH. Lung recruitment and breathing pattern during variable versus continuous flow nasal continuous positive airway pressure in premature infants: an evaluation of three devices. Pediatrics 2001;107:304–8.

38. Pandit PB, Courtney SE, Pyon KH, Saslow JG, Habib RH. Work of breathing during constant- and variable-flow nasal continuous positive airway pressure in preterm neonates. Pediatrics. 2001;108:682–5.

39. Mazzella M, Bellini C, Calevo MG, Campone F, Massocco D, Mezzano P, et al. A randomised control study comparing the Infant Flow Driver with nasal continuous positive airway pressure in preterm infants. Arch Dis Child Fetal Neonatal Ed 2001;85:F86–90.

40. Liptsen E, Aghai ZH, Pyon KH, Saslow JG, Nakhla T, Long J, et al. Work of breathing during nasal continuous positive airway pressure in preterm infants: a comparison of bubble vs variable-flow devices. J Perinatol 2005;25:453–8.

41. Boumecid H, Rakza T, Abazine A, Klosowski S, Matran R, Storme L. Influence of three nasal continuous positive airway pressure devices on breathing pattern in preterm infants. Arch Dis Child Fetal Neonatal Ed 2007;92: F298–300.

42. Pantalitschka T, Sievers J, Urschitz MS, Herberts T, Reher C, Poets CF. Randomised crossover trial of four nasal respiratory support systems for apnoea of prematurity in very low birthweight infants. Arch Dis Child Fetal Neonatal Ed. 2009;94:F245–8.

43. Yagui AC, Vale LA, Haddad LB, Prado C, Rossi FS, Deutsch AD, et al. Bubble CPAP versus CPAP with variable flow in newborns with respiratory distress: a randomized controlled trial. J Pediatr (Rio J) 2011;87:499–504.

44. Bober K, Œwietliñski J, Zejda J, Kornacka K, Pawlik D, Behrendt J, et al. A multicenter randomized controlled trial comparing effectiveness of two nasal continuous positive airway pressure devices in very-low-birth-weight infants. Pediatr Crit Care Med 2012;13:191–6.

45. Kirchner L, Wald M, Jeitler V, Pollak A. In vitro comparison of noise levels produced by different CPAP generators. Neonatology 2012;10:95–100.

46. Huckstadt T, Foitzik B, Wauer RR, Schmalisch G. Comparison of two different CPAP systems by tidal breathing parameters. Intensive Care Med. 2003;29:1134–40.

47. Stefanescu BM, Murphy WP, Hansell BJ, Fuloria M, Morgan TM, Aschner JL. A randomized, controlled trial comparing two different continuous positive airway pressure systems for the successful extubation of extremely low birth weight infants. Pediatrics 2003;112;1031–8.

48. Gupta S, Sinha SK, Tin W, Donn SM. A randomized controlled trial of post-extubation bubble continuous positive airway pressure versus infant flow driver continuous positive airway pressure in preterm infants with respiratory distress syndrome. J Pediatr 2009;154:645–50.

49. Bhatti A, Khan J, Murki S, Sundaram V, Saini SS, Kumar P. Jet Continuous positive airway pres-

sure versus bubble continuous positive airway pressure in preterm babies with respiratory distress: A randomized controlled trial. E-PAS. 2014:4680–5.

50. Manley BJ, Dold SK, Davis PG, Roehr CC. High-flow nasal cannulae for respiratory support of preterm infants: a review of the evidence. Neonatology 2012;102:300–8.

51. Yoder BA, Stoddard RA, Li M, King J, Dirnberger DR, Abbasi S. Heated, humidified high-flow nasal cannula versus nasal cpap for respiratory support in neonates. Pediatrics 2013;131:e1482–90.

52. Collins CL, Holberton JR, Barfield C, Davis PG. A randomized controlled trial to compare heated humidified high-flow nasal cannulae with nasal continuous positive airway pressure postextubation in premature infants. J Pediatr. 2013;162: 949–54.

53. Klingenberg C, Pettersen M, Hansen EA, Gustavsen LJ, Dahl IA, Leknessund A, et al. Patient comfort during treatment with heated humidified high flow nasal cannulae versus nasal continuous positive airway pressure: A randomised cross-over trial. Arch Dis Child Fetal Neonatal Ed 2014;99:F134–7.

54. Manley BJ, Owen LS, Doyle LW, Andersen CC, Cartwright DW, Pritchard MA, et al. High-flow nasal cannulae in very preterm infants after extubation. N Engl J Med 2013;369:1425–33.

55. De Paoli AG, Davis PG, Faber B, Morley CJ. Devices and pressure sources for administration of nasal continuous positive airway pressure (NCPAP) in preterm neonates. Cochrane Database Syst Rev 2008;1:CD002977.

56. Mazzella M, Bellini C, Calevo MG, Campone F, Massocco D, Mezzano P, et al. A randomised control study comparing the Infant Flow Driver with nasal continuous positive airway pressure in preterm infants. Arch Dis Child Fetal Neonatal Ed 2001;85:F86–90.

57. Rego MA, Martinez FE. Comparison of two nasal prongs for application of continuous positive airway pressure in neonates. Pediatr Crit Care Med. 2002;3:239–43.

58. Yong SC, Chen SJ, Boo NY. Incidence of nasal trauma associated with nasal prong versus nasal mask during continuous positive airway pressure treatment in very low birthweight infants: A randomised control study, Arch Dis Child Fetal Neonatal Ed 2005;90:F480–83.

59. Kieran EA, Twomey AR, Molloy EJ, Murphy JF, O'Donnell CP. Randomized trial of prongs or mask for nasal continuous positive airway pressure in preterm infants. Pediatrics. 2012;130: 1170–6.

60. Chandrasekaran A, Sachdeva A, Sankar MJ, Agarwal R, Deorari AK, Paul VK. Nasal mask versus nasal prongs in the delivery of continuous positive airway pressure in preterm infants—an open label randomized controlled trial. E-PAS. 2014:2936–512.

61. Horton D, Durand D. Use of a new nasal cannula to deliver nasal ventilation to NICU patients. Open forum abstracts; Journal of respiratory care 2012.

62. Nzegwu NI, Mack T, DellaVentura R, Dunphy L, Koval N, Levit O, et al. Systematic use of the RAM nasal cannula in the Yale-New Haven Children's Hospital Neonatal Intensive Care Unit: A quality improvement project. J Matern Fetal Neonatal Med 2014 ;30:1–4. [Epub ahead of print].

63. Ancora G, Maranella E, Grandi S, Pierantoni L, Guglielmi M, Faldella G. Role of bilevel positive airway pressure in the management of preterm newborns who have received surfactant. Acta Paediatr 2010;99:1807–11.

64. Lista G, Castoldi F, Fontana P, Daniele I, Cavigioli F, Rossi S, et al. Nasal continuous positive airway pressure (CPAP) versus bi-level nasal CPAP in preterm babies with respiratory distress syndrome: A randomised control trial. Arch Dis Child Fetal Neonatal Ed 2010;95:F85–9.

65. O'Brien K, Campbell C, Brown L, Wenger L, Shah V. Infant flow biphasic nasal continuous positive airway pressure (BP-NCPAP) vs infant flow NCPAP for the facilitation of extubation in infants' <1,250 grams: A randomized controlled trial. BMC Pediatr 2012;12:43–51.

66. Sea-PAP. A Lifesaving Innovation for Infant Respiratory Distress. Available from: http://www. seattlechildrens.org/research/developmental-therapeutics/labsprograms/neonatal-respiratory-support-technologies-team/sea-PAP/ Accessed June 25, 2014.

67. Diblasi RM, Zignego JC, Smith CV, Hansen TN, Richardson CP. Effective gas exchange in paralyzed juvenile rabbits using simple, inexpensive respiratory support devices. Pediatr Res 2010;68:526–30.

68. Thomas CW, Meinzen-Derr J, Hoath SB, Narendran V. Neurodevelopmental outcomes of extremely low birth weight infants ventilated with continuous positive airway pressure vs

mechanical ventilation. Indian J Pediatr. 2012;79: 218–23.

69. Vaucher YE, Peralta-Carcelen M, Finer NN, Carlo WA, Gantz MG, Walsh MC. SUPPORT Study Group of the Eunice Kennedy Shriver NICHD Neonatal Research Network. Neurodevelopmental outcomes in the early CPAP and pulse oximetry trial. N Engl J Med 2012;367:2495–504.

70. Report of the National Neonatal Perinatal Database. NNF India, 2002–2003.

71. Kumar A, Bhat BV. Epidemiology of respiratory distress of newborns. Indian J Pediatr 1996;63: 93–8.

72. Daga S, Mhatre S, Borhade A, Khan D. Home-made continuous positive airways pressure device may reduce mortality in neonates with respiratory distress in low-resource setting. J Trop Pediatr 2014;60:343–7.

73. Hendriks H, Kirsten GF, Voss M, Conradie H. Is continuous positive airway pressure a feasible treatment modality for neonates with respiratory distress syndrome in a rural district hospital? J Trop Pediatr 2014;60:348–51.

74. Kawaza K, Machen HE, Brown J, Mwanza Z, Iniguez S, Gest A, et al. Efficacy of a low-cost bubble CPAP system in treatment of respiratory distress in a neonatal ward in Malawi. PLoS One. 2014;9:e86327.

75. Martin S, Duke T, Davis P. Efficacy and safety of bubble CPAP in neonatal care in low and middle income countries: a systematic review. Arch Dis Child Fetal Neonatal Ed 2014;99:F495–504.

76. Kamath BD, Macguire ER, McClure EM, Goldenberg RL, Jobe AH. Neonatal mortality from respiratory distress syndrome: lessons for low-resource countries. Pediatrics 2011;127: 1139-46.

Point of Care Neonatal Ultrasound—Head, Lung, Gut and Line Localization

Chandra Rath, Pradeep Suryawanshi

Ultrasonography (USG) is no longer the exclusive domain of radiologists and cardiologists. With appropriate training, clinician performed ultrasound (CPU) is now practised widely in obstetrics, emergency medicine and adult intensive care, and is the standard practice in neonatology in many developed countries.[1] Cardiologists and radiologists undoubtedly have an indispensable role to play in clinical care, but it is unrealistic to expect 24-hour specialist cover, even in a resource-rich setting. Neonatal intensive care is a dynamic process, involving frequent evaluation, some in real time, which makes dependence on radiologist or cardiologist impractical. CPU has already proven its mettle in day-to-day management and the information obtained has often resulted in a management change.[2] In this review, we shall discuss the practical use of ultrasound for imaging the head, lung, and gut, and for vascular line localization. We also discuss the application to clinical decision making in resource-poor settings.

CRANIAL ULTRASONOGRAPHY

Role of cranial ultrasonography in neonatal intensive care unit (NICU) is for:

- Preterm infants for evaluation of germinal matrix hemorrhage-intraventricular hemorrhage (GMH-IVH) and follow-up.

- Unexplained cardiac failure (to rule out vascular abnormalities).
- Hypoxic ischemic encephalopathy (HIE).
- Congenital malformations.
- Neonatal seizures.
- Evaluation of suspected subgaleal hematoma
- Evaluation of antenatally detected abnormalities.

Preterm infants, especially those less than 32 weeks gestation, are at risk for GMH-IVH, and ischemic white matter injuries. Late preterm infants who are monochorionic twins, small for gestational age (SGA), and or have experienced events such as chorioamnionitis, fetal distress, acidosis, difficult delivery, or hypotension are also at risk for ischemic white matter injury. If these abnormalities are detected early via ultrasound, follow-up and early intervention can be planned appropriately. Serial ultrasounds may be necessary to detect white matter lesions, which may not be evident until 2 to 4 weeks after the ischemic event. There may be significant changes in USG findings between the first and second scan, possibly changing medical management and prognosis. Serial USG is also important in identifying significant post-hemorrhagic hydrocephalus for early intervention.

Procedure

Cranial USG is done through the anterior and posterior fontanelle, the mastoid foramen and poorly ossified parts of the temporal bone. The mastoid, temporal and posterior fontanelle views are supplementary to the absolutely necessary anterior fontenalle view. Usually 5–10 Hz 2D curved or linear array transducers are useful for cranial USG. Frequency of the probe may be increased for optimal visualization of superficial structures like subcortical white matter and venous sinuses; this will increase resolution at the expense of penetration. Similarly, lower frequency may be used for visualization of deeper structures in the posterior fossa. The transducers used should fit perfectly on the anterior fontanelle, as a large footprint makes the contact and image quality suboptimal, and small footprints reduce the diagnostic ability.

In this review, we shall focus on hemorrhage, parenchymal changes and hydrocephalous evaluation, which are most frequently encountered in day-to-day practice.

Germinal Matrix-Intraventricular Hemorrhage

GMH-IVH is one of the most common ultrasound findings in NICU. Studies performed in the 1980s suggested that >90% IVH cases in very low birth weight (VLBW) infants occurred within postnatal days 4 to 5.[3] Premature infants are relatively resistant to hemorrhage after this period, irrespective of the gestational age (GA) because of the shutdown in angiogenesis, making the vessels resistant to rupture despite fluctuation in cerebral blood flow.[4] A recently published review[5] which included studies from the antenatal steroid and surfactant era, concluded that 48% of cases of IVH occurred in the first 6 hours of life in VLBW infants, and suggested that early cranial USG may have prognostic, preventive and medicolegal implications. A small percentage of GMH-IVH may occur up to third week of life.

Observational studies from the 1990s showed that in the first 2 weeks of life, 12–51% of infants <1,500 grams or gestational age of <33 weeks had abnormalities on ultrasound out of which 6–20% were major (such as grades 3 and 4 IVH or bilateral cystic periventricular leukomalacia).[3] More severe IVH occurs in more premature infants. Although the American Academy of Neurology and the Practice Committee of the Child Neurology Society[3] suggested screening all preterms <30 weeks due to the incidence of severe IVH,[3] infants up to 34 weeks are also at increased risk of GMH-IVH. In a recent study by Ballardini, et al.[6] in late preterm infants (33–36 weeks), intracranial lesions were found in 13% of the neonates when ultrasound was undertaken within day 7 of life. The risk factors for detecting intracranial abnormalities were head circumference less than the 3rd percentile, the need for ventilation or surfactant, low APGAR score at fifth minute, and neurological abnormalities. However, severe grades of IVH and extreme periventricular leukomalacia (PVL) are rare in this gestational age.[6] In another study, Bhat, et al.[7] detected abnormal cranial ultrasonography in 6.8% preterm (30–34 weeks) newborns and recommended screening in infants born between 30 and 34 weeks of gestational age. They also detected severe intracranial anomalies in 1.5% of neonates in this gestational age group; however, inclusion of less than 40% of the eligible neonates,[8] born during the study period makes this data a little less meaningful. Vanderwalt, et al.[8] in a cost analysis study, concluded that cranial ultrasound screening of infants >32 weeks is not cost-effective.

There is no consensus for the optimal timing for cranial ultrasonography. Based on the above discussion, we propose a screening schedule for preterm neonates (Table 11.1). The incidence of severe intracranial abnormalities is low in neonates with gestational age greater than 30 weeks, and the proposed schedule may not be very cost-effective in resource-poor settings. IVH is often asymptomatic but the likelihood of signs increase with the severity of hemorrhage.

TABLE 11.1: Proposed cranial ultrasonography scanning protocol for preterm infants

< 28 wk or birth weight <1000 g or 28–31 + 6 wk and/or birth weight <1500 g on life support.	28–31+6 wk or birth weight 1000–1500 g without life support	32–34 wks with risk factors: Monochorionic twins, head circumference <3rd centile, ventilation and/or surfactant need, fetal distress, acidosis, 5 min APGAR score of <6, or hypotension
6 h of age	Day 3 to 1 wk	Day 5 to 1 wk and then as indicated
Day 3 to 1 wk	4 wks	
4 wk	TAE or discharge	
Term age equivalent (TAE) or discharge whichever occurs first		

One week after any "new" sick event such as sepsis, hypotension, necrotizing enterocolitis, etc. (If near term after the 1 week scan then as required).[9] In case of IVH other than GMH alone, weekly scans are indicated. Cranial USG anytime in case of clinical suspicion of IVH

Possible clinical signs are tense anterior fontanelle, pallor and associated drop in hematocrit, unresponsiveness; tonic seizures and decerebrate posturing; these should warrant immediate bedside cranial USG.

Approximately, 50–75% of preterm survivors with predominantly grade IV IVH develop cerebral palsy, intellectual disability, and/or hydrocephalus.[10,11] A recent Australian report on neurodevelopmental outcomes of extremely preterm infants revealed that grade I–II IVH, even in the absence of white matter injury or other late ultrasound abnormalities, is associated with adverse neurodevelopmental outcomes,[12] supporting the use of routine cranial USG to identify all silent GMH-IVH. A grading system developed by Papile and Burstein[13] is still widely used for prognostication where grade I is a bleeding confined to germinal matrix and looks as echogenic as choroid plexus in USG. The caudothalamic groove acts as a convenient landmark: echogenicity anterior to the groove represents blood as the choroid finishes at the groove. Grade II is grade I with intraventricular extension where blood can be seen as white bright spots/lines in the ventricles separate from choroid plexus, grade III is ventricle dilatation because of excessive blood inside it, and grade IV is extension of hemorrhage in to the parenchyma. It must be remembered here that Papile classification was originally developed using CT scan but there have been reports of its use in cranial USG with accuracy.[14]

Grade IV is interpreted as the result of an extension of the hemorrhage from the ventricle into the adjacent white matter. However, it is now postulated that large blood clots in the germinal matrix and ventricles impair the flow of blood from the medullary veins (which drain the cerebral white matter) into the terminal vein leading to venous infarction and possibly hemorrhagic infarction, i.e. periventricular hemorrhagic infarct (PVHI). Besides this compression theory, ependymal trauma and inflammation as a possible cause has also been proposed. Therefore, PVHI is not a simple extension of germinal matrix hemorrhage into adjacent brain parenchyma as assumed in the Papile classification.[15] PVHI is always associated with an ipsilateral GM-IVH. When GM-IVH is bilateral, it usually is larger on the side ipsilateral to the PVHI. A scoring system has been proposed using parameters like the extent of PVHI, midline shift and unilateral or bilateral PVHI. This scoring helps in better prognostication, as there is a strikingly significant relationship between high PVHI score and the likelihood to withdraw care, the development of early neonatal seizures, and abnormal neuromotor examination at 12 and 30 months of age.[16,17] Grade I-III IVH are easy to identify on cranial USG; however, clinicians may occasionally face difficulties in differentiating PVL from

PVHI as both lesions are initially echogenic with later cystic evolution. PVHI is an echo-dense lesion in the periventricular white matter which is unilateral or, if bilateral, obviously asymmetric. PVHI is also associated with a GMH-IVH lesion, which is usually ipsilateral or larger on the ipsilateral side. PVL develops in the first week of life as bilateral echo density at the lateral border of the lateral ventricle with minimal or no IVH. PVHI usually evolves into a single or few relatively large cysts, which communicate with the lateral ventricle where as PVL evolves in to multiple tiny cysts, which do not communicate with lateral ventricle. Bass, et al.[18] could differentiate between PVHI and PVL in 77% of their study subjects with cranial USG while 11% had mixed lesions.[18]

Once the diagnosis of GMH-IVH is made, we should look for cerebellar bleeding, as the external layer of the cerebellum is also a germinal zone. Bleeding in and around the cerebellum may lead to poor future neuro-developmental outcome. Early detection with the help of cranial USG through the mastoid foramen is important for prognostication and appropriate counselling of the family. Though small punctate cerebellar hemorrhages may not be seen well with cranial USG as compared to MRI, it remains a useful bedside tool.[19]

Post-hemorrhagic Ventricular Dilatation

The risk of developing post-hemorrhagic ventricular dilatation (PHVD) is considerable after a severe hemorrhage (grade III/IV). PHVD is defined as ventricular enlargement ≥97th centile for gestational age (GA),[20] and is recognized in about one-third of infants with GMH-IVH. About 35% of neonates who develop PHVD require some form of intervention.[21] Evaluation of progressive PVHD with clinical parameters such as serial measurement of head circumference, tense fontanelle, sunset phenomena of the eyes are not as reliable as serial cranial USG.[20,22,23] It is hard to distinguish post-hemorrhagic ventri-culomegaly from atrophic ventriculomegaly resulting from white matter loss. However, regardless of the mechanism, the extent of white matter loss has a direct correlation with the motor outcome.[24] The measurements commonly used in clinical practice (Fig. 11.1) are accurate compared to MRI.[25] Ventricular index is one of the most commonly used measurements and the reference value correlates well for term neonates. However, it may not increase during

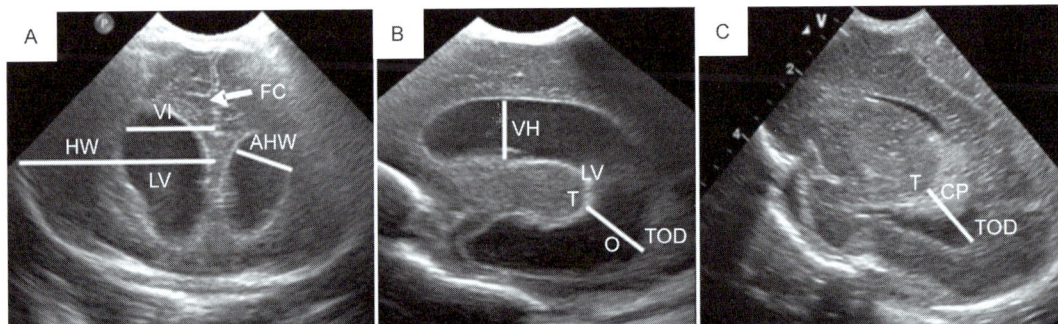

Fig. 11.1: Commonly used measurements used in evaluation of PHVD. (A) Coronal plane Ventricular Index (VI)—distance between the falx and the lateral wall of the anterior horn at the level of the third ventricle (4 mm above the 97th centile for GA is an indication for CSF drainage), FHR=VI/Hemispheric width (HW), AHW-Maximum diagonal width (values above 6mm significant). (B) Sagittal plane TOD— distance between the outermost point of the thalamus at its junction with the choroid plexus, to the outermost part of the occipital horn, Ventricular height (VH)-At the level of foramen of Monro. (C) Sagittal plane—TOD in a non-dilated ventricle, LV=Lateral ventricle, T=Thalamus, CP=Choroid plexus, O=Occipital horn of the lateral ventricle, FC=Falx cerebri

early hydrocephalus and the reference values for preterm infants show variation because of less representation of this population in the reference curves:[20,26–28] Another commonly used measurement, the anterior horn width (AHW), has the advantage of identifying early hydrocephalous[27] with a minimal variation with change in gestational age.[27–29] However, a recent study by Sondhi, *et al.*[30] demonstrated an evident increase in size with ongoing maturity. Thalamo-occipital distance (TOD), which essentially measures the occipital horn length of the lateral ventricle, may be a useful measurement and sometimes represent the only site of ventricular dilatation.[30] Absence of increased TOD is an important negative finding. However, difficult visualization, considerable variation in reference curves, and the presence of isolated dilation of the occipital horn in normal preterm infants makes this measurement clinically less meaningful.[27–31] Other measurements like ventricular height and frontal horn ratio are less valuable in clinical practice as no reference curves are available. Measurement of the 3rd and 4th ventricle may assist in differentiating communicating and non-communicating hydrocephalus; however, the absence of quality reference curves, inter-observer variability, and difficulties in measurements are the main drawbacks.[29,30]

Ventricular index and AHW are the most widely studied and used measurements in clinical practice. Vetricular index greater by 4 mm of the 97th centile for gestational age is associated with a poor prognosis.[21] A normal AHW is less than 3 mm, with the 95th percentile curve reaching 2 mm at 36 weeks and 3 mm at 40 weeks. A size of more than 6 mm is considered abnormal. The implications of AHW between 3 and 5 mm is not clear. Cranial USG is useful in the identification of PVHD and should be undertaken at least twice weekly to identify progression; however interventional decisions are usually a combination of clinical findings, history and ultrasound findings. Indian data regarding these measurements are scarce.[32, 33]

Periventricular Leukomalacia

PVL, which occurs as a consequence of preterm brain ischemia and/or inflammation, is of great diagnostic importance because of its association with cerebral palsy and abnormal development. PVL usually occurs in preterm infants ≤32 weeks gestation as they have poorly vascularized white matter, which contains oligodendro-cyte progenitors sensitive to ischemia and inflammation.[34] MRI has been reported to be a better modality than ultrasound in detecting white matter injury particularly in the diagnosis of punctate white matter lesion (PWML) and diffuse excessive high signal intensity.[35] However, serial USG has a definite role in evaluation of cystic PVL, a more severe form of white matter injury. The more extensive cysts tend to develop within 2–3 weeks following an insult, while the more localized cystic lesions may take as long as 3–6 weeks to develop.[36] Therefore, PVL diagnosed in the first week of life indicates an antenatal insult rather than a perinatal insult. Echogenicity in the brain equal to or greater than echogenicity in the choroid plexus, when persisting for more than 10–14 days, should alert the clinician about possible early PVL. Transient hyper-echoic lesions or periventricular halos might be seen in normal white matter of preterm infants. The pattern of distribution of PVL on ultrasound is typically dorsal and lateral to the external angles of the lateral ventricles. Any brain lesion, which causes brain parenchymal loss, may result in cyst formation. It has been suggested that PVHI and PVL can be differentiated by the location of the cysts. PVL has a predilection for periventricular arterial border zones, particularly in the region near the trigon of the lateral ventricles. PVHI is prominent more anteriorly with the lesion radiating from the periventricular region at the site of confluence of the medullary and terminal vein and assumes a triangular, fan-shaped appearance in the periventricular white matter.[14] The typical positions of various cystic lesions are depicted in **Fig. 11.2**. A classification for PVL has been suggested, though this is not widely accepted.[37]

Doppler Evaluation

Doppler imaging of the anterior cerebral artery (ACA) and middle cerebral artery (MCA) is easily done through the anterior fontanelle in the sagittal plane and through the temporal window in the axial plane. The peak systolic velocity (PSV), end diastolic velocity (EDV), resistive index (RI) and pulsitility index (PI) are the most common measurements used for monitoring intracranial hemodynamics. Measuring PI is useful as it minimizes the effect of vessel angulation and correlates well with acute changes in intra-cerebral perfusion pressure.[38] Age-dependent reference values are available, and the normal range for the RI is 0.65–0.90. Values <0.5 or >0.9 are abnormal. An increase in diastolic flow results in a decrease in the RI, and conversely a decrease in diastolic flow results in an increase in the RI. Various factors can influence RI; for example, presence of a patent ductus arteriosus (PDA), scanning pressure on the anterior fontanelle, IVH, PVL, hydrocephalus, pneumothorax and low arterial carbon dioxide can increase the RI. Similarly RI is decreased in asphyxia, vascular malformation, tachycardia and decreased cardiac output.[39] RI <0.5 in asphyxiated new-

borns in the first few days of life is associated with both immediate and long term poor outcome.[40–45] Unfortunately, some full-term neonates with significant asphyxia may not show this decreased RI and may instead have a normal or increased RI which may be due to a relative decrease in diastolic flow velocity. This decrease in diastolic flow velocity may be because of the presence of a significant PDA, myocardial dysfunction (such as in transient myocardial ischemia), or hypervolemia. Mean cerebral blood flow is mainly determined from the diastolic flow. As intracranial pressure (ICP) rises, the arterial flow is more affected during diastole than during systole, resulting in an increase in RI as happens in hydro-cephalus.[46] In individual infants, a tendency towards a correlation between ICP and flow variables was found when studied longi-tudinally.[47] However, it is doubtful whether the RI can be used as an indicator for the timing of intervention, because it can vary widely between individual preterm infants and accu-racy subjected to presence of other conditions, that may influence cerebral blood flow.

Cranial USG has many other applications in term and preterm infants which is beyond the scope of this review. It is excellent for the detection of IVH, ventriculomegaly, perforator stroke, sinovenous thrombosis and cystic PVL, but MRI is superior in detecting cortical abnormalities, posterior fossa lesions, subtler white matter injury, early watershed infarct

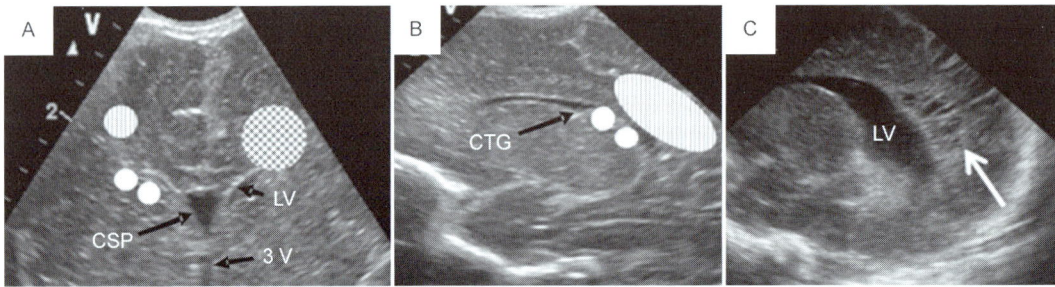

Fig. 11.2: Coronal view (A) Dotted area—site for subependymal cyst, connatal cyst, Striped–site for PVL, Chequerboard-site for PVHI. (B) Sagittal view—Striped–site for PVL, Dotted area–site for choroid plexus cyst. (C) White arrow showing cystic PVL. LV=Lateral ventricle, 3V=3rd Vetricle, CSP=Cavum septum pellucidum, CTG=Caudothalamic groove

events, microabscesses and involvement of posterior limb of internal capsule. Reviews of the studies directly comparing cranial USG with MRI with cerebral palsy as the outcome show that utility of MRI tends to be similar or higher compared with cranial USG.[48,49] In a recently published study, serial cranial USG seems highly effective in diagnosing all common preterm brain injuries, but may miss cerebellar abnormalities.[50] However, it will be interesting to see neurodevelopmental prediction with early MRI in few of the upcoming studies.

LUNG ULTRASOUND

Clinical signs and radiographs are routinely used to diagnose neonatal lung disease albeit they have low specificity and sensitivity for many common clinical conditions. Lung ultrasound is being increasingly used in Neonatal Intensive Care Unit (NICU) and adult ICU because of its high sensitivity and specificity.[51] It is easy to learn and can be performed with a basic ultrasound machine. Lung and pleura being superficial structures, USG requires a high-frequency linear array probe (>7.5 MHz). Micro convex probe may be used, however, linear probe displays a wider field. A basic USG setting with 2D, M mode and occasional color Doppler is all that is required to do lung ultrasound. Normal USG of lung shows 'A lines', which are parallel to straight solid pleural lines, are reverberation artefacts, and are equidistant from each other. On the other hand B-lines occur when sound waves pass through the pleural line encountering a mixture of air and water as in pulmonary oedema. These are discrete laser-like vertical hyper echoic lines that arise from the pleural line, extend to the bottom of the screen without fading, and move synchronously with lung sliding (Fig. 11.3). The pleural line slides from side to side with respiration and represents movement of the pleural surface with the respiratory cycle. This sign is known as sliding sign, a normal lung feature. Lung sliding can

also be observed using time motion mode (M mode) where the fixed superficial chest wall structures give rise to an appearance of water and the constantly moving underlying lung gives rise to a sandy appearance known as seashore sign (Fig. 11.3). The 'lung pulse' refers to the rhythmic movement of the pleura in synchrony with the cardiac rhythm. As the heart beats the movement of the heart is transmitted through the medium of the lung, which is demonstrated in M-mode as a regular motion artefact through the seashore pattern to the level of the pleura. In normal well-aerated lung, the 'lung pulse' is not present, as lung sliding becomes dominant and resistant to cardiac vibrations. The lung pulse is easily identified when the baby is not breathing.

Pneumothorax

USG is an invaluable tool for the assessment of pneumothorax, with accuracy approaching CT, and far exceeding plain radiography in adults.[52] It is of immense value in emergencies such as tension pneumothorax, as it is readily available at the bedside and can be done in less than a minute. Features of pneumothorax such as the absence of lung sliding, presence of lung point (a point where seashore sign changes in to stratosphere sign), presence of stratosphere sign on M mode (Fig. 11.3), absence of B-lines and absence of lung pulse are easy to identify with minimal training. In stratosphere sign parallel horizontal lines above and below the pleural line is noted and it resembles a barcode. In contrast to the seashore sign which is a normal lung sign, in stratosphere sign the grainy shore below the pleural line is not seen (which is due to the movement of the lungs with respiration), rather only sea (parallel lines) is noted and this denotes a static lung which is not moving with respiration because of pneumothorax (Fig. 11.3). Though studies in neonates are lacking, Lichtenstein, et al.[53] from his experience in NICU suggested that neonatal signs are no different from adult lung signs.

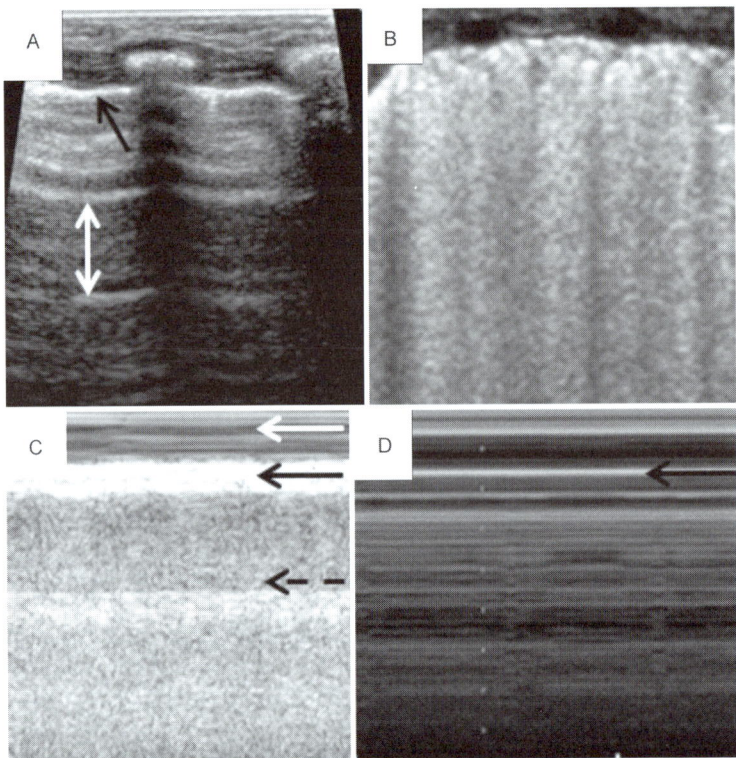

Fig. 11.3: (A) Normal lung ultrasound—Horizontal A lines shown by the white arrow equidistance from each other and the pleural line, black arrow showing the pleural line (PL). (B) Multiple vertical lines starting from the PL and almost coalescing with each other giving a white lung appearance. (C) Normal lung M mode-Seashore sign, black arrow denoting PL, white arrow showing the chest wall looking like water and the broken black arrow showing lung parenchyma looking like a sandy beach. (D) Stratosphere sign as seen in pneumothorax, there is no water and sandy part, it all looks like water

Pneumonia

Lung ultrasound is a clinically useful tool in diagnosing pneumonia; however, consolidation that does not reach the pleura cannot be visualised. In adults, lung consolidation extends to the pleura in 98.5% of cases and can be seen on USG.[52] Lung mass is smaller in the newborn and extension to the pleura may be much more frequent. Coarse and/or irregular disrupted pleural line, hepatisation of the lung tissue (echogenicity similar to liver), hyperechoic area of varying size and shape in the same lung field, irregular margin around consolidation, presence of dynamic airbronchogram, disappearance of lung sliding, mild pleural effusion and presence of lung pulse are few of the features which can be identified in pneumonia. The international consensus committee on lung ultrasound agreed that there is strong evidence that USG is an accurate tool in diagnosing lung consolidation when compared with chest radiography in pediatric age group.[54] Some neonatal studies have also shown USG to be a useful tool in recognizing neonatal pneumonia with good specificity and sensitivity.[55,56]

Pleural Effusion

Opacities detected by conventional radiography can be differentiated as consolidation or effusion only by an ultrasound scan. For pleural effusions, USG has a sensitivity of 93% and specificity of 97%.[57] USG can also be used to differentiate between transudate and exudate.[54] Visualization of internal echoes, mobile particles or septa, is highly suggestive of exudate; however, in case of an anechoic effusion, the only way to differentiate between transudate and exudate is to use thoracocentesis.

Extravascular Fluid

Presence of vertical 'B lines' represents extravascular fluid in lungs (Fig. 11.3). B lines can be used to monitor cardiac failure (systolic and diastolic), iatrogenic fluid overload (a sudden change from A to B line), or preload/afterload reduction therapy. However, B lines and white lung in neonates should be considered in the clinical context of the disease. B lines and white lung can also be seen in respiratory distress syndrome (RDS), transient tachypnea of the newborn (TTN), consolidation and atelectasis of any cause, meconium aspiration syndrome and broncho-pulmonary dysplasia.

Respiratory Distress Syndrome and Transient Tachypnea of the Newborn

USG is a useful tool in the management of RDS and TTN with good interobserver agreement. In TTN, very compact B lines in the inferior pulmonary fields and not so compact B lines in the superior lung field gives a characteristic sign called the double lung point, a sign with which we may use to differentiate it from RDS. The double lung point sign is also useful in management and prognosis, particularly in a resource-poor setting. Co-existence of lung consolidation, abnormal pleural line (thickness of >0.5 mm or blurred), bilateral white lung and disappearance of A lines are constant ultrasonography features of RDS with a specificity and sensitivity of 100%. Other features like pleural effusion, lung pulse and uniform bilateral involvement are infrequent associations. The most important indicator of RDS is consolidation, which is seen in all RDS patients but the extent and scope of consolidation varies with severity of RDS. Consolidation in moderate RDS is subpleural

and focal in nature whereas consolidation in severe RDS is more widespread and deep. Similarly lung pulse was present in all grade 3 and 4 RDS while it was absent in all grade 2 RDS.[58] In term and near term infants, USG at 1–2 hours of life has been shown to anticipate the need for respiratory support and severe respiratory distress with 100% specificity and 77.7% sensitivity.[59] In a recent study, lung ultrasound predicted need for intubation after 2 hours of life in preterm babies with a positive predictive value of 100%, and negative predictive value of 94.7%.[60] Another recent study predicted the need for surfactant administration on the basis of a scoring system which consists of oxygenation indices and lung ultrasound, with a sensitivity and specificity of 100% and 61% respectively.[61] The basic principle in all these studies is the abundance of B lines. A higher number of B lines appear as whiter lungs that need more support compared to a finding with more A lines.

USG is not yet completely ready to replace X-ray in neonatology. Few non-specific signs, paucity of neonatal research and publications are the drawbacks. However, this technology undoubtedly has the potential to replace X-ray as the most useful bedside lung disease diagnostic tool.

NECROTIZING ENTEROCOLITIS (NEC)

Identification and management of NEC is currently based on recommendations from the modified Bell's criteria.[62] Abdominal X-ray is the cornerstone in diagnosis and is able to detect bowel distension, bowel wall thickness, pneumatosis intestinalis, portal venous gas and free abdominal air. USG provides additional information about gut viability and free fluid in the abdomen. An 8–15 MHz linear probe should be used for bowel loop ultrasound.

Data on normal thickness of the bowel in preterm neonates is scarce; we suggest a thickness of 1.2 to 2 mm from personal experience. Normal term bowel wall thickness has been described as 1.1 to 2.6 mm. A normal bowel perfusion is 1–9 colour doppler signal dots per cm 2 (mean 3.8) in a setting of the lowest possible pulse repetition frequency and the highest Doppler gain settings without flash artefacts. The velocity was set at 0.029–0.11 m/sec.[63] Normal bowel wall is smooth with peristalsis.

A bowel wall thickness >2 mm should be considered suspicious and conversely; a thickness <1.0 mm indicates an abnormal thinning resulting from ischemia or necrosis. Increased bowel perfusion may present in different patterns such as ring-shape, Y-shaped and zebra-shaped. Absent bowel perfusion can be assumed when no color signal is detected at the slowest possible velocity (0.029 m/sec) and suggests a complete bowel wall necrosis with 100% sensitivity.[63] Intramural gas, a common finding though not pathognomonic of NEC, can be identified as highly echogenic dots in the bowel wall and may involve the whole circumference, in which case it is called the "circle sign" (Fig. 11.4). Intramural gas must be differentiated from intraluminal gas, which moves with compression of the abdomen with the ultrasound probe. The amount of intramural gas present does not always relate to the clinical severity of NEC and its disappearance does not correlate with clinical improvement.[64] In the absence of NEC, the commonest cause of portal venous gas is the passage small

amounts of gas through an umbilical venous catheter. Neither is the presence portal venous gas fatal, nor does its disappearance always herald clinical improvement. Portal venous gas has been reported in only 30% of the neonates with NEC, and is detected by ultrasound much earlier than it appears on X-ray.[65,66] Free abdominal gas secondary to perforation can been seen as a bright white hyper echogenicity between the diaphragm and liver which moves with abdominal compression. Detection of intraperitoneal fluid and or a mass may help in diagnosing perforated NEC. In a study by Silva, et al.[67] when three of the seven USG features (portal venous gas, intramural gas, increased wall echogenicity, bowel wall thickening or thinning, absent perfusion, free echogenic fluid) were present, there was a sensitivity of 0.82 and a specificity of 0.78 for poor outcome.

USG for NEC is not without drawbacks; inter-observer variability, large amount of bowel gas and tender unstable abdomen may hamper good USG evaluation. However, USG has an obvious advantage over routine X-ray in diagnosis and prognostication of NEC,[68] especially in neonates with clinical deterioration without X-ray changes.

LINE-LOCALIZATION

Though central line placement in NICU is a necessity, it is not without complication.

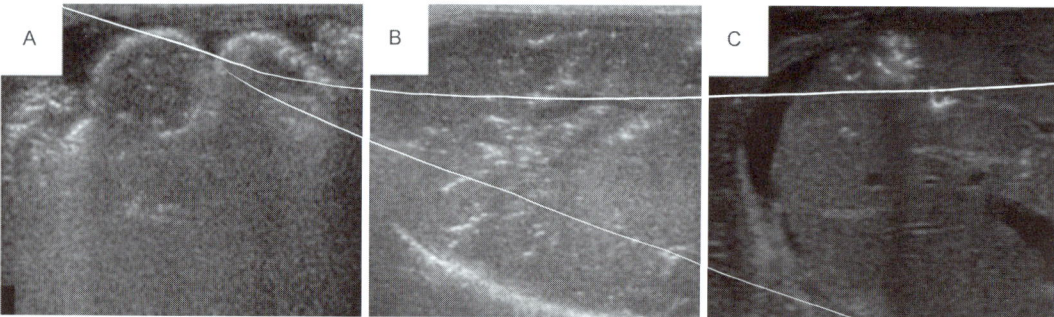

Fig. 11.4: (A) Extensive pneumatosis intestinalis (white dots) white arrow-bowel wall, (B) Extensive portal venous air in the liver USG (White dots), (C) Portal venous gas (White dots)

Identification of central line tip location may help in reducing the complications, and USG is one of the easiest bedside modality to do so. A recently published review[69] suggested considering USG as a potential alternative to X-ray in central line tip location in neonates. Two recent studies[70,71] could identify around 25% of the cases with abnormal tip position, which were reported to be normal in X-ray reporting. Ultrasound-guided umbilical catheter placement is a faster method to place catheters requiring fewer manipulations and X-rays when compared with conventional catheter placement.[72]

TRAINING AND MEDICO-LEGAL IMPLICATIONS

It is important to have a structured training program for clinicians in order to make them ultrasound literate. Few developed countries in the world have a structured training program for bedside echocardiography and fewer have it for bedside cranial ultrasound.[1,73] Most of these training programs require the clinician to undertake 75–250 studies under the guidance of the experts in an accredited center, and which might take anytime between 6 months to 24 months to complete. The course also includes hands on basic, advanced training courses and an online physics course. However, issues like different clinical needs, misdiagnosis, medicolegal liability and financial return for examination, need further discussion. Clinical need is a pertinent issue in the Indian scenario, as there are very few hospitals around the country catering to newborns that have in-house radiological and pediatric cardiology services. In reality, 24-hour presence of specialists to provide ultrasound services in the NICU is not achievable. It is here where clinician-performed ultrasound can be handy. However, the risk of misdiagnosis is a real and important concern, and some of this can be resolved by guidelines about when consultative referral should be mandatory. The other important step, which

can reduce misdiagnosis, is structured training and accreditation. There is a medico-legal vacuum as far as clinician-performed ultrasound is concerned. If a registered medical practitioner with 6 months training or 1 year experience in sonography or a gynecologist with experience are allowed to do ultrasound, we do not see any reason why adequately trained clinicians cannot do bedside USG for better patient management. The motivation to acquire point of care ultrasound skill should be to assist in clinical decision-making and clinicians should be careful in practicing outside the limits of their skills. Neonatologists with adequate training should be able to report his/her USG findings in the progress sheet for day-to-day clinical decision-making. It is important to mention in the report, whether clinician or an imaging specialist performs bedside ultrasound.

CONCLUSION

Head, lung and abdomen ultrasound are useful bedside clinical tools, which can be used as frequently as required without the risk of radiation exposure. Cranial USG is most commonly used to identify IVH, PVHD and cystic PVL with good efficacy. Lung ultrasound is useful in identifying pneumothorax, pleural effusion, pneumonia and plays a supportive role in the management of RDS. Bedside USG for NEC should be supplementary to usual management. Bedside USG has a definite role in line localization. Use of bedside USG in neonatology is on the rise with frequent new utility additions like endotracheal tube tip localization and is becoming an obligatory screening and diagnostic tool.

It must be emphasized here that clinician-performed USG is not here to replace the role of pediatric cardiologists and radiologists in neonatal practice. However, ultrasound-literate clinicians should be able to do USG in an acute clinical setting, document it and do appropriate intervention in absence of specialist expertise.

REFERENCES

1. Evans N, Gournay V, Cabanas F, Kluckow M, Leone T, Groves A, *et al*. Point-of-care ultrasound in the neonatal intensive care unit: international perspectives 2011;16:61–8.

2. El-Khuffash A, Herbozo C, Jain A, Lapointe A, McNamara PJ. Targeted neonatal echocardiography (TnECHO) service in a Canadian neonatal intensive care unit: a 4-year experience. J Perinatol 2013;33:687–90.

3. Ment LR, Bada HS, Barnes P, Grant PE, Hirtz D, Papile LA, *et al*. Practice parameter: neuroimaging of the neonate: report of the Quality Standards Subcommittee of the American Academy of Neurology and the Practice Committee of the Child Neurology Society. Neurology 2002;58:1726–38.

4. Praveen B. Pathogenesis and prevention of intraventricular hemorrhage. Clin Perinatol 2014;41:47–67.

5. Al-Abdi SY, Al-Aamri MA. A systematic review and meta-analysis of the timing of early intraventricular hemorrhage in preterm neonates: Clinical and research implications. J Clin Neonatol 2014;3:76–88.

6. Ballardini E, Tarocco A, Baldan A, Antoniazzi E, Garani G, Borgna-Pignatti C. Universal cranial ultrasound screening in preterm infants with gestational age 33–36 weeks. A retrospective analysis of 724 newborns. Pediatr Neurol. 2014; 51:790–4.

7. Bhat V, Karam M, Saslow J, Taylor H, Pyon K, Kemble N, *et al*. Utility of performing routine head ultrasound in preterm infants with gestational age 30–34 weeks. J Matern Fetal Neonatal Med 2012;25:116–9.

8. Van der walt C, Vazzalwar R, Schweig L, Donovan R. IVH Screening By Cranial Ultrasound for All Preterm Infants [3]30 Weeks Is Not Cost Effective. In: Proceedings of the AAP Experience National Conference and Exhibition: Perinatal Pediatrics Scientific Posters Presentations; 2013 October 25; Orlando. Florida; 2013. Available from: https://aap.confex.com/aap/2013/webprogram/Paper 21331.html. Accessed July 15, 2015.

9. Andre P, Thebaud B, Delavaucoupet J, Zupan V, Blanc N, d'Allest AM, *et al*. Late-onset cystic periventricular leukomalacia in premature infants: a threat until term. Am J Perinatol 2001;18:79–86.

10. Sherlock RL, Anderson PJ, Doyle LW. Neurodevelopmental sequelae of intraventricular haemorrhage at 8 years of age in a regional cohort of ELBW/ very preterm infants. Early Hum Dev 2005;81:909–16.

11. Luu TM, Ment LR, Schneider KC, Katz KH, Alan WC, Vohr BR. Lasting effects of preterm birth and neonatal brain hemorrhage at 12 years of age. Pediatrics 2009;123:1037–44.

12. Bolisetty S, Dhawan A, Abdel-Latif M, Bajuk B, Stack J, Lui K. Intraventricular hemorrhage and neuro-developmental outcomes in extreme preterm infants. Pediatrics 2014;133:55–62.

13. Burstein J, Papile LA, Burstein R. Intraventricular hemorrhage and hydrocephalus in premature newborns: A prospective study with CT. Am J Roentgenol 1979;132:631–5.

14. Khan IA, Wahab S, Khan RA, Ullah E, Ali M. Neonatal intracranial ischemia and hemorrhage: Role of cranial sonography and CT scanning. J Korean Neurosurg Soc 2010;47:89–94.

15. Volpe JJ. Intracranial Hemorrhage. In: Volpe JJ. Neurology of the Newborn. 5th Ed. Saunders; Philadelphia 2008;11:517–88.

16. Bassan H, Benson CB, Limperopoulos C, Feldman HA, Ringer SA, Veracruz E, *et al*. Ultrasonographic features and severity scoring of periventricular hemorrhagic infarction in relation to risk factors and outcome. Pediatrics 2006; 117:2111–8.

17. Bassan H, Limperopoulos C, Visconti K, Mayer DA, Feldman HA, Avery L, *et al*. Neurodevelopmental outcome in survivors of periventricular hemorrhagic infarction. Pediatrics 2007; 120:785–92.

18. Bass WT, Jones MA, White LE, Montgomery TR, Karlowicz MG. Ultrasonographic differential diagnosis and neurodevelopemental outcome of cerebral white matter lesions in premature infants. J Perinatol 199;19:330–6.

19. Steggerda SJ, Leijser LM, Wiggers-de Bruïne FT, van der Grond J, Walther FJ, van Wezel-Meijler G. Cerebellar injury in preterm infants: incidence and findings on US and MR images. Radiology 2009;252:190–9.

20. Levene MI. Measurement of the growth of the lateral ventricles in preterm infants with real-time ultrasound. Arch Dis Child 1981;56:900–4.

21. De Vries LS, Liem KD, van Dijk K, Smit BJ, Sie L, Rademaker KJ, *et al*. Early versus late treatment of posthaemorrhagic ventricular dilatation: results of a retrospective study from five neonatal intensive care units in The Netherlands. Acta Paediatr 2002;91:212–7.

22. Ingram MC, Huguenard AL, Miller BA, Chern JJ. Poor correlation between head circumference and

cranial ultrasound findings in premature infants with intraventricular hemorrhage. J Neurosurg Pediatr 2014;14:184–9.

23. Muller WD, Urlesberger B. Correlation of ventricular size and head circumference after severe intra-periventricular haemorrhage in preterm infants. Childs Nerv Syst 1992;8:33–5.

24. Brouwer A, Groenendaal F, van Haastert I, Rademaker K, Hanlo P, de Vries LS. Neurodevelopmental outcome of preterm infants with severe intraventricular hemorrhage and ther-apy for post-hemorrhagic ventricular dilatation. J Pediatr 2008;152:648–54.

25. Leijser LM, Srinivasan L, Rutherford MA, Counsell SJ, Allsop JM, Cowan FM. Structural linear measurements in the newborn brain: accuracy of cranial ultrasound compared to MRI. Pediatr Radiol 2007;37:640–8.

26. Grasby DC, Esterman A, Marshall P. Ultrasound grading of cerebral ventricular dilatation in preterm neonates. J Paediatr Child Health 2003; 39:86–90.

27. Liao MF, Chaou WT, Tsao LY, Nishida H, Sakanoue M. Ultrasound measurement of the ventricular size in newborn infants. Brain Dev 1986;8:262–8.

28. Brouwer MJ, de Vries LS, Groenendaal F, Koopman C, Pistorius LR, Mulder EJH, et al. New reference values for the neonatal cerebral ventricles. Radiology 2012;262:224–33.

29. Davies MW, Swaminathan M, Chuang SL, Betheras FR. Reference ranges for the linear dimensions of the intracranial ventricles in preterm neonates. Arch Dis Child Fetal Neonatal Ed 2000;82:F218–23.

30. Sondhi V, Gupta G, Gupta PK, Patnaik SK, Tshering K. Establishment of nomograms and reference ranges for intracranial ventricular dimensions and ventriculo-hemispheric ratio in newborns by ultrasonography. Acta Paediatr 2008;97:738-44.

31. Reeder JD, Kaude JV, Setzer ES. The occipital horn of the lateral ventricles in premature infants. An ultrasonographic study. Eur J Radiol 1983;3: 148–50.

32. Chowdhary V, Culati P, Arora S, Thirupuram S. Cranial sonography in preterm infants. Indian Pediatr 1992;27:411–5.

33. Soni JP, Gupta BD, Soni M, Singh RN, Purohit NN, Gupta M, et al. Normal parameters of ventricular system in healthy infants. Indian Pediatr 1995;32:549–55.

34. Blumenthal I. Periventricular leucomalacia: A review. Eur J Pediatr 2004;163:435–42.

35. Hart AR, Whitby EW, Griffiths PD, Smith MF. Magnetic resonance imaging and developmental outcome following preterm birth: review of current evidence. Dev Med and Child Neurol 2008;50:655–63.

36. De Vries LS, van Haastert IL, Rademaker KJ, Koopman C, Groenendaal F. Ultrasound abnormalities preceding cerebral palsy in high-risk preterm infants. J Pediatr 2004;144:815–20.

37. De Vries LS, Eken P, Dubowitz LM. The spectrum of leukomalacia using cranial ultrasound. Behav Brain Res 1992;49:1–6.

38. Seibert JJ, McCowan TC, Chadduck WM, Adametz JR, Glasier CM, Williamson SL, et al. Duplex pulsed doppler US versus intracranial pressure in the neonate. Clinical and experimental studies. Radiology 1989;171:155–60.

39. Bulas DI. Transcranial doppler: Applications in neonates and children. Ultrasound Clin 2009;4: 533–51.

40. Liu J, Cao HY, Huang XH, Wang Q. The pattern and early diagnostic value of Doppler ultrasound for neonatal hypoxic-ischemic encephalopathy. J Trop Pediatr 2007;53:351–4.

41. Nishimaki S, Iwasaki S, Minamisawa S, Seki K, Yokota S. Blood flow velocities in the anterior cerebral artery and basilar artery in asphyxiated infants. J Ultrasound Med 2008;27:955–60.

42. Argollo N, Lessa I, Ribeiro S. Cranial Doppler resistance index measurement in preterm newborns with cerebral white matter lesion. J Pediatr (Rio J) 2006;82:221–6.

43. Ilves P, Lintrop M, Metsvaht T, Vaher U, Talvik T. Cerebral blood-flow velocities in predicting outcome of asphyxiated newborn infants. Acta Paediatr 2004;93:523–8.

44. Kirimi E, Tuncer O, Atas B, Sakarya ME, Ceylan A. Clinical value of color doppler ultrasonography measurements of full-term newborns with perinatal asphyxia and hypoxic ischemic encephalopathy in the first 12 hours of life and long-term prognosis. Tohoku J Exp Med 2002; 197:27–33.

45. Ilves P, Talvik R, Talvik T. Changes in doppler ultrasonography in asphyxiated term infants with hypoxic-ischaemic encephalopathy. Acta Paediatr 1998;87:680–4.

46. Mackamee LR, Gonzales JI, Chance GW. Cerebral blood flow velocity profiles in intraventricular haemorrhage progressing to hydrocephalus. Pediatr Res 1998;43:224A.

47. Maertzdorf WJ, Vles JSH, Beuls E, Mulder ALM, Blanco CE. Intracranial pressure and cerebral blood flow velocity in preterm infants with post-

haemorrhagic ventricular dilatation. Arch Dis Child Fetal Neonatal Ed 2002;87:3 F185–8.

48. Soo HK, Lana V, Laura RM, Petra SH. The role of neuroimaging in predicting neurodevelopmental outcomes of preterm neonates. Clin Perinatol 2014;41:257–83.

49. deVries LS, Benders MJ, Groenendaal F. Imaging the premature brain: ultrasound or MRI? Neuroradiology 2013;55:13–22.

50. Plaisier A, Raets MMA, Ecury-Goossen GM, Govaert P, Feijen-Roon M, Reiss IK, et al. Serial cranial ultrasonography or early MRI for detecting preterm brain injury? Arch Dis Child Fetal Neonatal Ed 2015;100:F293–F300.

51. Lichtenstein DA, Mauriat P. Lung ultrasound in the critically Ill neonate. Curr Pediatr Rev 2012: 8:217–23.

52. Lichtenstein D. Lung ultrasound in the critically ill. Clin Intensive Care 2005;16:79–-87.

53. Lichtenstein DA. Ultrasound examination of the lungs in the intensive care unit. Pediatr Crit Care Med 2009;10:693–8.

54. Volpicelli G, Elbarbary M, Blaivas M, Lichtenstein DA, Mathis G, Kirpatrick AW, et al. International Liaison Committee on Lung Ultrasound (ILC-LUS) for International Consensus Conference on Lung Ultrasound (ICC-LUS). International evidence-based recommendations for point of-care lung ultrasound. Intensive Care Med 2012; 38:577–91.

55. Hadeel M. Seif El Dien , Dalia AK ElLatif A. The value of bedside Lung Ultrasonography in diagnosis of neonatal pneumonia. Egyptian J Radiol Nuclear Med 2013;44:339–47.

56. Liu J, Liu F, Liu Y, Wang HW, Feng ZC. Lung Ultrasonography for the diagnosis of severe neonatal pneumonia. Chest 2014;146:383–8.

57. Lichtenstein D, Goldstein I, Mourgeon E, Cluzel P, Grenier P, Rouby JJ. Comparative diagnostic performances of auscultation, chest radiography and lung ultrasonography in ARDS. Anesthesiology 2004;100:9–15.

58. Liu J, Cao HI, Wang HW, Kong XY. Role of lung ultrasound in diagnosis of respiratory syndrome in newborn infants. Iran J Pediatr 2015;25:e323.

59. Raimondi F, Migliaro F, Sodano A, Umbaldo A, Romano A, Vallone G, et al. Can neonatal lung ultrasound monitor fluid clearance and predict the need of respiratory support? Crit Care 2012;16:R220.

60. Raimondi F, Migliaro F, Sodano A, Ferrara T, Lama S, Vallone G, et al. Use of neonatal chest ultrasound to predict noninvasive ventilation failure. Pediatrics 2014;134:e1089–94.

61. Brat R, Yousef N, Klifa R, Reynaud S, Aguilera SS, De Luca D. Lung ultrasonography score to evaluate oxygenation and surfactant need in neonates treated with continuous positive airway pressure. JAMA Pediatr 2015;169:e151797.

62. Walsh MC, Kliegman RM. Necrotizing enterocolitis: treatment based on staging criteria. Pediatr Clin North Am 1986;33:179–201.

63. Faingold R, Daneman A, Tomlinson G,Babyn PS, Manson DE, Mohanta A, et al. Necrotizing enterocolitis: assessment of bowel viability with color doppler US. Radiology 2005;235:587–94.

64. Leonidas JC, Krasna IH, Fox HA, Broder MS. Peritoneal fluid in necrotizing enterocolitis: a radiologic sign of clinical deterioration. J Pediatr 1973;82:672–5.

65. Kim WY, Kim WS, Kim IO, Kwon TH, Chang W, Lee EK, et al. Sonographic evaluation of neonates with early-stage necrotizing enterocolitis. Pediatr Radiol 2005;35:1056–61.

66. Kirks DR, O'Byrne SA. The value of the lateral abdominal roentgenogram in the diagnosis of neonatal hepatic portal venous gas (HPVG). Am J Roentgenol Radium Ther Nucl Med 1974;122: 153–8.

67. Silva CT, Danemann A, Navarro OM, Moore AM, Moineddin R, Gerstle JT, et al. Correlation of sonographic findings and outcome in necrotizing enterocolitis. Pediatr Radiol 2007;37:274–82.

68. Garbi Gautel A, Brevaut Malaty V, Panual M, Michel F, Merrot T, Gire C. Prognostic value of abdominal sonography in necrotizing enterocolitis of premature infants born before 33 weeks gestational age. J Pediatr Surg 2014;49:508–13.

69. Perin G, Scarpa MG. Defining central venous line position in children: tips for the tip. J Vasc Access 2015;16:77–86.

70. Jain A, McNamara PJ, Ng E, El-Khuffash A. The use of targeted neonatal echocardiography to confirm placement of peripherally inserted central catheters in neonates. Am J Perinatol 2012;29:101–6.

71. Tauzin L, Sigur N, Joubert C, Parra J, Hassid S, Moulies ME. Echocardiography allows more accurate placement of peripherally inserted central catheters in low birthweight infants. Acta Paediatr 2013;102:703–6.

72. Fleming SE, Kim JH. Ultrasound-guided umbilical catheter insertion in neonates. J Perinatol 2011;31:344–9.

73. Stanojevic M. Training of ultrasound in neonatology: Global or local? Donald School J Ultrasound Obstet Gynecol 2013;7:338–45.

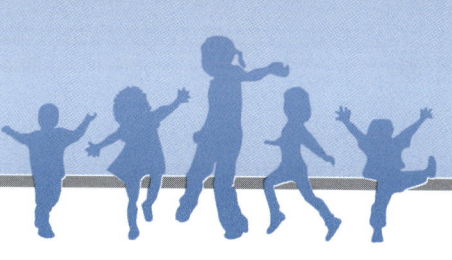

Hyperinsulinemic Hypoglycemia in Infancy

Shrenik Vora, Suresh Chandran, Victor Samuel Rajadurai, Khalid Hussain

Hyperinsulinemic hypoglycemia has increasingly been recognized as a cause of intractable hypoglycemia in neonates and infants. Hyperinsulinemic hypoglycemia occurs due to unregulated insulin secretion from β-cells of pancreas in relation to blood glucose levels.[1] Small for gestational age (SGA) infants and macrosomic infants born to diabetic mothers (IDM) are the two most common groups of infants at risk of hypoglycemia in the neonatal period.[2] Glucose is the principal energy source for the neonatal brain and hypoglycemia is known to cause irreversible neuronal injury when it is recurrent and severe; so prompt recognition and treatment of these infants with hyperinsulinemic hypoglycemia is paramount.[3] Hyperinsulinemic hypoglycemia can be transient, prolonged or persistent (congenital). Knowledge of blood glucose homeostasis and appropriate investigations for intermediary metabolites during an episode of hypoglycemia is the cornerstone for diagnosis and management of hyperinsulinemic hypoglycemia. The management of medically unresponsive hyperinsulinemic hypoglycemia still remains a challenge. Knowledge of the genetic mutations, newer imaging modalities like Fluorine 18L-3, 4-dihydroxyphenylalanine positron emission tomography (18F-DOPA-PET) scan and availability of histological differentiation of focal and diffuse forms of persistent hyperinsulinemic hypoglycemia has streamlined the management of congenital hyperinsulinemic hypoglycemia (CHI).[4] The purpose of this review is to provide an overview of physiology of insulin secretion, controversies regarding definition of hypoglycemia, spectrum of clinical presentation, and recent advances in diagnosis and management of different forms of hyperinsulinism.

GLUCOSE HOMEOSTASIS

Normoglycemia is maintained by a balance between the insulin secretion following food intake and response of the counter regulatory hormones (glucagon, growth hormone, adrenaline and cortisol) in the face of hypoglycemia. Insulin promotes peripheral uptake of glucose and counter regulatory hormones increase hepatic glucose output by glycogenolysis followed by gluconeogenesis. Liver glycogen stores in a healthy full-term infant last for 10–12 hours from birth. Endocrine changes occur soon after birth with a decrease in plasma levels of insulin and increase of catecholamine and glucagon.[5] Hepatic glucose production in a full-term infant is 4–6 mg/kg/ min and the infant switches on the endogenous production of glucose following birth until exogenous nutritional supply is established. The newborn infant has essential enzymes needed for gluconeogenesis from alanine, pyruvate, glycerol, and lactate. Soon after birth hepatic glycogenolysis provides glucose whereas β-oxidation of fatty acids and lactate generation due to proteolysis provide an adequate substrate for gluconeogenesis.[6] Infants with disorders of glycogenolysis present after 4–5 hours of fast whereas infants with disorders of gluconeogenesis become hypoglycemic after an overnight fast. On the contrary, infants with hyperinsulinism present with hypoglycemia at any time after the last feed.[7]

Insulin Release from β-cells of Pancreas

Knowledge of insulin secretion by β-cells of pancreas in response to plasma glucose helps to understand the pathogenesis and management of hyperinsulinemic hypoglycemia. As shown in Fig. 12.1, the metabolism of glucose, amino acids and fatty acids results in the generation of metabolic coupling factors like ATP and β-ketoglutarate, which are involved in regulating insulin exocytosis. Under normal physiological conditions, each of these coupling factors plays a key role in regulating insulin secretion precisely to keep fasting blood glucose concentrations between 3.5–5.9 mmol/L. As blood glucose level rises after feed or glucose infusion, it triggers insulin secretion from pancreatic β-cells. The GLUT2 transporters present on pancreatic β-cells facilitate the uptake of glucose. Glycolytic phosphorylation by glucokinase (GK) enzyme follows leading to a rise in the ATP:ADP ratio. Functional integrity of the pancreatic ATP sensitive potassium (KATP) channel depends on the interactions between the pore-forming inward rectifier potassium channel subunit (KIR6.2) and the regulatory sulfonylurea receptor 1(SUR1), encoded by KCNJ11 and ABCC8 genes, respectively. The increase in the cytosolic ATP:ADP ratio activates plasma membrane SUR1, which leads to the closure of KATP channel. This in turn depolarizes the membrane allowing calcium ions to flow in to the cell via voltage-gated calcium channels.

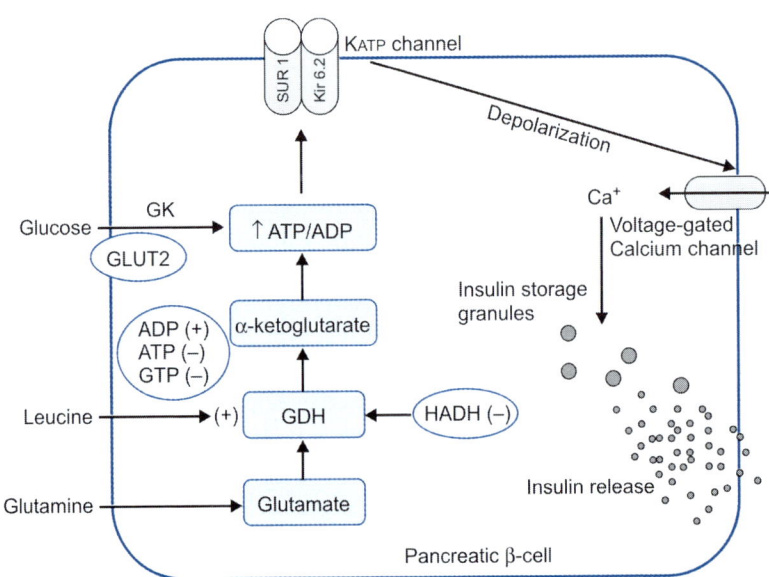

Fig. 12.1: Glucose and protein mediated insulin secretion from β-cells of pancreas.

GDH: Glutamate dehydrogenase; HADH: L3-hydroxyacyl-CoenzymeA dehydrogenase; GK: Glucokinase; SUR 1: Sulfonylurea receptor; Kir 6.2: Potassium channel inwardly rectifier; GLUT2: Glucose transporter 2

Following this, the insulin storage granules undergo exocytosis resulting in release of insulin.[8] Insulin secretion is also regulated by metabolic signals arising from lipid and amino acid metabolism mediated through its effect on glutamate dehydrogenase (GDH).[9]

DEFINITION OF HYPOGLYCEMIA

Definition of hypoglycemia and screening guidelines in neonatal period remain controversial. Following severance of the umbilical cord at birth, glucose supply from the mother to the neonate ceases leading to a rapid fall in neonatal glucose concentration. Glucose level decreases reaching a nadir at 1 hour of age and then stabilizes by 3 hours of age spontaneously or in response to milk feeds in healthy full-term infants.

In a comprehensive review of the literature in 1997, an expert panel of the World Health Organization concluded that there are numerous approaches to defining normoglycemia, including the statistical, metabolic, neurophysiological, and, perhaps most importantly, the neurodevelopmental approach. These different approaches towards definition of normoglycemia contribute to the controversy that surrounds this issue.[10] Current consensus by world experts on hyperinsulinism states that hypoglycemia cannot be defined as a specific plasma glucose concentration due to inability to identify a single value that causes brain damage and brain responses varies by the presence of alternative fuels like ketones.[11] Currently the most common practice is to screen the at-risk infants, which includes IDM and neonatal conditions like SGA (birth weight <10th centile), large for gestational age (LGA, birth weight >90th centile), perinatal asphyxia, prematurity, infection, and dysmorphic infants suggestive of Beckwith-Wiedemann syndrome. This has led to the development of guidelines designed to identify infants "at-risk" and the implementation of an "operational threshold" for physicians to consider intervention.[12]

In 2011, clinical report of the American Academy of Pediatrics recommended screening of "at-risk" infants within first hours of birth. The macrosomic IDM, late-preterms (34 to 36+6 weeks gestation) and SGA infants should be fed every 2–3 hours with estimation of pre-feed glucose levels for multiple feed-fast cycles for at least 24 hours. Further monitoring of blood sugar levels should be continued only if plasma glucose levels remain below 2.5 mmol/L. Symptoms in infants with blood glucose value less than 2.2 mmol/L warrant parenteral glucose infusion. In asymptomatic infants, a practical approach based on age, risk factors and mode of feeding can be considered when treatment is planned. Any infant with persistent or recurrent hypoglycemia should be screened for hyperinsulinism.[13] Hyperinsulinemic hypoglycemia is defined as inappropriately elevated plasma insulin concentration in the presence of hypoglycemia (<3.5 mmol/L) in infants receiving glucose infusion rate (GIR) of more than 8 mg/kg/min, with suppressed ketone bodies and free fatty acids and a positive glycemic response to parenteral glucagon. In infants with suspected hyperinsulinemic hypoglycemia, due to lack of alternative energy fuels the blood glucose levels should be maintained >3.5 mmol/L.[14]

TYPES OF HYPERINSULINEMIC HYPOGLYCEMIA

Hyperinsulinemic hypoglycemia can be transient, prolonged or persistent (congenital).

Transient Hyperinsulinemic Hypoglycemia

This is observed often in IDM, SGA infants and in infants who had perinatal asphyxia, polycythemia and Rh isoimmunization. There is no clear definition of the precise duration of transient hypoglycemia. Hyperinsulinemic hypoglycemia usually presents soon after the birth and settles within a few days responding to increment of feeds or to increasing glucose infusion rate until the β-cell insulin secretion is normalized.[15]

Prolonged Hyperinsulinemic Hypoglycemia

Some of the SGA infants develop a syndrome of prolonged hyperinsulinemic hypoglycemia requiring high GIR to maintain normo-glycemia and responding to medical treatment with KATP channel agonist (diazoxide). The etiology of prolonged hyperinsulinemic hypoglycemia in SGA infants could be due to a lack of supply of exogenous substrate, depletion of hepatic glycogen stores, defective gluconeogenesis, hyper-insulinism due to transient alteration in the regulation of β-cell insulin secretion, increased sensitivity to insulin or adrenocortical insufficiency. No genetic cause has been identified in prolonged hyperinsulinemic hypoglycemia and in most of the cases, resolution is observed in several weeks to months. The incidence of prolonged hyperinsulinemic hypoglycemia is reported to be as high as 1:12,000 births. There are few reports where the prolonged hyperinsulinemic hypoglycemia was diagnosed as late as 2 weeks after birth (range: 2–180 days) and hence there is a risk involved in early discharge of these SGA infants.[16]

Congenital Hyperinsulinism (CHI)

CHI is a heterogeneous condition presenting with hyperinsulinism, hypoketonemia, and hypo-fattyacidemia with severe and persistent hypoglycemia. The etiopathogenesis of CHI can be due to two major defects known as channelopathies and metabolopathies. Channelopathies refer to defects in the pancreatic β-cell ATP-sensitive KATP channel that lead to unregulated insulin secretion, the commonest genetic cause being autosomal recessively inherited inactivating mutation in ABCC8 and KCNJ11 (chromosome11p15.1) genes.[17] Metabolopathies cause congenital hyperinsulinemic hypoglycemia either by altering the concentration of intracellular signaling molecules (such as ATP/ADP) or by accumulation of intermediary metabolites, triggering insulin release. The commonest cause for metabolopathies is Hyperinsulinism-Hyperammonemia (HI/HA) syndrome. The

incidence of CHI is estimated to be 1:40,000–50,000 in the general population, but in familial forms it may be as high as 1:2500 in populations with substantial consanguinity.[18]

Genetics of Congenital Hyperinsulinism

Genetic defects in key genes regulating insulin secretion causes CHI. Mutations in nine genes –ABCC8, KCNJ11, GLUD1, GCK, HADH, SLC16A1, HNF4A, HNF1A, UCP2—have been identified to cause CHI, altering the β-cell function.[19]

Histologically, focal and diffuse forms have been reported. Diffuse forms are inherited in an autosomal recessive or dominant manner and focal forms are sporadic in nature.

CHI due to channelopathies: Recessive inactivating mutations in ABCC8 and KCNJ11 genes are the most common causes of CHI and these mutations are found in 50% of the patients. These mutations alter the function of KATP channel, causing unregulated insulin secretion. This results in severe CHI and is unresponsive to KATP channel agonist, diazoxide. Histologically, recessive KATP channel mutation is characterized by large β-cells with enlarged nuclei. A milder form of CHI has been reported with dominant inactivating mutations in ABCC8 and KCNJ11 genes. These milder forms are also reported to be mostly unresponsive to diazoxide. In ABCC8 gene about 150 homozygous, compound heterozygous and heterozygous inactivating mutations and in KCNJ11 around 24 mutations have been reported.[20]

Focal lesions due to KATP mutations are confined to restricted areas of pancreas. Chromosome 11p15.5 (in close proximity to KATP channel gene 11p15.1) has maternally expressed tumor suppressors H19 and CDK1C and paternally expressed growth factor gene, IGF2. Genetically focal lesion arises following a paternally inherited, monoallelic mutation in one of the KATP channel genes. During the development of pancreas, when segmental paternal uniparental disomy occurs as a somatic mutation, KATP channel activity is lost in the β-cell. These cells also lose maternally expressed tumor suppressor activities of H19 and CDK1C and the activity of paternally expressed IGF2 is doubled, promoting the growth of abnormal β-cells. Histology reveals focal enlargement of β-cell with large nuclei. Generally (96.2%) focal lesions are unresponsive to diazoxide but are curable by limited excision.[7,18,21]

HI/HA syndrome: It is the second commonest form of CHI, caused by activating missense mutation of the GLUD1 gene, which encodes the mitochondrial enzyme GDH. GDH is expressed in pancreatic β-cells, liver, kidney and brain. GLUD1 gene mutations lead to a gain of GDH function by reducing its sensitivity to allosteric inhibition by GTP and ATP, resulting in activation of insulin secretion by the amino acid leucine. Mechanism of hyperammonemia in HI/HA syndrome is unclear, may be due to increased hepatic GDH activity and ammonia synthesis or due to abnormal muscle catabolism. Recently, renal ammoniagenesis has been implicated as a source of HA.[22] Hyperammonemia, a characteristic biochemical marker of HI/HA syndrome, is typically mild to moderate in infants and is not associated with lethargy or coma. Some of these patients may not have hyperammonemia and it could be due to mosaicism for the mutation in the liver, where the mutation is absent or seen in <50% in hepatocytes. Infants with HI/HA syndrome experience both fasting and postprandial hypoglycemia following leucine intake usually after first few months of life. Diazoxide remains the mainstay of treatment in patients with HI/HA syndrome.[23]

Hydroxyacyl Coenzyme A Dehydrogenase (HADH) gene mutation: Short-chain-3-hydroxyacyl-CoA dehydro-genase (SCHAD), encoded by the gene HADH, catalyses the penultimate reaction of the β-oxidation cycle.[24] HADH is expressed in pancreatic β-cells, indicating a vital role in insulin secretion. In patients with HADH gene mutation, "protein

to protein" interaction is lost between GDH and SCHAD causing leucine-induced hyperinsulinemic hypoglycemia via a novel pathway not involving GTP regulation of GDH. The clinical phenotype of HADH mutations varies from mild to severe neonatal hyperinsulinemic hypoglycemia with raised levels of fatty acid metabolites responding to diazoxide.[25]

Glucokinase—Cytosolic enzyme defects: Glucokinase (GCK) is a glycolytic enzyme and plays an important role as a glucose sensor in the pancreatic β-cell controlling glucose regulated insulin secretion. Heterozygous activating mutations have been reported to cause CHI and inactivating monoallelic mutations causing mild form of diabetes (GCK-MODY). Inappropriate insulin secretion following heterozygous activating mutations of glucokinase resulted from increased affinity of the enzyme for glucose, raising the ATP: ADP ratio in the β-cell.[26] Affected patients present with fasting hypoglycemia and can be symptomatic anytime from infancy to adulthood. Mostly this form of hyperinsulinemic hypoglycemia is diazoxide-responsive but cases requiring octreotide and subtotal pancreatec-tomy have been reported.

Mutations in mitochondrial uncoupling protein 2 (UCP2) gene: UCP2 acts as a negative regulator of insulin secretion of β-cells. It has been shown that UCP2 uncouples mitochondrial oxidative phosphorylation from ATP generation. Loss of function mutation of UCP2 gene has been reported to cause transient hyperinsulinemic hypoglycemia or mild fasting diazoxide responsive CHI .[26, 27]

HNF4A/HNF1A gene mutations: HNF4A gene encodes for a transcription factor HNF4a (hepatocyte nuclear factor 4a), a member of the nuclear hormone receptor superfamily. Mutations in HNF4A gene are uncommon causes of hyperinsulinemic hypoglycemia, which can be either transient or persistent. HNF4A is required in the pancreatic β-cell for the regulation of the pathway of insulin secretion, heterozygous mutations of which cause maturity-onset diabetes of the young type 1 (MODY1).[28] Exact mechanism of hyper-insulinemic hypoglycemia due to HNF4A gene mutations is unclear. The possible mecha-nisms might be a reduction in expression of the potassium channel subunit (Kir 6.2) or reduction in expression of nuclear PPARa (peroxisome proliferator-activated receptor a), which can shift energy metabolism in cells towards fatty acid oxidation (FAO). Similar to HNF4A, HNF1A mutations can cause hyper-insulinism in newborn and infancy, and diabetes in later life.[29]

Exercise-induced hyperinsulinemic hypogly-cemia (SLC16A1 gene mutation): This is a dominantly inherited form of CHI charac-terized by inappropriate insulin secretion following anaerobic exercise or pyruvate load. In normal physiological status, lactate and pyruvate transport into the α-cell is mediated by monocarboxylase transporter 1(MCT1), which is encoded by the SLC16A1 gene. Under normal circumstances, MCT1 expression in the pancreatic α-cell is very low, minimizing the effects of pyruvate and lactate on insulin secretion. Increased levels of MCT1 due to promoter-activating mutations in SLC16A1 gene permits entry of circulating lactate and pyruvate into the β-cell, leading to an increase in ATP generation, triggering insulin release by closure of KATP channel and depolari-zation of the cell. Affected children become hypoglycemic typically 30–45 minute after a period of intensive anaerobic exercise due to lactate and pyruvate accumulation.[19,30] Exercise-induced hyperinsulinemic hypogly-cemia is not observed in neonates and reported cases are limited to older children and adults.

Other causes of hyperinsulinemic hypogly-cemia: Rarely, hyperinsulinemic hypogly-cemia is also seen associated with overgrowth syndromes like Beckwith-Wiedemann and Sotos syndromes and metabolic conditions like congenital disorder of glycosylation (CDG) and tyrosinemia. Beckwith-Wiedemann syndrome, the most common syndrome associated with hyperinsulinemic hypoglycemia is characterized by overgrowth, macroglossia, hemi-hypertrophy and abdominal wall defects. The hypoglycemia can be asymptomatic transient to rarely pro-longed, extending beyond neonatal period.[31] CDG type Ib (phosphomannose-isomerase deficiency), perhaps causing abnormal glycosylation of KATP channel, causes hyperinsulinism and that may explain the response of hyperinsulinemic hypoglycemia in these infants to diazoxide.[32] The mechanism of hyperinsulinemic hypoglycemia in tyrosinemia type 1 is still unclear but may be due to accumulation of toxic metabolites causing islet-cell hyperplasia.[33]

CLINICAL PRESENTATION

Patients with hyperinsulinemic hypoglycemia present during the newborn period most often during the first 24–48 hours of life. However, different studies showed median age of presentation ranging from hours to weeks. Symptoms of hypoglycemia are mostly non-specific such as lethargy, poor feeding, apnea, jitteriness, irritability, high-pitched cry, exag-gerated reflexes, seizures and coma. Presentation of persistent hyperinsulinemic hypoglycemia is more severe needing higher concentrations of glucose to maintain the blood glucose level.[34] High index of suspicion, early diagnosis and aggressive management is essential to prevent unexplained deaths and brain injury due to hypoglycemia.

Neonatal Hypoglycemic Brain Injury (NHBI): Hypoglycemia, being a surrogate marker of neuronal energy deficiency, is a major cause of brain injury. Speculated mechanisms of cellular injury includes; excitatory neurotoxins active at N-methyl-D-aspartate receptors, increased mitochondrial free radical gene-ration and initiation of apoptosis. Several neuroprotective mechanisms are believed to play a role to guard against these neuronal injuries by substitution of alternative cerebral substrates like lactate, ketone bodies, pyruvate, amino acids, free fatty acids and glycerol.[35] It has been postulated that immature newborn brain requires decreased cerebral energy fuels as compared to children and adults. Also limited glycogen stores in astrocytes provide immediate supply of glucose to the neurons. These mechanisms can protect the brain for limited periods and permanent damage occurs if recurrent protracted hypoglycemia prevails.[36] An increased risk of cerebral palsy, development delay and low mental scores at 18 months of age has been shown in infants with recurrent hypoglycemia lasting for five or more days. Pathological changes of NHBI include swelling of the neuronal and glial cells, necrosis, gyrus atrophy and white matter demyelination.[37] Neonatal hypoglycemic brain injury predominantly affects parieto-occipital regions as evidenced by MRI scans.[38]

DIAGNOSIS

A detailed history related to pregnancy (diabetes/diet/insulin), delivery (asphyxia), gestational age and birth weight (SGA/LGA/macrosomia) is essential. Parental consanguinity, family history of diabetes, and history of siblings having infantile seizures may indicate inherited cause of the hypoglycemia. A thorough physical examination of the infant to look for dysmorphic features (e.g. omphalocele, hemihypertrophy, macroglossia), evidence of hypopituitarism (e.g. cleft lip/palate, micropenis, short stature), adrenal insufficiency (e.g. hyperpigmentation, weight loss) and disorders of glycogenesis (e.g. hepatosplenomegaly) has to be carried out. Sudden cardio-respiratory arrest and acidosis with hypoglycemia in an otherwise healthy infant might point towards a metabolic disorder.[39] As mentioned previously, "at-risk" groups of infants should be screened for hypoglycemia in relation to the risk factors specific to the individual case. Any patient with recurrent or persistent hypoglycemia

despite GIR of >8 mg/kg/min is indicative of hyperinsulinemic hypoglycemia. The key feature of hyperinsulinemic hypoglycemia is detectable serum insulin and/or C-peptide levels during episodes of hypoglycemia along with hypoketonemia and hypofattyacidemia. When diagnosis is in doubt, a positive glycemic (>1.5 mmol/L) response to glucagon or octreotide therapy gives a supportive evidence of hyperinsulinemic hypoglycemia.[40] Harris, et al.[41] showed a good correlation between continuous interstitial glucose monitoring and blood glucose measurements. Reports suggest that continuous interstitial glucose monitoring can potentially be advantageous in measuring the duration, severity, and frequency of low glucose concentrations in high-risk infants and can help identify and prevent unwanted periods of hypoglycemia or hyperglycemia.[42] To aid in the diagnosis, further assessment of plasma and urine metabolic profile (Box 12.1) and genetic testing need to be done in some infants presenting with more subtle forms of CHI, after liaising with local tertiary centres.[43] Additional provocation tests (leucine/protein

Box 12.1: Investigations for suspected hyperinsulinemic hypoglycemia	
Urine	*Blood*
Reducing substances	Glucose
Ketone bodies	Insulin/C-peptide
Amino acids	Ketone bodies
Organic acids	Free fatty acids
	Amino acids
	Lactate
	Ammonia
	Bicarbonate
	Blood gas analysis
	Inborn error of metabolism (IEM) screen
	Acyl carnitine profile
	Cortisol
	Growth hormone
	Insulin Growth Factor Binding Protein 1 (IGFBP1)

loading or exercise testing) are indicated in those patients with protein/leucine sensitivity and exercise-induced hypoglycemia.

MANAGEMENT OF HYPERINSULINEMIC HYPOGLYCEMIA

The management of patients with hyper-insulinemic hypoglycemia can be extremely complicated, particularly in prolonged and persistent hyperinsulinemic hypoglycemia. They will require frequent blood glucose monitoring and the insertion of a central venous catheter to deliver concentrated dextrose infusion. Ideally, these patients should be managed at specialized centers that have the necessary multidisciplinary team experience and expertise.[44] Expert review suggests that the goal of treatment for "at-risk" infants without suspected CHI should be to maintain blood glucose levels >2.8 mmol/L for those aged <48 hours and >3.3 mmol/L for those aged >48 hours. For neonates with suspected CHI, recommendation is to keep blood glucose levels >3.9 mmol/L.[11]

The treatment of hyperinsulinemic hypo-glycemia involves medical therapy, and surgery in some cases. The mainstay of initial medical treatment is the provision of adequate carbohydrate to maintain normoglycemia, i.e. blood sugar level between 3.5–6 mmol/L. Sometimes, to ensure regular frequent feeds, feeding via naso-gastric tube or feeding gastrostomy may be needed. Symptomatic hypoglycemia is treated with "minibolus" of intravenous 10% dextrose at 2 mL/kg to achieve normoglycemia and higher dextrose concentrations should be avoided as bolus to prevent rebound hypoglycemia by further stimulating insulin secretion. This is followed by gradually increasing GIR depending on blood sugar levels by using intravenous glucose at high concentrations.[45]

Diazoxide, a KATP channel agonist, is the mainstay of medical treatment in prolonged hyperinsulinemic hypoglycemia. It prevents α-cell membrane depolarization and inhibits insulin secretion by keeping KATP channels open. It is given orally in the dose of 5–20 mg/kg/day in 3 divided doses. When using dia-zoxide in infants having hepatic dysfunction or hypoalbuminemia, use lower doses of 3 mg/kg/day as it is highly protein bound (>90%). Also lower doses are safer in SGA infants as they are very sensitive to diazoxide.[46] Diazoxide is usually combined with thiazide diuretics to counteract its most common side effect of fluid retention in neonates.[1] Hypertrichosis is another important common complication of diazoxide which usually reverts following cessation of therapy. Diazoxide responsiveness is noted when infant can fast appropriately for age, maintains normal glucose levels and shows rise in serum fatty acids and ketone bodies at the end of fast.[36,40] Nifedipine, a calcium channel blocker, has been used in few diazoxide unresponsive cases of CHI, but vast majority of such patients fail to show any response.[47]

Octreotide, a somatostatin analogue causing inhibition of insulin release by acti-vation of somatostatin receptor-5, stabilizing KATP channel and inhibition of calcium mobilisation is used in resistant cases. It is given as 6–8 hourly subcutaneous injections in a dose of 5–25 mcg/kg/day.[48] Recently, few articles suggest once-a-month intramuscular treatment with long-acting release octreotide (Lanreotide) as a simple, cost-effective and efficient alternative to thrice daily octreotide.[49] Glucagon is primarily used for management of acute symptomatic hypoglycemia as subcutaneous injection at dose of 0.5–1 mg in cases where intravenous access is difficult. It is also used as continuous intravenous infu-sion at dose of 1–20 mcg/kg/hour for short-term stabilization of glucose control in combination with octreotide in patients with hyperinsulinemic hypoglycemia. It activates adenylate cyclase via G-protein-coupled receptor thereby increasing glycogenolysis and gluconeogenesis.[50] Recent advances have shown the effectiveness of the mammalian target of rapamycin (mTOR) inhibitor, Sirolimus in infants with severe diffuse form of hyperinsulinemic hypoglycemia that had been unresponsive to maximal doses of diazoxide and octreotide.[51] Once glucose levels are stabilized, reduce and stop intravenous glucose infusion followed by glucagon and octreotide. The maintenance dose of octreotide is reduced in patients with severe hepatic impairment. These children with CHI are always at increased risk of infection due to central line related sepsis and prolonged/multiple hospitalizations.

Molecular testing for mutations in genes responsible for CHI becomes necessary if hypoglycemia is diazoxide-unresponsive.[52]

Confirmed cases of CHI should be differentiated into focal and diffuse forms using 18F-DOPA-PET scan to make surgical decision.[53] Laparoscopic excision is curative in focal forms whereas near total pancreatectomy is needed in diffuse disease.[54] Decision for surgery also includes dependence on high GIR requirement along with unresponsiveness to medications. In immediate post-operative period, some children may develop transient hyperglycemia needing insulin administration. Many children have persistent hypoglycemia following surgery needing on-going diazoxide therapy,

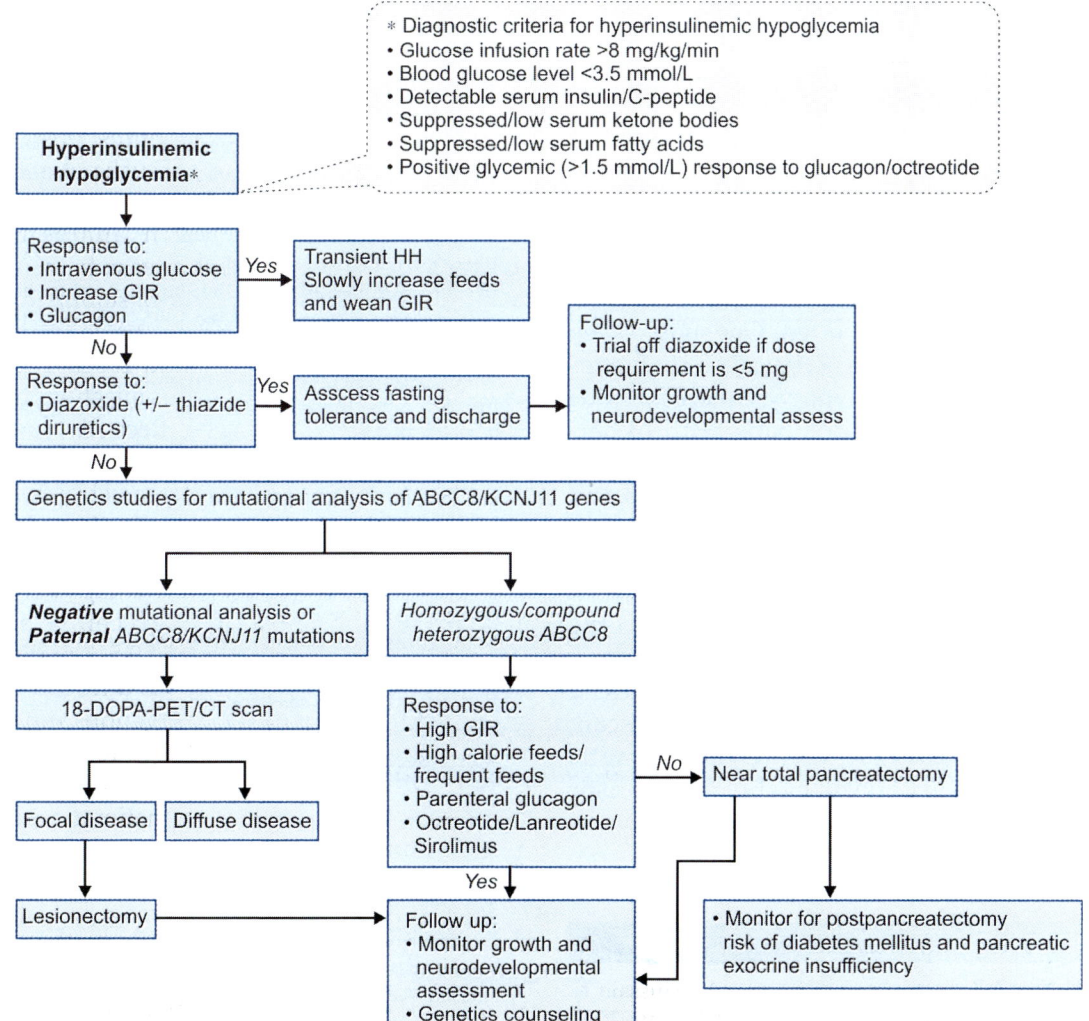

Fig. 12.2: Suggested outline for diagnosis and management of hyperinsulinemic hypoglycemia

before developing diabetes later on. Near total pancreatectomy leads to post-operative diabetes and exocrine pancreatic insufficiency in most of the infants with diffuse persistent hyperinsulinemic hypoglycemia.[55] Infants on treatment for CHI should have long-term developmental follow up due to high risk of neurodevelopmental delay, cerebral palsy and epilepsy.[35, 36] All the familial forms of CHI should undergo genetic counseling. **Fig. 12.2** suggests outline for the diagnosis and management of hyperinsulinemic hypoglycemia.

CONCLUSION

Being an important cause of hypoglycemia in infancy, early diagnosis and aggressive management of hyperinsulinemic hypoglycemia is the cornerstone for prevention of hypoglycemia induced neuronal injury. Molecular basis of the various forms of hyperinsulinemic hypoglycemia involving defects in key genes, which regulate insulin secretion, are beginning to be understood and being increasingly reported. One should keep in mind, the spectrum of clinical presentations of hyperinsulinemic hypoglycemia. Diazoxide unres-ponsiveness in a baby with hyperinsulinemic hypoglycemia warrants genetic studies to look for common mutations and trials with newer drugs like lanreotide and sirolimus appears promising. However, the management of hyperinsulinemic hypoglycemia still remains a challenge to the neonatologists and endocrinologists, even in developed countries; due to lack of facilities for genetic studies and 18F-DOPA-PET scan. Novel insights in identifying genetic mechanisms in CHI will modify the futuristic approach to diagnosis and treatment of hyperinsulinemic hypoglycemia.

REFERENCES

1. Arya VB, Senniappan S, Guemes M, Hussain K. Neonatal hypoglycemia. Indian J Pediatr 2014; 81:58–65.

2. Straussman S, Levitsky LL. Neonatal hypoglycemia. Curr Opin Endocrinol Diabetes Obes 2010;17:20–4.

3. Menni F, de Lonlay P, Sevin C, Touati G, Peigne´ C, Barbier V, et al. Neurologic outcomes of 90 neonates and infants with persistent hyperinsulinemic hypoglycemia. Pediatrics 2001;107:476–9.

4. Hussain K, Blankenstein O, De Lonlay P, Christesen HT. Hyperinsulinaemic hypoglycaemia: biochemical basis and the importance of maintaining normoglycaemia during management. Arch Dis Child 2007;92:568–70.

5. Hawdon J. Glucose homeostasis in the healthy fetus and neonate. In: Rennie JM, (Ed) Metabolic and Endocrine Disorders. Textbook of Neonatology. London: Elsevier, Churchill Livingstone 2005;851–52.

6. Henquin JC. Triggering and amplifying pathways of regulation of insulin secretion by glucose. Diabetes 2000;49:1751–60.

7. Yorifuji T. Congenital hyperinsulinism: Current status and future prospectives. Ann Pediatr Endocrinol Metab 2014;19:57–68.

8. Inagaki N, Gonoi T, Clement JP, Namba N, Inazawa J, Gonzalez G, et al. Reconstitution of IKATP: An inward rectifier subunit plus the sulfonylurea receptor. Science 1995;270:1166–70.

9. Zhang T, Li C. Mechanisms of amino acid-stimulated insulin secretion in congenital hyperinsulinism. Acta Biochim Biophys Sin (Shanghai) 2013;45:36–43.

10. World Health Organization. Hypoglycaemia of the Newborn. Review of the Literature. Geneva: WHO, 1997;WHO/CHD/97.1.

11. Thornton PS, Stanley CA, De Leon D, Harris D, Haymond MW, Hussain K, et al. Recommendations from the Pediatric Endocrine Society for Evaluation and Management of Persistent Hypoglycemia in Neonates, Infants, and Children. J Pediatr 2015; 167:238–45.

12. Tin W. Defining neonatal hypoglycaemia: a continuing debate. Semin Fetal Neonatal Med. 2014; 19:27–32.

13. Adamkin DH, Committee on Fetus and Newborn. Postnatal glucose homeostasis in late-preterm and term infants. Pediatrics 2011;127: 575–79.

14. Kapoor RR, Flanagan SE, James C, Shield J, Ellard S, Hussain K. Hyperinsulinaemic hypoglycaemia. Arch Dis Child 2009;94:450–7.

15. Vanhaltren K, Malhotra A. Characteristics of infants at risk of hypoglycaemia secondary to

being 'infant of a diabetic mother'. J Pediatr Endocrinol Metab 2013;26:861–5.

16. Chong JH, Chandran S, Agarwal P, Rajadurai VS. Delayed presentation of prolonged hyperinsulinaemic hypogly-caemia in a preterm small-for-gestational age neonate. BMJ Case Rep. 2013. Doi:10.1136/bcr-2013-200920.

17. Bellanne´-Chantelot C, Saint-Martin C, Ribeiro MJ, Vaury C, Verkarre V, Arnoux JB, et al. ABCC8 and KCNJ11 molecular spectrum of 109 patients with diazoxide-unresponsive congenital hyperinsulinism. J Med Genet. 2010;47:752–59.

18. James C, Kapoor RR, Ismail D, Hussain K. The genetic basis of congenital hyperinsulinism. J Med Genet 2009;46:289–99.

19. Mohammed Z, Hussain K. The genetics of hyperinsulinemic hypoglycemia. NeoReviews. 2013;14: 179–88.

20. Verkarre V, Fournet JC, de Lonlay P, Gross-Morand MS, Devillers M, Rahier J, et al. Paternal mutation of the sulfonylurea receptor (SUR1) gene and maternal loss of 11p15 imprinted genes lead to persistent hyperinsulinism in focal adenomatous hyperplasia. J Clin Invest 1998;102: 1286–91.

21. Flanagan SE, Clauin S, Bellanne´-Chantelot C, de Lonlay P, Harries LW, Gloyn AL, et al. Update of mutations in the genes encoding the pancreatic b-cell K (ATP) channel subunits Kir6.2 (KCNJ11) and sulfonylurea receptor 1 (ABCC8) in diabetes mellitus and hyperinsulinism. Hum Mutat 2009; 30:170–80.

22. Stanley CA, Lieu YK, Hsu BY, Burlina AB, Greenberg CR, Hopwood NJ, et al. Hyperinsulinism and hyperammonemia in infants with regulatory mutations of the glutamate dehydrogenase gene. N Engl J Med 1998;338:1352–7.

23. MacMullen C, Fang J, Hsu BY, Kelly A, de Lonlay-Debeney P, Saudubray JM, et al. Hyperinsulinism/hyperammonemia syndrome in children with regulatory mutations in the inhibitory guanosine triphosphate-binding domain of glutamate dehydrogenase. J Clin Endocrinol Metab 2001;86:1782–7.

24. Hussain K, Clayton PT, Krywawych S, Chatziandreou I, Mills P, Ginbey DW, et al. Hyperinsulinism of infancy associated with a novel splice site mutation in the SCHAD gene. J Pediatr 2005;146:706–8.

25. Chandran S, Yap F, Hussain K. Molecular mechanisms of protein induced hyperinsulinaemic hypoglycaemia. World J Diabetes 2014; 5:666–77.

26. Cuesta-Muñoz A, Huopio H, Otonkoski T, Gomez-Zumaquero JM, Näntö-Salonen K, Rahier J, et al. Severe persistent hyperinsulinemic hypoglycemia due to a de novo glucokinase mutation. Diabetes 2004;53:2164–8.

27. Gonzalez Barroso MM, Giurgea I, Bouillaud F, Anedda A, Bellanne Chantelot C, Hubert L, et al. Mutations in UCP2 in congenital hyperinsulinism reveal a role for regulation of insulin secretion. PLoS One 2008;3:e3850.

28. Gupta RK, Vatamaniuk MZ, Lee CS, Flaschen RC, Fulmer JT, Matschinsky FM, et al. The MODY1 gene HNF 4alpha regulates selected genes involved in insulin secretion. J Clin Invest 2005;115:1006–15.

29. Pearson ER, Boj SF, Steele AM, Barrett T, Stals K, Shield JP, et al. Macrosomia and hyperinsulinaemic hypo-glycaemia in patients with heterozygous mutations in the HNF4A gene. PLoS Med 2007;4:e118.

30. Otonkoski T, Kaminen N, Ustinov J, Lapatto R, Meissner T, Mayatepek E, et al. Physical exercise-induced hyperinsulinemic hypoglycemia is an autosomal-dominant trait characterized by abnormal pyruvate induced insulin release. Diabetes 2003;52:199–204.

31. Munns CF, Batch JA. Hyperinsulinism and Beckwith-Wiedemann syndrome. Arch Dis Child Fetal Neonatal Ed 2001;84:F67–9.

32. Sun L, Eklund EA, Chung WK, Wang C, Cohen J, Freeze HH. Congenital disorder of glycosylation id presenting with hyperinsulinemic hypogly-cemia and islet cell hyperplasia. J Clin Endocrinol Metab 2005;90:4371–5.

33. Baumann U, Preece MA, Green A, Kelly DA, McKiernan PJ. Hyperinsulinism in tyrosinaemia type I. J Inherit Metab Dis 2005;28:131–35.

34. Kapoor RR, Flanagan SE, Arya VB, Shield JP, Ellard S, Hussain K. Clinical and molecular characterisation of 300 patients with congenital hyperinsulinism. Eur J Endocrino 2013;168: 557–64.

35. Vannucci RC, Vannucci SJ. Hypoglycemic brain injury. Semin Neonatol 2001;6:147–55.

36. Chandran S, Rajadurai VS, Alim AH, Hussain K. Current perspectives on neonatal hypoglycemia, its management, and cerebral injury risk. Research and Reports in Neonatology. 2015;5: 17–30.

37. Mazor-Aronovitch K, Gillis D, Lobel D, Hirsch HJ, Pinhas-Hamiel O, Modan-Moses D, et al. Long-term neurodevelopmental outcome in

conservatively treated congenital hyperinsu-linism. Eur J Endocrinol 2007;157:491–7.

38. Wang L, Fan G, Ji X, Sun B, Guo Q. MRI findings of brain damage due to neonatal hypoglycemia. Zhonghua Fang She Xue Za Zhi 2009,43:42–5.

39. Deshpande S, Ward Platt M. The investigation and management of neo-natal hypoglycaemia. Semin Fetal Neonatal Med 2005;10:351–61.

40. Senniappan S, Arya VB, Hussain K. The mole-cular mechanisms, diagnosis and management of congenital hyperinsulinism. Indian J Endocr Metab 2013;17:19–30.

41. Harris DL, Battin MR, Weston PJ, Harding JE. Continuous glucose monitoring in newborn babies at risk of hypoglycemia. J Pediatr 2010; 157:198–202.

42. Saif M, Kapoor A, Kochar IP, Jindal R. Conti-nuous glucose monitoring system for congenital hyperinsulinemia. Indian Pediatr 2013;50:421–2.

43. Hussain K. Investigations for neonatal hypogly-caemia. Clin Biochem 2011;44:465–6.

44. Hussain K, Blankenstein O, De Lonlay P, Christesen HT. Hyperinsulinaemic hypogly-caemia: biochemical basis and the importance of maintaining normoglycaemia during manage-ment. Arch Dis Child 2007;92:568–70.

45. Aynsley-Green A, Hussain K, Hall J, Saudubray JM, Nihoul-Fékété C, De Lonlay-Debeney P, et al. Practical management of hyperinsulinism in infancy. Arch Dis Child Fetal Neonatal Ed 2000; 82:F98–107.

46. Tas E, Mahmood B, Garibaldi L, Sperling M. Liver injury may increase the risk of diazoxide toxicity: a case report. Eur j Pediatr 2015;174:403–6.

47. Hussain K. Diagnosis and management of hyperinsulinaemic hypoglycaemia of infancy. Horm Res 2008;69:2–13.

48. Kim-Hanh Le Quan Sang, Jean-Baptiste Arnoux, Asmaa Mamoune, Saint-Martin C, Bellanné-Chantelot C, Valayannopoulos, et al. Successful treatment of congenital hyperinsulinism with long-acting release octreotide. Eur J Endocrino 2012;166:333–9.

49. Modan-Moses D, Koren I, Mazor-Aronovitch K, Pinhas-Hamiel O, Landau H. Treatment of congenital hyperinsulinism with Lanreotide acetate (Somatuline Autogel). J Clin Endocrinol Metab 2011; 96:2312–7.

50. Moens K, Berger V, Ahn JM, Van Schravendijk C, Hruby VJ, Pipeleers D, et al. Assessment of the role of interstitial glucagon in the acute glucose secretory responsiveness of in situ pancreatic beta-cells. Diabetes 2002;51:669–75.

51. Senniappan S, Alexandrescu S, Tatevian N, Shah P, Arya V, Flanagan S, et al. Sirolimus therapy in infants with severe hyperinsulinemic hypogly-cemia. N Engl J Med 2014;370:1131–7.

52. Hussain K, Aynsley-Green A. Hyperinsulinaemic hypoglycaemia in preterm neonates. Arch Dis Child Fetal Neonatal Ed. 2004;89:F65–7.

53. Mohnike K, Blankenstein O, Christesen HT, de Lonlay J, Hussain K, Koopmans KP, et al. Pro-posal for a standardized protocol for 18-F DOPA-PET (PET/CT) in congenital hyperinsulinism. Horm Res 2006;66:40–2.

54. Bax KN, van der Zee DC. The laparoscopic approach towards hyperinsulinism in children. Sem Ped Surg 2007;16:245–51.

55. Leibowitz G, Glaser B, Higazi AA, Salameh M, Cerasi E, Landau H. Hyperinsulinemic hypogly-cemia of infancy (nesidioblastosis) in clinical remission: High incidence of diabetes mellitus and persistent beta-cell dysfunction at long-term follow-up. J Clin Endocrinol Metab 1995;80: 386–92.

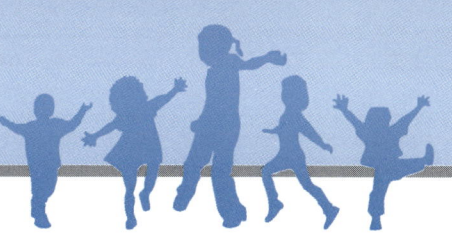

Subclinical Hypothyroidism in Children

M Shriraam, M Sridhar

Subclinical hypothyroidism (SCH) is a biochemical condition characterized by serum levels of Thyroid Stimulating Hormone (TSH) above the statistically defined upper limit of reference range, with normal concentration of thyroid hormones, and without clinical features of hypothyroidism.[1] SCH is a common disorder with a prevalence of 1–10% in adults and about 2% in children; epidemiological studies concerning childhood and adolescence are scarce.[2–4] SCH is mostly detected incidentally as patients exhibit few or no signs of thyroid dysfunction. The abnormalities most frequently associated in the pediatric population are goiter, poor school performance, weight gain, increased cholesterol levels, impaired growth velocity, anemia, excessive sleepiness, weakness, and impaired psychomotor and cognitive development.[4, 5]

NORMAL TSH LEVEL

TSH is secreted in a pulsatile manner and shows diurnal variation. The levels may vary based on the time of sampling as well as its relation to food.[6] Most of the commercially available kits use third generation TSH assays like radioimmunoassay, chemiluminescence or electrochemiluminescence method. There is no biological reference range derived from

these kits based on studies in pediatric population in India. The reference range given in the kit by the manufacturers of these assays vary. TSH above the laboratory reference ranges are considered abnormal by most pediatricians. These factors add to the difficulty in interpreting the TSH values and in decision-making for the clinician.[7] Two large population studies from India by Marwaha, *et al.*[8,9] reported normograms for TSH in Indian children. In study amongst children 5–16 yrs, the mean and 97th percentile for TSH (radioimmunoassay method) was, 3.17 and 7.5, respectively. This gives us a range of 1.33–5.01 mIU/L as normal values for our population. Almost 12% of the reference population had TSH values above the normal range provided by the test kit manufacturer. Such patients need long-term follow up for development of overt hypothyroidism.

ETIOLOGY

SCH is most commonly (50–80% of cases) caused by chronic autoimmune thryoiditis, which is typically characterized by high titers of thyroid peroxidase antibodies, thyroglobulin antibodies and rarely TSH-receptor blocking antibodies.[10] There are many causes of potentially reversible/irreversible

Box 13.1: Differential diagnosis of elevated TSH after infancy

- Reversible
  - Autoimmune thyroiditis
  - Recovering from acute illness
  - Recovering from subacute thyroiditis
  - Antithyroid drugs
  - Simple obesity
  - Cortisol deficiency
  - Laboratory error
- Irreversible
  - Autoimmune thyroiditis
  - Thyroid dysgenesis
  - Subtotal/hemi thyroidectomy
  - Neck radiotherapy,
  - Reidel's thyroiditis

subclinical hypothyroidism[11] (Box 13.1). Nonthyroidal causes include diabetes mellitus, cystic fibrosis, celiac disease, and chronic renal failure.[12]

Mutations in several proteins involved in TSH action have been demonstrated. Loss of function mutations in the TSH receptor gene have been demonstrated.[13,14] Dual oxidase 2 (DUOX2), phosphodiesterase 8B and thyroidperoxidase mutations have also been reported as causes of mild elevations of TSH.[15–17] Congenital conditions are commonly associated with SCH. SCH is also associated with Down syndrome; present in up to 32% of these patients. Anti-thyroid antibodies were not more likely to be found in this group than in patients with a normal TSH.[18] Almost one-third patients with William syndrome also have SCH with negative anti-thyroid antibodies.[19]

Abnormal sialylation of the carbohydrate moiety of TSH with resultant reduced metabolic clearance may also contribute to elevated TSH in occasional cases of hypothyroidism.[20]

EPIDEMIOLOGY

Large scale population studies focussing on the prevalence of SCH among children, especially from India are limited. With the difficulty in defining normal TSH, the prevalence reported in different studies may vary depending on the cut-off value. The sample selection in many of the studies is strictly not representative of the general pediatric population. In some follow-up studies, a mildly elevated TSH has been documented to normalize after few months.[21] Persistently elevated TSH over a period of time may be the best indicator to assess the true prevalence of SCH in the pediatric population.

Marwaha, *et al.*[22] conducted a large nation-wide survey on the thyroid status after 2 decades of salt iodization in India. The prevalence of subclinical and overt hypothyroidism was 6.1% and 0.4%, respectively among the study population (total population of 38961 children). TSH elevation was found more common among children with goiter. The prevalence of goitre among the studied population was 15.5%, much above 5% prescribed by WHO. Further, thyroid autoimmunity, as defined by positive thyroperoxidase antibody titers, was observed in 3.6% of the study population and was more common among girls. In another study from Chandigarh, India, goiter prevalence was 15.1% and that of SCH was 2.6%. The population studied was iodine sufficient in that study with prevalence of autoimmunity not significantly different from the controls.[23] A study from USA, done primarily to assess cognitive parameters among adolescents with thyroid disorders, the prevalence of SCH was 1.7%.[4] Lazar, *et al.*[21] in a retrospective analysis from an insurance-based large database of children between 6 months to 16 years of age, reported a prevalence of elevated TSH (5.5–10.0 mIU/6) to be 2.9%.[21] Transiently elevated TSH may occasionally be diagnosed as part of newborn screening program. In a large series from China, the incidence was 1 in 8809 neonates.[24] The TSH elevation was treated with thyroxine replacement, considering its critical role in neurocognitive development, with a favourable outcome at 2–3 years follow up. Long term follow-up of these children was not available to know whether the TSH rise was transient or persisted beyond 3 years of age. SCH is observed more commonly in obese children when compared with normal weight controls; excess adipose tissue is hypothesized to signal elevation in TSH.[25]

Children with Down syndrome are at increased risk up to 28 times the normal population for hypothyroidism. Autoimmune predisposition or dysgenesis may contribute to thyroid dysfunction among children with this chromosomal anomaly.[26] In this setting, SCH may warrant treatment as the progression to overt hypothyroidism is more likely.

Type 1 diabetes predisposes children to thyroid dysfunction. In a study by Soliman, et al.[27] the prevalence of SCH in children (mean age 10 yrs) with type I diabetes was 11.2%. Other conditions which may be associated with elevated risk for SCH include anti-epileptic drug usage and celiac disease.

CLINICAL ISSUES

Most patients with SCH exhibit few or no signs or symptoms of hypothyroidism. It has been suggested that some patients have functional, clinical, or biochemical manifestations of hypothyroidism that are more common than age-matched controls.[28] Goiter is the most common manifestation.[12] The abnormalities found most commonly in the pediatric population include weight gain, increased cholesterol levels, impaired growth velocity, anemia, sleepiness, weakness, and impaired psychomotor and cognitive development.[5]

NATURAL PROGRESSION OF SCH AND EFFECTS OF INTERVENTION

There are very few prospective studies evaluating the natural progression of SCH in pediatric age group (Table 13.1). In a study from India, a cohort of 32 children with SCH and autoimmune thyroiditis (AIT) and goiter were followed. Development of overt hypothyroidism (12.5% in this cohort) was insidious, and was not accompanied by symptoms and signs.[29] In a larger study on 323 children with either Hashimoto or idiopathic SCH followed up for 3 years, 13.5% of SCH developed overt hypothyroidism. The study could not detect predictive factors for progression of SCH to overt hypothyroidism in idiopathic SCH.[30] Wasniewska, et al.[31] followed up 92 patients with idiopathic SCH over 2 years, and none of them developed overt hypothyroidism. Lazar, et al.[21] studied 3510 patients with SCH over 5 years and showed that 73.6% of them normalized TSH. Elevated antibodies [thyroid peroxidise (TPOab) and thryoglobulin antibodies (TGab)] may predict future overt hypothyroidism and TPOab > TGab may predict impending thyroid failure in AIT.[32, 33] Leonardi, et al.[35] studied 44 Italian children 'false positive' to neonatal screening for congenital hypo-thyroidism; 28 of them had SCH on re-testing at 2–3 years of age. Twenty of these 28 children were treated with replacement therapy and then withdrawn from therapy 2–3 months prior to re-evaluation. Out of the 28 children with SCH, TSH was normal in 9 children (32%) and persistently elevated in the remaining 19 (62%) at 4.1–6.6 yrs of age. At 7.2–9.5 yrs of age, TSH remained normal in 9 children who previously normalized their thyroid function, returned to normal in 5 out of 19 of the children with previous elevated TSH and persisted above normal in remaining fourteen childrens.

Effect of Treating Children with SCH

This aspect has been even less investigated and a summary of the evidence is presented in Table 13.2. Wasniewska, et al.[37] compared thyroxine treated and untreated SCH over 2 years and found no significant changes in TSH values in both groups. Cetinkaya, et al.[38] treated 39 children with short stature and SCH; improvement in height was significant in pre-pubertal as compared to pubertal age group, with no progression to overt hypothyroidism in any in the cohort. Chase, et al.[39] noted a

TABLE 13.1: Natural history and progression of SCH in pediatric case series

Authors Year; Place	Number of patients	Level of evidence/ Type of study	Period of follow-up	Key results	Comments
Radetti, et al.[32] 2012; Italy	323	Retrospective cross-sectional	3 years	13.5% of SCH developed OH	There were no predictors in pts of SCH.
Wasniewska, et al.[31] 2009; Italy	92 with SCH	Prospective observational	2 years	38 normalized TSH54 remained SCH11 had increase of TSH more than 10 miu/mL	None developed OH. Natural progression in idiopathic SCH is a progressive decrease over time of TSH in majority.
Lazar, et al.[21] 2009; Israel	121052 of which 2.9% had SCH	Prospective observational	5 years	In SCH group 73.6% normalized TSH, 2% increase >10 miu/mL, and 0.03% had OH	Female patients with >7.5 miu/mL of TSH are at greater risk of sustained raise.
Gopalakrishanan, et al.[29] 2008; India	98 of which 32 had SCH	Longitudinal study	24 months	4/32 patients with SCH developed OH	Important to monitor TFT. Development of OH is insidious and may not be accompanied by symptoms and clinical signs.
Leonardi, et al.[35] 2008; Italy	44	Prospective observational	8 years	14 had SCH at end of the study. None developed OH	Newborn false positive TSH have an increased risk of developing SCH
Radetti, et al.[30] 2006; Italy	160 of which 55 were SCH Rest euthyroid	Prospective observational	5 years	16/55 SCH normalized TFT. 16 remained SCH 23 had twofold rise above the normal limit	Presence of goitre and elevated TGAb, together with increase in TPOab and TSH may predict future OH. At 5 yrs 50% of all participants remained euthyroid.
Zois, et al.[33] 2006; Greece	29 with AIT of which 7 had SCH	Prospective observational	5 years	All 7 continued to be in SCH None of the 29 developed OH	TPOab > TGab increase predicted impending thyroid failure in AIT. Thyroid hypoechogenicity seem to predict the same
Jaruatanasirikul, et al.[34] 2001; Thailand	46 of which 8 had SCH	Prospective observational	6 years	4/8 SCH normalized TSH 4/8 developed OH	No clinical or biochemical marker at baseline predicted course of SCH
Moore, et al.[36] 1996; UK	18 with SCH and AIT	Prospective observational	5.8 years	7/18 were euthyroid 10 remained SCH1 became OH	Expectant management is recommended in majority of SCH with minimally elevated TSH

SCH–Subclinical hypothyroidism, TFT–Thyroid function tests, TPOab–thyroid peroxidise antibodies, TGab–thyroglobulin antibodies, TSH–Thyroid stimulating hormone, OH–Overt hypothyroidism, AIT–autoimmune thyroiditis

TABLE 13.2: Studies reporting effect of replacement therapy in childhood SCH

Authors	Patients	Type of study	Follow-up	Results	Comments
Wasniewska, et al.[37]	69 treated SCH vs 92 untreated SCH	Case control	2 y	Significant difference was not found	TSH value changes between treated and untreated groups were similar. Therapy is unable to prevent the risk of further TSH increase after treatment withdrawal
Aijaz, et al.[5]	11 SCH children	Interventional	91 d	Short term thyroxine therapy showed no neuropsychological benefits as compared to normal population	Thyroxine therapy showed no positive effect on neuropsychological function in children with SCH
Cetinkaya, et al.[38]	2067 total, 39 SCH	Interventional	12 mo	Showed improvement in growth velocity; no hyperthyroidism noted after replacement.	Short stature can be associated with SCH. Thyroid hormone replacement improves the height in such patients
Chase, et al.[39]	25 diabetic children with SCH	Case control	2 y	Pre-pubertal diabetics showed increased growth velocity than postpubertal diabetics	Higher the initial TSH value showed increased growth velocity

SCH–Subclinical hypothyroidism, TFT–Thyroid function tests, TSH–Thyroid stimulating hormone, OH–Overt hypothyroidism, AIT–autoimmune thyroiditis, TRH–thyrotrophin releasing hormone

similar significant height increase in the prepubertal age group as compared to the pubertal age group when children with SCH and type 1 diabetes were given thyroxine replacement therapy. Aijaz, et al.[5] studied short term thyroxine replacement therapy and its effects in neuropsychological outcome and concluded no significant change.

MANAGEMENT OF SCH

Based on available literature, SCH seems to be a benign condition which requires periodic follow-up and monitoring of thyroid function tests. Expectant management is the norm for this condition. Natural progression to OH does occur but lot less frequently than expected. There appeared to be no long-term effects of untreated SCH on growth, puberty or neurocognitive function; however, there is a lack of high-quality evidence.

We propose an algorithm (Fig. 13.1) for management of subclinical hypothyroidism in pediatric age group. The first step in our setting on patients with elevated TSH, especially below 10 mIU/L, is to repeat the test on another day, preferably from another laboratory with a different kit. SCH in adults is associated with dyslipidemia and subtle cardiac dysfunction, with reasonable benefit of treatment of SCH on those parameters. However, pediatric studies focussing on the same are scarce and more research is needed on these issues in this age group.

Girls, goiter, family history of thyroid disorder, other autoimmune problems, markedly elevated TPO titers (at least 3 times the upper limit of normal and symptoms which may correlate with hypothyroidism are risk factors; a clinical decision to start on thyroxine may be taken if any or combination of above is present.

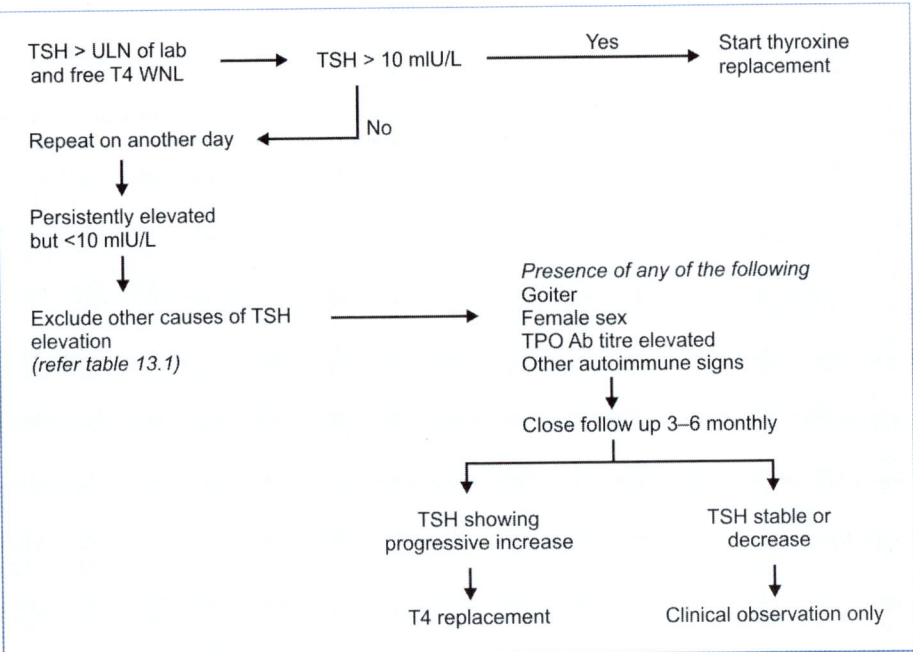

Fig. 13.1: Approach to subclinical hypothyroidism (SCH) in children

CONCLUSION

SCH is a biochemical entity commonly faced by practising pediatricians. Several factors including clinical condition of the child and laboratory factors influencing TSH levels should be considered while interpreting the results. Clinical decision to treat marginal elevation in TSH should be made keeping in mind that more often TSH normalizes without treatment if followed up over a period of time. Even if the decision to treat the slightly elevated TSH is made, a clear plan should be made to stop treatment and reassess after 1–2 years to see if the treatment is required lifelong.

REFERENCES

1. Surks MI, Ortiz GH, Sawin CT. Subclinical thyroid disease: Scientific review and guidelines for diagnosis and management. JAMA 2004;291: 228–38.
2. Canaris GJ, Manowitz NR, Mayor G, Ridgway EC. The Colorado thyroid disease prevalence study. Arch Intern Med 2000;160:526–34.
3. Paoli-Valeri M, Maman-Alvardo D, Jiménez-Lopez V. Frequency of subclinical hypothyroidism among healthy children and those with neurological conditions in the state of Mérida, Venezuela. Invest Clin 2003;44:209–18.
4. Wu T, Flowers JW, Tudiver F. Subclinical thyroid disorders and cognitive performance among adolescents in the United States. BMC Pediatr 2006;6:12.
5. Aijaz NJ, Flaherty EM, Preston T. Neurocognitive function in children with compensated hypothyroidism: lack of short term effects on or off thyroxin. BMC Endocr Disord 2006;6:2.
6. Scobbo RR, Vondohlen TW, Hassan M, Islam S. Serum TSH variability in normal individuals: the influence of time of sample collection. WV Med J 2004;100:138–42.
7. Sarkar R. TSH comparison between chemiluminescence (Architect) and electrochemiluminescence (Cobas) immunoassays: An Indian population perspective. Indian J Clin Biochem 2014;29: 189–95.
8. Marwaha RK, Tandon N, Desai AK, Kanwar R, Aggarwal R, Sastry A, et al. Reference range of thyroid hormones in healthy school-age children: Country-wide data from India. Clin Biochem. 2010;43:51–6.

9. Marwaha RK, Tandon N, Desai A, Kanwar R, Grewal K, Aggarwal R, et al. Reference range of thyroid hormones in normal Indian school-age children. Clin Endocrinol(Oxf). 2008;68:369–74.

10. Palmieri EA, Fazio S, Lombardi G. Subclinical hypothyroidism and cardiovascular risk: A reason to treat? Treat Endocrinol 2004;3:233–44.

11. Papi G, Uberti ED, Betterle C. Subclinical Hypothryoidism. Curr Opin Endocrinol Diabetes Obes. 2007;14:197–208.

12. Cooper DS. Clinical practice. Subclinical hypothyroidism. N Engl J Med 2001;345:260–5.

13. Narumi S, Muroya K, Abe Y, Yasui M, Asakura Y, Adachi M, et al. TSHR mutations as a cause of congenital hypothyroidism in Japan: A population-based genetic epidemiology study. J Clin Endocrinol Metab 2009;94:1317–23.

14. Nicoletti A, Bal M, De Marco G, Baldazzi L, Agretti P, Menabo S, et al. Thyrotropin-stimulating hormone receptor gene analysis in pediatric patients with non-autoimmune subclinical hypothyroidism. J Clin Endocrinol Metab. 2009; 94:4187–94.

15. De Marco G, Agretti P, Montanelli, Dicosmo C, Bagattini B, De Servi M, et al. Identification and functional analysis of novel dual oxidase 2 (DUOX2) mutations in children with congenital or subclinical hypothyroidism. J Clin Endocrinol Metab 2011;96:E1335–9.

16. Grandone A, Perrone L, Cirillo G, Di Sessa A, Corona AM, Amato A, et al. Impact of phosphodiesterase 8B gene rs4704397 variation on thyroid homeostasis in childhood obesity. Eur J Endocrinol 2012;166:255-60.

17. Turkkahraman D, Alper OM, Aydin F, Yildiz A, Pehlivanoglu S, Luleci G, et al. Final diagnosis in children with subclinical hypothyroidism and mutation analysis of the thyroid peroxidise gene (TPO). J Pediatr Endocrinol Metab 2009;22: 845–51.

18. Rubello D, Pozzan GB, Casara D, Girelli ME, Boccato S, Rigon F, et al. Natural course of subclinical hypothyroidism in Down's syndrome: Prospective study results and therapeutic considerations. J Endocrinol Invest 1995;18:35–40.

19. Schaub RL, Hale DE, Rose SR. The spectrum of thyroid abnormalities in individuals with 18q deletions. J Clin Endocrinol Metab 2005;90: 2259–63.

20. Persani L, Borgato S, Romoli R, Asteria C, Pizzocaro A, Beck-Peccoz P. Changes in the degree of sialylation of carbohydrate chains modify the biological properties of circulating thyrotropin isoforms in various physiological and pathological states. J Clin Endocrinol Metab 1998;83:2486–92.

21. Lazar L, Frumkin RB, Battat E, Lebenthal Y, Phillip M, Meyerovitch J. Natural history of thyroid function tests over 5 years in a large pediatric cohort. J Clin Endocrinol Metab. 2009; 94:1678–82.

22. Marwaha RK, Tandon N, Garg MK, Desai A, Kanwar R, Sastry A, et al. Thyroid status two decades after salt iodization: country-wide data in school children from India. Clin Endocrinol (Oxf) 2012;76:905–10.

23. Das S, Bhansali A, Dutta P, Aggarwal A, Bansal MP, Garg D, et al. Persistence of goitre in the post-iodization phase: micronutrient deficiency or thyroid autoimmunity? Indian J Med Res 2011; 133:103–9.

24. Xiao Chen X, Feng Qin Y, Lian Zhou X, Lai Yang R, Hua Shi Y, Qing Mao H, et al. Diagnosis and treatment of subclinical hypothyroidism detected by neonatal screening. World J Pediatr 2011;7: 350–4.

25. Torun E, Cindemir E, Özgen IT, Öktem F. Subclinical hypothyroidism in obese children. Dicle MedJ 2013;40:5–8.

26. Cebeci AN, Güven A, Yýldýz M. Profile of hypothyroidism in Down's syndrome. J Clin Res Pediatr Endocrinol 2013;5:116–20.

27. Soliman GZA, Bahagt NM, EL-mofty Z. Prevalence of thyroid disorder in Egyptian children with type I diabetes mellitus and the prevalence of thyroid antibodies among them. Thyroid Disorders Ther 2013;2:1.

28. Zulewski H, Müller B, Exer P, Miserez AR. Estimation of tissue hypothyroidism by a new clinical score: Evaluation of patients with various grades of hypothyroidism and controls. J Clin Endocrinol Metab 1997;82:771-6.

29. Gopalakrishnan S, Chugh PK, Chhillar M. Goitrous autoimmune thyroiditis in a pediatric population: A longitudinal study. Pediatrics 2008;122:e670-4.

30. Radetti G, Gottardi E, Bona G, Corrias A, Salardi S, Loche S, et al. The natural history of euthyroid Hashimoto's thyroiditis in children. J Pediatr 2006;149:827–32.

31. Wasniewska M, Salerno M, Cassio A, Corrias A, Aversa T, Zirilli G, et al. Prospective evaluation of the natural course of idiopathic subclinical hypothyroidism in childhood and adolescence. Eur J Endocrinol 2009;160:417–21.

32. Radetti G, Maselli M, Buzi F, Corrias A, Mussa A, Cambiaso P, *et al.* The natural history of the normal/mild elevated TSH serum levels in children and adolescents with Hashimoto's thyroiditis and isolated hyperthyro-tropinaemia: A 3-year follow-up. Clin Endocrinol (Oxf) 2012;76:394–8.

33. Zois C, Stavrou I, Svarna E, Seferiadis K, Tsatsoulis A. Natural course of autoimmune thyroiditis after elimination of iodine deficiency in northwestern Greece. Thyroid 2006;16:289–93.

34. Jaruratanasirikul S, Leethanaporn K, Khuntigij P, Sriplung H. The clinical course of Hashimoto's thryoiditis in children and adolescents: 6 years longitudinal follow-up. J Pediatr Endocrinol Metab 2001;14:177–84.

35. Leonardi D, Polizzotti N, Carta A, Gelsomino R, Sava L, Vigneri R, *et al.* Longitudinal study of thyroid function in children with mild hyper-thyrotropinemia at neonatal screening for conge-nital hypothyroidism. J Clin Endocrinol Metab 2008;93:2679–85.

36. Moore DC. Natural course of subclinical hypothyroidism in childhood and adolescence. Arch Pediatr Adolesc Med 1996;150:293–7.

37. Wasniewska M, Corrias A, Aversa T, Valenzise M, Mussa A, De Martino L, *et al.* Comparative evaluation of therapy with L-Thyroxine versus no treatment in children with idiopathic and mild subclinical hypothyroidism. Horm Res Paediatr 2012;77:376–81.

38. Cetinkaya E, Aslan A, Vidinlisan S, Ocal G. Height improvement by L-thyroxine treatment in subclinical hypothyroidism. Pediatr Int 2003;45:534–7.

39. Chase HP, Garg SK, Cockerham RS, Wilcox WD, Walravens PA. Thyroid hormone replacement and growth of children with subclinical hypo-thyroidism and diabetes. Diabet Med 1990;7:299–303.

Metabolic Liver Diseases Presenting as Acute Liver Failure in Children

Seema Alam, Bikrant Bihari Lal ▬▬

Inborn errors of metabolism, where hepatomegaly and/or abnormal liver functions form part of the clinical disease, are collectively referred to as Metabolic liver diseases (MLD). MLD can have varied presentations in infants and children, most common of them being: (i) organomegaly, (ii) encephalopathy due to hyperammonemia and/or primary lactic acidemia, (iii) pediatric acute liver failure (ALF), (iv) cirrhosis with or without portal hypertension, and (v) cholestatic liver disease. A high index of suspicion for MLD is important as urgent intervention such as dietary manipulation or disease-specific treatment may be life-saving. The outcome of patients undergoing liver transplantation for MLD has improved considerably over the last decade. Moreover, it is important to establish the correct diagnosis, so that appropriate genetic counselling can be offered to the family. MLD merit special attention in differential diagnosis of pediatric ALF, especially in infants and young children in whom they constitute 13–43% of all cases (Table 14.1).[1–9]

The Pediatric ALF study group definition can be used to define acute liver failure in infants and children.[6] The group enlists criteria for defining ALF as follows: (i) children with no known evidence of chronic liver disease (CLD), (ii) biochemical evidence of acute liver injury, and (iii) hepatic-based coagulopathy defined as International normalized ratio (INR) ≥1.5 not corrected by vitamin K in the presence of clinical hepatic encephalopathy or INR ≥2 regardless of the presence or absence of clinical hepatic encephalopathy. Neonatal liver failure is defined as "failure of the synthetic function of liver within 4 weeks of birth".[10] Presence of encephalopathy is not mandatory for defining acute liver failure in infants as it is often very difficult to recognize. Moreover, encephalopathy may be a very late event in the course of the disease.[1,5] We have previously reported that average jaundice to encephalopathy interval is significantly higher in pediatric ALF due to MLD group vis-à-vis other etiologies.[1] Another important difference is that complete absence of evidence of CLD cannot be kept as prerequisite, especially when the etiology is a suspected MLD.[4] MLD patients may have variable degrees of liver damage before clinical presentation, and overt signs and stigmata of chronic liver disease may be present.

METABOLIC CAUSES OF ACUTE LIVER FAILURE

MLD are an important causes of pediatric ALF, especially in neonates, infants and young children. MLD account for 13–43% of acute

TABLE 14.1: Studies evaluating prevalence and spectrum of metabolic liver diseases among patients with pediatric acute liver failure

Study (Place) : Age (No.)	Infants/Young children	Older children
Alam, et al.[1] (India); 0–3 y (n = 40); > 3 y (n = 57)	MLD-13, 33%: Galactosemia, 4; Tyrosinemia, 3; HFI, 2; UCD, 2; Respiratory Chain defect, 1; Gluconeogenetic defect, 1. Indeterminate-4, 10%	MLD-6, 10%: Wilson's disease, 6. Indeterminate-7, 12%
Rajanayagam, et al.[2] (Australia); Infants (n = 24); >1 y (n = 30)	MLD-1, 4.1%: Mitochondriopathy, 1. Indeterminate-8, 33%	MLD-6, 20%: Wilson's disease, 5; Mitochondriopathy, 1. Indeterminate-9, 30%
Brett, et al.[3] (Portugal); <2 y (n = 28);	MLD-12, 43%: Respiratory Chain Defect, 3; Tyrosinemia, 2; CDG, 2; Galactosemia, 2; UCD, 1; FAOD, 1; HFI, 1. Indeterminate-5, 18%	NA
Sundaram, et al.[4] PALF Study Group (USA/UK/Canada); <3 months (n = 148);	MLD-28, 18.9%: Galactosemia, 12; Respiratory Chain Defect, 5; Tyrosinemia, 3; Niemann Pick Type C, 3; Mitochondriopathy, 3; UCD, 2. Indeterminate-56, 38%	NA
Dhawan, et al.[5] (UK); Neonates (n = 31); Older children (n =100)	MLD- 4, 13%: Galactosemia, Tyrosinemia, Mitochondriopathy	MLD-18, 18%
PALF Study Group[6]; 0–3 y (n = 127); >3 y (n = 221)	MLD-23, 18%: Respiratory Chain defect, 7; FAOD, 4; Tyrosinemia, 4; Galactosemia, 2; Alpha-1 antitrypsin deficiency, 1; HFI, 1; Niemann Pick C, 1; UCD, 1. Indeterminate-68, 53%	MLD-13, 6%: Wilson's disease, 9; Mitochondriopathy, 2; UCD, 1; Reye's Syndrome, 1. Indeterminate-101, 46%
Durand, et al.[7] (France); Infants (n = 80)	MLD-34, 42.5%: Respiratory Chain Defects, 17; Tyrosinemia, 2; UCD, 2; Galactosemia, 2; HFI, 2. Indeterminate-13, 16%	NA
Kaur, et al.[8] (India); Children 0–18 y (n = 43)	NA	MLD-4, 9.2 %: Galactosemia, 4.6%; Wilson's disease, 4.6%; Indeterminate-4, 9.3%
Lee, et al.[9] (UK) 0–17 y (n = 97)	NA	MLD 15, 15.4%: Mitochondriopathy, 4; Tyrosinemia, 2; Wilson's Disease, 2; Other MLD, 7.

MLD=Metabolic Liver Disease, HFI=Hereditary fructose intolerance, UCD=Urea cycle defect, CDG=Congenital disorders of glycosylation, FAOD=Fatty acid oxidation defect

liver failure in younger children, while accounting for only 5–20% of ALF in older children[1–9] (Table 14.1). Studies which focus on infants and young children have higher prevalence of MLD as compared to the studies which include older children. The proportion of cases with indeterminate etiology are higher (38–53%)[4–6] in studies, where the proportion of MLD cases is lower (13–19%). On the other hand, the studies with higher prevalence (33–43%) of MLD among pediatric ALF[1,3,7] had much smaller proportion (13–18%) of cases remaining indeterminate. Narkewicz, et al.[11] retrospectively analyzed the workup of children labelled as indeterminate in pediatric ALF study group, and found that 54% of these children had not been screened for some common metabolic disorders, before assigning them as indeterminate. In an earlier Indian study, 4 children among 67 with fulminant liver failure were reported to be non A, non E, but MLD was not reported.[12] However, this series included only one infant, and the definition used for ALF was different. With advent of better diagnostic protocols, MLDs are more frequently diagnosed now.[1]

Some of the authors have earlier listed neonatal hemochromatosis as a MLD. Being a gestation-associated alloimmune disorder, it has now been excluded from the list of MLDs. Galactosemia, tyrosinemia, mitochondriopathies and fatty acid oxidation defect (FAOD) are the commonest metabolic diseases presenting as ALF in infants. Wilson's disease is the commonest MLD presenting as ALF among older children, others being mitochondriopathies, FAOD and urea cycle defects.

PATHOPHYSIOLOGY

In disorders such as galactosemia, tyrosinemia and Urea cycle defects, the pathogenesis of MLD can be attributed to a defect in the intermediary metabolic pathway leading to the accumulation of toxic metabolites (formed in one of the preceding steps) which leads to liver failure. These conditions present after a symptom-free interval before clinical signs of 'intoxication' appear. Acute attacks may be preceded by catabolic states, fever, intercurrent illnesses and specific food intake. Most of these disorders are treatable and require emergency removal of the toxin by using special diets, extracorporeal procedures, drugs or vitamins.[13] Another pathogenetic mechanism is an energy deficiency state. The mitochondrial energy defects encompass the congenital lactic acidemias, respiratory chain disorders, pyruvate oxidation defects and FAOD. Cytoplasmic energy defects include disorders of glycolysis, glycogen metabolism, gluconeogenesis and the pentose phosphate pathways. The metabolic defects with energy-deficient states present early and can even have prenatal onset. In lysosomal disorders (Wolman disease and cholesteryl ester storage disorder), peroxisomal disorders (Zellweger syndrome) and congenital defect of glycosylation, liver failure occurs due to involvement of cellular organelles.

SUSPECTING MLD AS CAUSE OF ALF

Box 14.1 enumerates the important points in history that should raise the suspicion of a metabolic disorder. Children with MLD presenting as ALF tend to be younger. A strong family history of consanguinity, recurrent abortions, sibling deaths and previously affected children are strong pointers to the possible etiology of MLD. History of recurrent diarrhea and vomiting, failure to thrive and developmental delay are other indicators suggesting MLD.[1,3] Patients with MLD tend to have a longer jaundice to encephalopathy interval. Neurological involvement in form of hypotonia, myopathy, seizures, ophthalmoplegia, psychomotor dysfunction or presence of multisystem involvement should raise the suspicion of a mitochondrial depletion syndrome.[14]

A meticulous dietary history can help guide the clinician. Onset of liver dysfunction on milk feeds points towards diagnosis of galactosemia, whereas onset of symptoms after introduction of complementary foods (containing fructose or sucrose) points towards hereditary fructose intolerance that can also present in those receiving fructose in form of honey, syrups or formula milk containing fructose or sorbitol. Aversion to sugars and sweet foods in older children also suggests this disorder. Some MLD have their typical age of presentation and age-appropriate differential diagnosis should be considered (Table 14.2). Encephalopathy is difficult to diagnose in children and could be disproportionately more severe to the liver dysfunction in urea cycle defects and primary lactic acidemias. Developmental delay, cardiomyopathy, renal tubulopathy in a

TABLE 14.2: Categorization of metabolic liver diseases by age of presentation

0–6 m	Galactosemia, Tyrosinemia type 1, Mitochondrial cytopathy and Wolman's disease
6 m–3 y	Tyrosinemia type I, FAOD, Mitochondrial cytopathy, Galactosemia, HFI, UCD and CDG
Older children	Wilson's disease, FAOD, Mitochondrial Cytopathy, HFI, UCD and CDG

hypotonic child with convulsive disorder with or without treatment with valproic acid could be a setting for mitochondrial disorders.

Children with MLD have much higher bilirubin, more severe synthetic dysfunction, hypoglycemia and hyperammonemia as compared to those with ALF not related to MLD.[1,3] Children with MLD tend to have a much higher bilirubin, but lower transaminases, gamma-glutamyl transferases (GGT) and INR as compared to the viral causes of ALF.[4]

APPROACH TO MLD PRESENTING AS ALF

The algorithmic diagnostic approach to an infant or young child with ALF and suspected MLD is depicted in Fig. 14.1. For an older child, the etiological list includes only WD, HFI, mitochondrial defect and FAOD. Except WD, all others have been covered in the above mentioned algorithm. WD should be suspected in a patient with ALF who have KF ring on slit-lamp examination, Coombs negative hemolytic anemia, low serum uric acid levels (<2.5 mg/dL), low serum alkaline phosphatase (SAP) activity (SAP: bilirubin ratio <4) and increased AST:ALT ratios.[15] As per European Association for Study of Liver (EASL) guidelines, serum ceruloplasmin <10 mg/dL is contributory for definitive diagnosis of WD,[16] but ceruloplasmin, being an acute phase reactant, can be falsely normal in children with acute liver failure. Hence, 24 hours urinary copper (>100 µg/day) and KF ring are important for diagnosis of WD in setting of ALF.

A careful history and examination should narrow down the differential diagnosis and establish the degree of liver dysfunction. The time of onset of the symptoms and the rapidity of progression can give a clue to diagnosis. First line metabolic screen should be done in all cases of pediatric ALF, that includes three consecutive samples of urinary non-glucose reducing substances, ketones, arterial blood gas analysis, and serum lactate, serum alpha-feto protein and blood ammonia levels.

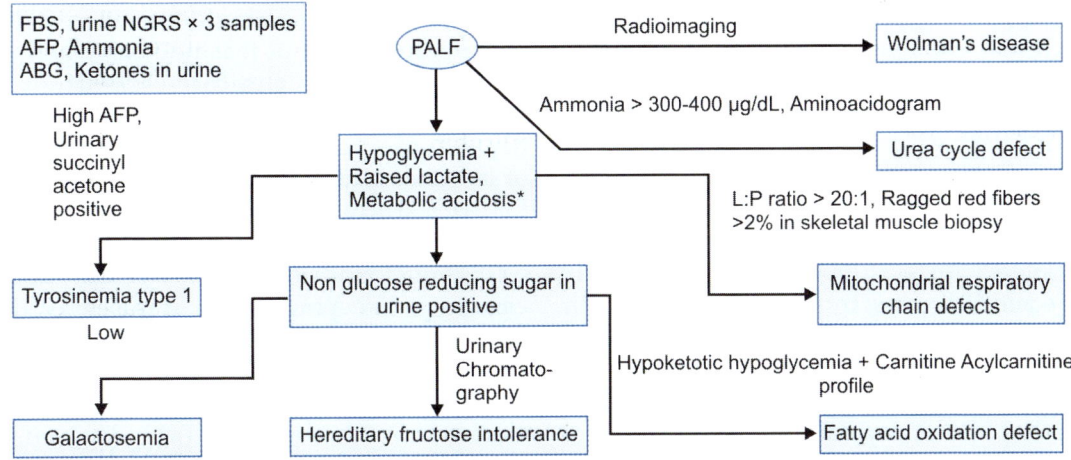

PALF: Pediatric acute liver failure, MLD: Metabolic liver disease, FBS: Fasting blood sugar, NGRS: Non glucose reducing sugar, AFP: Alphafeto protein, L:P: Lactate:Pyruvate, ABG: Arterial blood gases, GALT : Galactose-1-PO4 Uridyltransferase. *Hypoglycemia/acidosis/raised lactate may occur in ALF with non MLD also due to liver injury/sepsis/hypotension.

Fig. 14.1: Approach to a child with Acute liver failure and suspected Metabolic liver disease

Non-glucose reducing substances in urine can be identified by testing for reducing substances in urine by Benedict test, and then demonstrating absence of glucose by dipstick method. If suspecting galactosemia, it should be ensured that the child was on galactose-containing diet when the urinary samples were examined. In liver failure, blood sugar may be low and lactate may be high due to advanced liver disease. On the basis of the metabolic screen, we can narrow down on the possible etiology of the MLD. The specific diagnostic tests for the common MLDs presenting as pediatric ALF is shown in Table 14.2. It is important to remember that galactose-1-phosphate uridyl transferase (GALT) assay is not reliable if the child has received blood transfusion in the preceding three months. In such cases, it is advisable to continue the galactose free diet, till we can get reliable results of the GALT assay.

MANAGEMENT

With improvement in supportive management, the outcome of pediatric ALF has improved considerably. Liver transplantation may be life-saving for children who fail to respond to conservative management. Whenever MLD is a strong possibility, all feeds should be withdrawn for 24–48 hours awaiting first line investigations. The dietary modifications can be modelled on the basis of differentials considered based on history and examination. Appropriate feeds can be introduced based on final diagnosis. The main aim of withholding feeds is to stop further accumulation of potentially toxic metabolites, but at the same time further catabolic breakdown of body stores should be avoided as it can worsen liver failure. Intravenous infusion of 10% dextrose with required electrolytes is appropriate for most cases. The exception is congenital lactic acidosis and mitochondrial disorders where a 5% dextrose-based solution should be used as high carbohydrate supply may exacerbate the lactic acidosis. Restriction of protein to 0.5–1 g/kg/day (half in form of essential amino acids) is recommended for management of urea cycle defects. If FAOD has been excluded, then intralipid should be added at 1 g/kg/day to boost energy intake.

Supportive management for pediatric ALF includes glucose for maintaining normoglycemia, correction of coagulopathy in case of bleeding, antibiotics for sepsis, and maintenance of fluid and electrolyte balance. Although most data is from cirrhotics, but among anti-ammonia measures, polyethylene glycol 3350 was more effective than lactulose with resolution of encephalopathy in 90% and 50% cases, respectively.[17] A systemic review states that there is insufficient evidence to support or refute the use of non-absorbable disaccharides (Lactulose and Lactitol) for hepatic encephalopathy. Antibiotics (Rifaximin and Neomycin) were superior to non-absorbable disaccharides in improving encephalopathy, but it is unclear whether this difference is clinically important.[18] Algorithmic approach of management of hepatic encephalopathy also mentions usage of lactulose and rifaximin.[19] In a report from US ALF study group, lactulose increased survival time but had no effect on overall outcome.[20] Sodium benzoate has been encouraged keeping in view it is as effective as lactulose but 10 times less expensive.[21] Sodium Benzoate is recommended for use in HE due to urea cycle defects.[22] Definitive management for common MLD is depicted in Table 14.3.

TABLE 14.3: Confirmatory tests and management of common metabolic liver diseases

Disorder	Confirmatory test	Management
Galactosemia	Galactose-1-PO_4 Uridyl-transferase assay	Galactose-free diet
Hereditary Fructose Intolerance	Fructo-aldolase B assay in liver tissue* Urine chromatography to show fructose Mutational analysis	Fructose-free diet
Tyrosinemia type 1	Urinary succinylacetone	NTBC* + Low tyrosine and phenylalanine diet **
Urea Cycle Defect (UCD)	Plasma aminoacidogram to show the levels of citrulline and arginine based on which the type of UCD can be decided Orotic acid estimation in urine to diagnose OTC**deficiency	Ammonia scavengers, protein free diet with essential amino acids supplementation
Fatty Acid Oxidation Defect	Carnitine—acyl carnitine profile	Avoid prolonged fasting Breastfeeding in MCAD MCT rich diet in VLCAD and LCHAD Carnitine in carnitine transporter deficiency Bezafibrate* in VLCAD
Respiratory chain disorder	Analysis of oxidative phosphorylation complexes I–IV from intact mitochondria isolated from fresh skeletal muscle* Oral Coenzyme Q for CoQ10 deficiency	Normocaloric and low carbohydrate diet Avoidance of certain drugs Carnitine in carnitine deficiency
Wilson Disease	24 hour urine copper KF ring Serum Ceruloplasmin SAP : Bilirubin ratio <4 AST/ALT ratio >4	Chelation therapy with D-Penicillamine started at 10 mg/kg/d and increased to 20 mg/kg/d, Zinc and Pyridoxine

NTBC: 2-nitro-4-trifluoro-benzoyl-cyclohexane-1,3-dione, OTC: Ornithine transcarbamylase, MCAD: Medium chain Acyl-CoA Dehydrogenase, MCT: Medium Chain Triglyceride, VLCAD: Very long chain Acyl-CoA Dehydrogenase, LCHAD: Long chain 3-hydroxyacyl-CoA Dehydrogenase, CoQ10: Coenzyme Q 10, SAP: Serum alkaline phosphatase, AST: Aspartate aminotransferase, ALT: Alanine aminotransferase, KF ring: Kayser Fleischer ring. *These tests and therapeutic options are not available in India; **OTC samples are being sent outside the country by Indian laboratories; *Low Tyrosine and Phenylalanine diet is being marketed in India but not manufactured

LIVER ASSIST DEVICES

The role of the support device (artificial or bio-artificial) in ALF has an objective to either support the patient until the native liver recovers, or to bridge the patient to liver transplantation. Artificial support therapies (plasma exchange, hemodialysis and Molecular Adsorbents Recirculating System) provide detoxification support without the use of cellular material. Molecular Adsorbents Recirculating System has been reported to be more beneficial than combined plasma exchange and hemodialysis.[24] In another study, it was found to be beneficial in decreasing ammonia levels in adolescents but there were no benefits in infants in whom the device was poorly tolerated.[25] There is scarcity of data regarding the role of liver assist devices in management of MLD. Intermittent and continuous hemodialysis are effective modalities for the acute management of urea cycle defects and organic acidemia.[26] The pre-procedure physiological condition of the patient is the main determinant of outcome.[27] Moreover, most of the artificial liver assist devices help during hepatic encephalopathy but do not improve overall survival in ALF. Bio-artificial systems use cellular material to provide detoxification and liver's synthetic functions. A variety of such systems have been tested in non-randomized trials, but are not recommended outside clinical trials.

LIVER TRANSPLANTATION

The advent of successful liver transplantation has revolutionized management of children with MLD who fail to respond to conservative management. Galactosemia, HFI, tyrosinemia type 1 and urea cycle defects may not respond to medical therapy and dietary restrictions if diagnosed late, and in an emergency liver transplantation may prove to be life-saving. Although individually rare, when considered together, MLD represents approximately 15–25% of indications for pediatric liver transplantation.[28] MLD are the second most common indication for liver transplantation after biliary atresia.[29] UCD, alpha-1-anti-trypsin deficiency, cystic fibrosis, WD and tyrosinemia type 1 are the common MLD requiring liver transplantation in children. Post-transplant survival for children with MLD is comparable to those with other diseases with a better graft survival than those with other diseases.[29] A better outcome of liver transplantation in MLD could be attributed to the fact that many children with MLD underwent liver transplantation to correct an enzymatic defect, and did not have structural (parenchymal) liver disease.

Liver transplantation has been successfully done in many cases of tyrosinemia, galacto-emia, mitochondriopathies and UCD presenting as ALF.[28–30] Liver transplantation is usually contraindicated in diseases with severe multisystemic involvement, e.g. mitochondrial defect with severe neurological involvement/cardiomyopathy. A rapid assessment of the severity of extrahepatic involvement in a child with mitochondriopathy and decompensating liver is mandatory, so as to take a decision about the usefulness of liver transplantation in such a case. Suitability of heterozygous parents as donors is another important issue to be resolved.

Although Wilson disease presenting with encephalopathy is invariably fatal and can be treated only by liver transplantation, the decision to list a child with this disorder without encephalopathy is very difficult.[5,31] Revised King's score for this disorder[31] had been previously shown to be efficacious in predicting the survival with native liver.[31,32] However, doubts have been raised recently over the ability of this score to predict mortality without liver transplantation.[33] Survival is difficult to predict and continued investigations for predictors of outcome in Wilson disease are necessary.

Hepatocyte transplantation is moderately successful for MLD presenting as ALF, as a bridge to liver transplantation.[34] Hepatocyte transplantation holds promise as an alternative to organ transplantation and numerous animal studies indicate that transplants of isolated liver cells can correct metabolic deficiencies of the liver. Stem cell based technology is a new biotechnology approach to treat patients with MLD. Adult liver stem cells can differentiate into hepatocyte like cells and can be infused in the recipient's liver to activate a missing metabolic function. The percentage of liver cell replacement considered as necessary to significantly improve metabolic disorders is around 5% of the total liver mass, while 10% could normalize the function.[35,36]

GENETIC COUNSELING

Parents who have a child with MLD must undergo genetic couseling. The probability of the next sibling being affected from the disease should be explained, and prenatal testing and counseling should be offered where available. The parents must be explained about the nature of the illness and risk of occurrence in future pregnancies. Prenatal diagnosis of tyrosinemia is possible by analysis of succinylacetone in amniotic fluid supernatant and by assay of fumaryl acetoacetate hydrolase in cultured amniotic fluid cells or chorionic villus material.[37] Similarly, a GALT assay can be planned early for the next child of parents who already have a child suffering from galactosemia.

CONCLUSION

Metabolic liver diseases account for 13–43% of cases of ALF in infants and young children. Many of these conditions are potentially curable with dietary modifications or medications if recognized early. A high index of suspicion in presence of red flag symptoms and signs is need of the hour. A protocol-based approach will identify the etiology in most of the patients. Liver transplantation has markedly improved the outcome of MLD in children.

REFERENCES

1. Alam S, Lal BB, Khanna R, Sood V, Rawat D. Acute liver failure in infants and young children in a specialized pediatric liver centre in India. Indian J Pediatr 2015 Jan 6. [Epub ahead of print].
2. Rajanayagam J, Coman D, Cartwright D, Lewindon PJ. Pediatric acute liver failure: Etiology, outcomes, and the role of serial pediatric end-stage liver disease scores. Pediatr Transplant 2013;17:362–8.
3. Brett A, Pinto C, Carvalho L, Garcia P, Diogo L, Gonçalves I. Acute liver failure in under two year-olds–are there markers of metabolic disease on admission? Ann Hepatol 2013;12:791–6.
4. Sundaram SS, Alonso E, Narkewicz MR, Zhang S, Squires RH and Pediatric Acute Liver Failure Study Group. Characterization and outcome of young infants with acute liver failure. J Pediatr 2011;159:813–8.
5. Dhawan A. Etiology and prognosis of acute liver failure in children. Liver Transplant 2008;14: S80–S4.
6. Squires RH, Shneider BL, Bucuvalas J, Alonso E, Sokol RJ, Narkewicz MR, et al. Acute liver failure in children: The first 348 patients in pediatric acute liver failure study group. J Pediatr 2006; 148:652–8.
7. Durand P, Debray D, Mandel R, Baujard C, Branchereau S, Gauthier F, et al. Acute liver failure in infancy: A 14-year experience of a pediatric liver transplantation center. J Pediatr 2001;139: 871–6.
8. Kaur S, Kumar P, Kumar V, Sarin SK, Kumar A. Etiology and prognostic factors of acute liver failure in children. Indian Pediatr 2013;50:677-9.
9. Lee WS, McKiernan P, Kelly DA. Etiology, outcome and prognostic indicators of childhood fulminant hepatic failure in the United Kingdom. J Pediatr Gastroenterol Nutr 2005;40:575–81.
10. Shanmugam NP, Bansal S, Greenough A, Verma A, Dhawan A. Neonatal liver failure- etiologies and management- state of the art. Eur J Pediatr 2011;170:573–81.
11. Narkewicz MR, DellOlio D, Karpen SJ, Murray KF, Schwarz K, Yazigi N, et al. Pattern of diagnostic evaluation for the causes of pediatric acute liver failure: an opportunity for quality improvement. J Pediatr 2009;155:801–6.
12. Poddar U, Thapa BR, Prasad A, Sharma AK, Singh K. Natural history and risk factors in fulminant hepatic failure. Arch Dis Child 2002;87: 54–6.

13. Boles RG, Buck EA, Blitzer MG, Platt MS, Cowan TM, Martin SK, et al. Retrospective biochemical screening of fatty acid oxidation disorders in postmortem livers of 418 cases of sudden death in the first year of life. J Pediatr 1998;132:924–33.

14. Dimmock DP, Zhang Q, Dionisi-Vici C, Carrozzo R, Shieh J, Tang LY, et al. Clinical and molecular features of mitochondrial DNA depletion due to mutations in deoxyguanosine kinase. Hum Mutat 2008;29:330–1.

15. Korman JD, Volenberg I, Balko J, Webster J, Schiodt FV, Squires RH, et al. Screening for Wilson disease in acute liver failure: a comparison of currently available diagnostic tests. Hepatology 2008;48:1167–74.

16. Eurpean Association for Study of Liver. EASL Clinical Practice Guidelines: Wilson's disease. J Hepatol 2012;56:671–85.

17. Rahimi RS, Singal AG, Cuthbert JA, Rockey DC. Lactulose vs polyethylene glycol 3350–electrolyte solution for treatment of overt hepatic encephalopathy: The HELP randomized clinical trial. JAMA Intern Med 2014;174:1727–33.

18. Als-Nielsen B, Gluud LL, Gluud C. Non-absorbable disaccharides for hepatic encephalopathy: Systematic review of randomised trials. BMJ 2004;328:1046.

19. Leise MD, Poterucha JJ, Kamath PS, Kim WR. Management of hepatic encephalopathy in the hospital. Mayo Clin Proc 2014;89:241–53.

20. Alba L, Hay JE, Angulo P, Lee WM. Lactulose therapy in acute liver failure. J Hepatol 2002;36:33A.

21. Sushma S, Dasarathy S, Tandon RK, Jain S, Gupta S, Bhist MS. Sodium benzoate in the treatment of acute hepatic encephalopathy: A double-blind randomized trial. Hepatology 1992;16:138–44.

22. Batshaw ML, Brusilow S, Waber L, Blom W, Brubakk AM, Burton BK, et al. Treatment of inborn errors of urea synthesis: activation of alternative pathways of waste nitrogen synthesis and excretion. N Engl J Med 1982;306:1387–92.

23. Schaefer B, Schaefer F, Engelmann G, Meyburg J, Heckert KH, Zorn M, et al. Comparison of Molecular Adsorbents Recirculating System (MARS) dialysis with combined plasma exchange and haemodialysis in children with acute liver failure. Nephrol Dial Transplant 2011;26:3633–9.

24. Liu JP, Gluud LL, Als-Nielsen B, Gluud C. Artificial and bioartificial support systems for liver failure. Cochrane Database Syst Rev 2004;1: CD003628.

25. Bourgoin P, Merouani A, Phan V, Litalien C, Lallier M, Alvarez F, et al. Molecular absorbent recirculating system therapy (MARS) in pediatric acute liver failure: A single center experience. Pediatr Nephrol 2014;29:901–8.

26. Lai YC, Huang HP, Tsai IJ, Tsau YK. High-volume continuous venovenous hemofiltration as an effective therapy for acute management of inborn errors of meta-bolism in young children. Blood Purif 2007;25:303–8.

27. Westrope C, Morris K, Burford D, Morrison G. Continuous hemofiltration in the control of neonatal hyperammonemia: A 10-year experience. Pediatr Nephrol 2010;25:1725–30.

28. Mazariegos G, Shneider B, Burton B, Fox IJ, Hadzic N, Kishnani P, et al. Liver transplantation for pediatric metabolic diseases. Mol Genet Metab 2014;111:418–27.

29. Arnon R, Kerkar N, Davis MK, Anand R, Yin W, González-Peralta RP, et al. Liver transplantation in children with metabolic diseases: The studies of pediatric liver transplantation experience. Pediatr Transplant 2010;14:796–805.

30. Stevenson T, Millan MT, Wayman K, Berquist WE, Sarwal M, Johnston EE, et al. Long-term outcome following pediatric liver transplantation for metabolic disorders. Pediatr Transplant 2010; 14:268–75.

31. Dhawan A, Taylor RM, Cheeseman P, De Silva P, Katsiyiannakis L, Mieli-Vergani G. Wilson's disease in children: 37-year experience and revised King's score for liver transplantation. Liver Transplant 2005;11:441–8.

32. Devarbhavi H, Singh R, Adarsh CK, Sheth K, Kiran R, Patil M. Factors that predict mortality in children with Wilson disease associated acute liver failure and comparison of Wilson disease specific prognostic indices. J Gastroenterol Hepatol 2014;29:380–6.

33. Fischer RT, Soltys KA, Squires RH, Jaffe R, Mazariegos GV, Shneider BL. Prognostic scoring indices in Wilson disease: A case series and cautionary tale. J Pediatr Gastroenterol Nutr 2011;52:466–9.

34. Hughes RD, Mitry RR, Dhawan A. Current status of hepatocyte transplantation. Transplantation 2012;93:342–7.

35. Sokal EM. Treating inborn errors of liver meta-bolism with stem cells: Current clinical development. J Inherit Metab Dis 2014;37:535–9.

36. Cantz T, Sharma AD, Ott M. Concise review: Cell therapies for hereditary metabolic liver diseases concepts, clinical results and future developments. Stem Cells 2015;33:1055–62.

37. De-Laet C, Dionisi-Vici C, Leonard JV, McKiernan P, Mitchell G, Monti L, et al. Recommendations for the management of tyrosinemia type 1. Orphanet J Rare Dis 2013;8:8.

Pediatric Inflammatory Bowel Disease

Akshay Kapoor, Vidyut Bhatia, Anupam Sibal

Inflammatory bowel disease (IBD) is a perplexing disease characterized by chronic mucosal inflammation. It results from a complex interplay of various factors including genetic and environmental, and adaptive immunity of the host. Crohn's disease (CD) and Ulcerative colitis (UC) are the two broad phenotypes of IBD. CD is characterized by its ability to involve any part of the gastro-intestinal tract in a discontinuous fashion. The inflammation associated with CD is often transmural and granulomatous. UC on the other hand tends to involve the rectum and the adjoining colonic mucosa to a variable extent; albeit in a continuous fashion. The inflammation in UC is usually superficial when compared with CD. The term indeterminate colitis or IBD-U is used when the clinical and histopathological features are unable to distinguish between CD and UC.[1] Early onset IBD is important as researchers believe that it has a distinct phenotype when compared with adult onset IBD. Moreover, the genetically attributable risk is considered to be higher in early onset IBD, as exposure to environmental factors is proportionately less.

EPIDEMIOLOGY

Multiple studies have shown that 25% of all IBD cases have their onset in children less than 18 years of age.[2] However, the incidence of the disease seems to be increasing internationally. A systematic review of international trends in pediatric IBD revealed a statistically significant increase in the period 1950–2009. The SPIRIT registry from Spain collected data in 2100 pediatric patients with IBD (1996–2009). It showed a collective increase in incidence of IBD from 0.97 to 2.8/100,000 inhabitants <18 years/year in the study period. The median age at diagnosis was 12 years and the increase in CD cases was more than UC cases, with males being majorly affected[3] A similar registry from Italy (1996–2003) showed a similar rise in the overall incidence of IBD cases from 0.89 to 1.39/10 in children <18 years of age. However, in this registry UC cases showed a greater increase than CD cases.[4] The incidence of IBD in a prospective study (<16 years) from UK was 5.2/100000 individuals/year. The proportion of CD was 60%, while the proportion of UC was 28%. The mean age at diagnosis was 12 years. Studies from other European countries have shown incidence rates of 0.6–6.8/100000 individuals/year for CD and 0.8–3.6 for UC. An evaluation of North American studies revealed an incidence of 3–4/100000 individuals/year. Although studies and data are lacking from South American, African and Asian nations, temporal trends are obvious from the studies in the western hemisphere.[5] There is a male preponderance in pediatric CD (1.5:1), while UC affects both sexes equally. CD is more common in children as compared to UC (2.8:1) when compared with adult data (0.85:1). CD in children presents more commonly as ileocolonic or colonic disease. UC presents commonly (85–90%) as pancolitis.[6] Pediatric CD is predominantly an inflammatory disease; stricturing and penetrating variants are rarely seen at presentation. UC, as mentioned previously presents with a more severe phenotype which requires surgery more often as compared to the adult phenotype.[7]

Data from India is limited. The first case series on CD was published from Southern India in 2005, detailing 10 children (5–15 years) with Crohn's disease.[8] There was female preponderance (9 out of 10), and interestingly, 50% of the children had received antitubercular therapy prior to diagnosis. Another tertiary referral center from Southern India reported 34 children with IBD (23 with CD and 11 with UC). These cases accounted for 7% of the total IBD load presenting to that centre. The proportion of IBD was 0.03% of all pediatric cases presenting to the outpatient department, and the median delay in diagnosis was 15 months.[9] A recent questionnaire-based survey from seven centers across India in 221 children and adolescents with IBD showed that children with IBD in India have features similar to adult-onset IBD. UC was present in 42% of these children while CD was found in 55%; the rest were classified as indeterminate colitis. These children shared similarities with adult-onset IBD in terms of distribution of the disease. However, as in other reports on IBD in children, growth failure and more severe forms of the disease were commonly observed. The UC cases had complications like toxic megacolon and bleeding in 12%, while 27% of CD cases had complications (fistulae, strictures, perforation). Biological agents were used in less than 1% of UC cases and in 12% of CD cases.[10]

Genetics and Environmental Influence

Pediatric IBD has alerted researchers to the possibility of genetic susceptibility playing a role in disease pathogenesis. Epidemiological studies have highlighted a familial association in 25–30% cases of pediatric IBD. The NOD2 gene for CD and the MHC region on 6p for UC were two of the first genes to be implicated in disease causation. With the availability of Genome wide association scanning (GWAS) using single nucleotide polymorphisms (SNP), more than 100 genes have been implicated in IBD.[11]

Studies in twins have not shown a very strong concordance. The concordance rate for CD in monozygotic twins is between 35–63%, while for UC, it is 16–18%. Concordance rate in dizygotic twins is around 4%. This suggests a greater role of the environment in IBD causation. The cold chain hypothesis and the hygiene hypothesis were formulated to explain the increased incidence of IBD as a by-product of alteration of the gut microbiota due to refrigeration and increased cleanliness.[12] Refrigeration altered the bacteria in the diet and supported the growth of disease causing organisms; while increased cleanliness, smaller families and less exposure to animals made children in developed countries more susceptible to IBD. This altered/impaired immunological tolerance in response to low bacterial load forms the basis of hygiene hypothesis, wherein alteration between the balance of Th1 and Th2 helper cells was proposed as a mechanism of increasing IBD.[13]

To summarize, IBD manifests in a genetically susceptible individual when he/she is exposed to certain environmental triggers (infections, diet, domestic hygiene, smoking, etc.) which evoke an aberrant adaptive immune response.

CLINICAL PRESENTATION

A diagnosis of IBD should always be entertained in children with persistent (>1 month) or recurrent (>2 in 6 months) gastrointestinal symptoms. Abdominal pains, chronic diarrhea, rectal bleeding and weight loss are some of the common symptoms seen in IBD patients. In children with UC, rectal bleeding, chronic diarrhea and abdominal pain are more common; while weight loss is a prominent feature of CD (58% *vs* 35%). The classic triad of pediatric CD; abdominal pain, chronic diarrhea and weight loss is seen in only one-fourth of the cases; 25% of the children may present with only nonspecific symptoms–vague abdominal discomfort, lethargy and anorexia.[2] Perianal lesions in the form of skin tags, sentinel piles and fistulae are more common in CD. Impaired growth velocity and growth failure are more commonly seen in CD patients. Impairment of growth parameters can precede the intestinal mucosal lesion by months to years. Extra-intestinal manifestations of IBD may be the presenting feature in 6–17% of the patients. Arthropathy, skin manifestations and aphthous stomatitis are commonly seen. Primary sclerosing cholangitis (PSC) is more commonly associated with UC.[14]

DIAGNOSIS

The diagnosis of IBD is not straightforward. It rests on an accurate history and thorough clinical examination, supplemented by a supportive biochemistry, serology, accurate and complete endoscopy and characteristic histopathology (Fig. 15.1). Radiological examination in the form of a barium meal, CT/MRI enteroclysis or PET scan may further aid in the diagnosis.

History and Examination

A complete history should be obtained with regard to the frequency and type of stools, the presence of blood/pus per-rectum, and

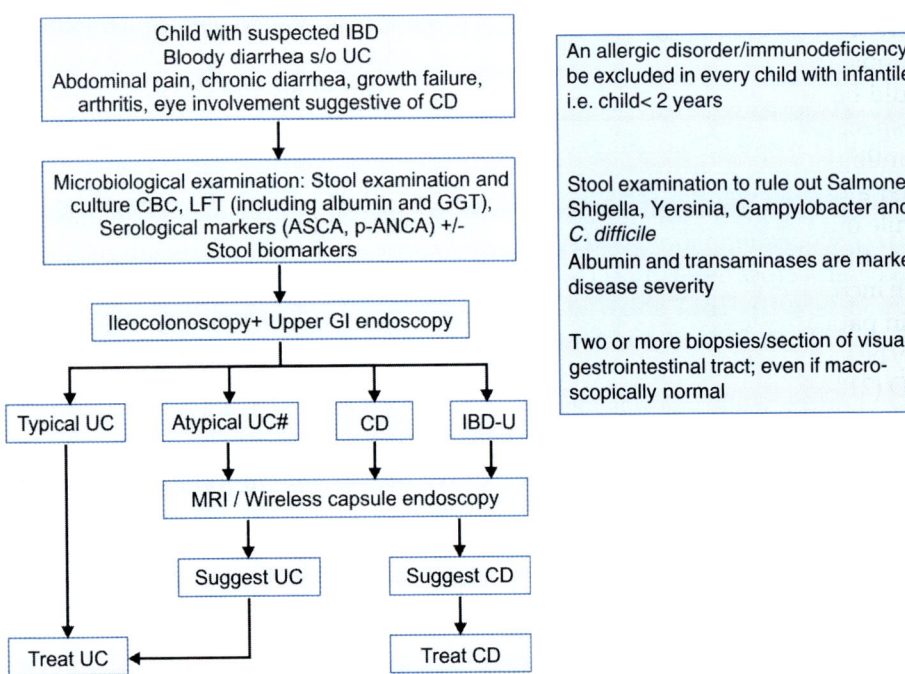

CD: Crohn's disease; IBD: Inflammatory bowel disease; UC: ulcerative colitis. #Atypical UC includes the following phenotypes: Rectal sparing, Cecal Patch, UGI involvement, Short duration, acute severe colitis

Fig. 15.1: Diagnostic algorithm in a child with suspected IBD (adapted from ESPGHAN Revised Porto Criteria for the Diagnosis of Inflammatory Bowel Disease in Children and Adolescents 2014)

associated abdominal pain, nausea, vomiting, lethargy and weight loss. Always ask for presence of nocturnal emergency and tenesmus. In infants with suspected UC, ask about the type of feeds being given to the child, as allergic colitis is a close differential. Record family history of IBD and history of antibiotic usage. Look for extra-intestinal manifestations like joint swelling, oral ulcers, skin lesions or visual problems. Chart height and weight centiles, including BMI. Carry out tanner staging for sexual maturity in all pre-pubertal and pubertal children. Perform abdominal examination for any tenderness, masses, lumps, or distension. Examine the perianal area for any skin tags, abscess, sentinel piles or fistulae.[15,16]

Investigations

A complete blood count with ESR, liver function tests (including albumin), iron status and CRP should be done in all cases of suspected IBD. Stool culture is necessary to rule out infectious diarrhea. *Clostridium difficile* toxin should be investigated in a fresh stool sample, especially if the child has received multiple antibiotics. However, it is pertinent to note that a documented enteric infection does not rule out the possibility of IBD.[15]

Anemia, thrombocytosis, hypoalbuminemia with increased ESR and CRP values are expected in patients with IBD. However, the values may be falsely normal in mild UC (54%) or mild CD (21%).

Serological Markers and Stool Tests

Antibodies to anti-Saccharomyces cerevisiae (ASCA) are associated with 60% cases of CD; while perinuclear antineutrophil cytoplasmic antibodies (p-ANCA) are associated with 60% of cases with UC. As, there is considerable overlap among the antibodies with each other and for other diseases like tuberculosis, they cannot be used in isolation to diagnose IBD. Additional markers like anti-*E. coli* outer membrane porin C antibody (anti-OmpC), anti-

bodies to bacterial flagellin (anti-CBir1) and anti-glycan antibodies are being studied.[17,18]

Non-invasive stool markers like fecal calprotectin and lactoferrin are increasingly been recognized as useful markers of small and large bowel inflammation in IBD patients.[19,20] Serial values may be of more benefit than single values as mucosal inflammation needs time to subside. Values of more than 100–150 μg/g of stool may differentiate IBD from functional causes. Stool markers need to be interpreted with caution in settings where invasive enteric infections are prevalent.

Endoscopy and Histopathology

Ileocolonoscopy and upper gastrointestinal endoscopy (UGI) are absolutely essential for diagnosis of IBD. The EECO and ESPGHAN guidelines recommend UGI endoscopy even in suspected UC cases to rule out CD. UGI involvement in CD cases is estimated to vary between 30–80%. Esophageal involvement was seen in 27% cases while gastro-duodenal involvement in 56% of the cases from the Pediatric IBD Collaborative research group registry.[21-23] The characteristic clinical, macroscopic and microscopic findings for CD and UC are given in Table 15.1.

The recently adapted Paris classification for Pediatric IBD, which was derived from the adult Montreal classification, has elucidated both the macroscopic and microscopic features of UC and CD in children. As the disease location and disease severity are determinants of the treatment strategy and the ultimate outcome, a uniform classification ameliorates any ambiguity in disease differentiation, phenotype and severity. The Paris classification for CD and UC are given in Tables 15.2 and 15.3, respectively.[21,24]

Imaging Studies

Fluoroscopy, CT, MRI and nuclear medicine scans are available to image the bowel in pediatric IBD. The Porto criteria formulated in 2005 advocated small bowel imaging (Barium

TABLE 15.1: Clinical differences between ulcerative colitis and Crohn's disease

Feature	Crohn's disease	Ulcerative colitis
Fever and weight loss	More common	Less common
Disease extent	Anywhere in the GI tract from mouth to anus; rectum is rarely involved.	Limited to colorectal mucosa, usually beginning at the rectum and spreading upwards to the cecum
Inflammation	Transmural; can lead to fistula. Patchy areas of inflammation (Skin lesions)	Mucosali, no fistula. Continous area of inflammation.
Perianal involvement	Fistulas, anal fissures and skin tags common	Not as common
Stenosis	Common	Rare
Feature	Crohn's disease	Ulcerative Colitis
Typical features on endoscopy	Discontinuous inflammation with intervening normalcy. Ulceration, structuring and fistulae, Cobblestoning.	Continuous inflammation with variable proximal extension from rectum. Erythema, friability and ulceration. Loss of vascular pattern, pseudopolyp formation
Typical features on histology	Submucosal/Transmural inflammation; Chronic ileitis/colitis; Non pericrypt granuloma; Focal biopsy changes; Patchy distribution; Crypt distortion and abscess	Mucosal inflammation Chronic colitis with crypt distortion and crypt abscess; Goblet cell depletion; Lymphoplasmacytosis; Plasma cell metaplasia

TABLE 15.2: Paris classification of Crohn's disease

Age at diagnosis	A1a	< 10 years
	A1b	10–<17 years
	A2	17–40 years
	A3	> 40 years
Location	L1	Distal 1/3 ileum +/− limited cecal disease
	L2	Colonic disease
	L3	Ileocolonic disease
	L4	Isolated Upper GI disease
	L4a	Esophageal disease
	L4b	Gastroduodenal disease
Behavior	B1	Non stricturing, nonpenetrating
	B2	Stricturing
	B3	Penetrating
	B2B3	Stricturing and penetrating
	P	Perianal disease modifier
Growth	G0	No evidence of growth delay

Source: Crohn's & Colitis Foundation of America

TABLE 15.3: Paris classification of ulcerative colitis

Extent	E1	Ulcerative proctitis
	E2	Left sided colitis distal to splenic flexure
	E3	Extensive colitis distal to hepatic flexure
	E4	Pancolitis, proximal to hepatic flexure
Severity	S0	Never severe
	S1	Ever severe

Source: Crohn's & Colitis Foundation of America

enterography are emerging as modalities with better resolution and delineation of the lumen and folds, with MR having less radiation exposure.[25] The use of PET scan to find areas of increased functional uptake and identify metabolically active tissue is still experimental. Video capsule endoscopy (VCE) is helpful in children, where ileal intubation is unsuccessful or not possible. It is also useful in classifying patients of IC. The drawbacks include inability to make a tissue diagnosis and the possibility of a retained capsule in stricturing CD.[26–29]

meal follow through) in IBD patients, especially those with CD, to rule out structuring and fistulae.[21] CT enterography and MR

While small bowel imaging using fluoro-scopy may show superficial mucosal disease better than any other modality, extra-luminal disease is poorly visualized. CT scan has greater resolution and can show extramural disease and its attendant complications; its use in pediatrics is limited due to the risk associated with ionizing radiation. MRI is costly and time consuming when compared to the other modalities, but can be used when soft tissue characterization is required (perianal CD). Pediatric CT protocols are now available to limit the total radiation dose being given to children.[30]

In countries and settings where tuberculosis (TB) is endemic, all efforts should be made by the treating clinician to distinguish it from CD, which is its closest differential. The fact that treatment approaches of the two diseases are diametrically opposite (antibacterials in TB *vs* immunomodulators in CD), it is all the more important to differentiate between the two. Colonoscopic features which suggest CD include perianal lesions, longitudinal ulcers, aphthous ulcers and cobblestoning. Features suggestive of TB include transverse ulcers, involvement of fewer colonic segments, a patulous ileocecal valve and pseudopolyp formation. Radiological features of CD include symmetric concentric bowel wall thickening with transmural enhancement. Segmental intestinal stenoses and fistulae formation is nearly always associated with CD. Extramural features like mesenteric vascular stranding and fibrofatty proliferation are pathogno-monic of CD. Intestinal TB is characterized by asymmetric bowel wall thickening with predominant involvement of the ileocecal area and large necrotic lymphnodes in the mesentry. Tissue diagnosis is mandatory for confirming either disease. Caseating granulo-mas are specific for TB while non-caseating epitheloid cell granulomas are more often found (though not specific) in CD.[31,32] **Fig. 15.1** shows schematic diagram to evaluate a child with IBD is regretted.

TREATMENT AND MONITORING STRATEGIES

The treatment protocols in IBD are aimed at mucosal healing, with consequent reduction in complications and increased quality of life. The goals of therapy are to maximize efficacy, minimize toxicity, prevention of compli-cations, and maintaining/re-establishing growth velocity and pubertal growth.

The treatment paradigm in pediatric IBD as in the adult world is the 'Step-up' approach, wherein medications with milder toxicity are used as first line therapy, before moving onto more aggressive therapies with higher toxicity. The Pediatric Ulcerative Colitis Activity Index (PUCAI) is a validated score to assess disease activity in UC. It has the advantage of being non-invasive and can be calculated easily in clinical practice **(Table 15.4)**. Studies have documented its high correlation with colonoscopy findings.[33,34]

PUCAI score <10 indicates remission; 10–34: mild disease activity; 35–64: moderate disease activity; >65: severe disease activity. A clinically significant response to therapy is a fall of more than 20 points. A similar score known as the Pediatric Crohn's Disease Activity index (PCDAI) is available for disease monitoring in CD **(Table 15.5)**. The PCDAI score can range from 0–100, with higher scores signifying more active disease. A score of <10 is consistent with inactive disease, 11–30 indicates mild disease, and >30 is moderate-severe disease. A decrease of 12.5 points is taken as evidence of improvement.

Ulcerative Colitis

The treatment can be divided into induction of remission and maintenance. The therapies available to induce remission include 5–aminosalicylic acid (5-ASA), corticosteroids, anti-tumor necrosis factor (TNF) therapy and calcineurin inhibitors. The drugs that can be used to maintain remission include 5-ASA, thiopurines, anti-TNF therapy and a few selected probiotics.

TABLE 15.4: The pediatric ulcerative colitis activity index

Item	Points
Abdominal pain	
No pain	0
Pain can be ignored	5
Pain cannot be ignored	10
Rectal Bleeding	
None	0
Small amount, in <50% stools	10
Small amount with most stools	20
Large amount, >50% of stool content	30
Stool consistency of most stools	
Formed	0
Partially formed	5
Completely unformed	10
Number of stools per 24 hours	
0–2	0
3–5	5
6–8	10
>8	15
Nocturnal stools (any episode causing awakening)	
No	0
Yes	10
Activity level	
No limitation of activity	0
Occasional limitation of activity	5
Severe restricted activity	10

Source: Turner D, Otley AR, Mack D, et al. Development and evaluation of a Pediatric Ulcerative Colitis Activity Index (PUCAI): A prospective multicenter study. Gastroenterology. 2007;133:423–32

Most guidelines recommend oral 5-ASA regimes as first line therapy during induction in mild-to-moderate UC. These are also to be used as maintenance therapy regardless of other treatments. Combination of oral and rectal 5-ASA compounds has been shown to be more effective than an oral drug alone. Topical 5-ASA (enemas) can be used as monotherapy in children with proctitis alone. Mesalazine and sulfasalazine are the 5-ASA agents of choice. A wide variety of ASA preparations are available in the market including azo-compounds (sulfasalazine, olsalazine), controlled release (Pentasa), pH-dependent (Salofalk, Asacol); however, there is no difference in the mucosal healing rate of the different compounds.[35]

Oral steroids (in a single daily dose) are effective agents in inducing remission in UC; however, they are not to be used in maintenance phase. These are recommended in moderate UC with systemic symptoms or severe UC without symptoms, and they can also be used in children who fail to achieve remission with optimal dose of 5-ASA agents. The dose of prednisolone is 1–2 mg/kg/day (max: 40 mg/day) for 2–4 weeks till remission is achieved. It can then be tapered gradually over the next 4–8 weeks. Children with severe colitis require hospitalization with vitals monitoring, complete blood counts and abdominal X-ray. Intravenous steroids, hydrocortisone (2 mg/kg four times a day) or methyl prednisolone (2 mg/kg/day), should be given in such cases. Failure to respond requires rescue therapy with either intravenous cyclosporine or infliximab.[34]

Antibiotics have no role in either induction of remission or maintenance in UC. Intravenous antibiotics like third generation cephalosporins and metronidazole can be considered if infection is suspected, especially in cases of toxic megacolon. Probiotics (VSL#3 and *E. coli* Nissle) can be considered as adjuvant therapy in patients with mild UC and residual activity not responding to standard therapy.

Immunomodulators [Azathioprine (AZA) and Mercatopurine (MP)] are indicated only for maintenance of remission. The scenarios for their potential use include: 5-ASA intolerance, frequently relapsing disease or steroid dependant disease. They can also be given after inducing remission with steroids in acute severe colitis. If calcineurin inhibitors like cyclosporin/tacrolimus were used in acute severe colitis, the patients would ultimately need AZA/MP. The therapeutic effect of the thiopurines is delayed and may take 2–3 months to reach full effect. Western literature recommends assay of thiopurine methyl-

TABLE 15.5: The pediatric Crohn's disease activity index

Items	Points
Abdominal pain	
None	0
Mild (brief episodes, not interfering with activities)	5
Moderate/severe (frequent or persistent, affecting with activities)	10
Stools	
0–1 liquid stools, no blood	0
2–5 liquid or up to 2 semi-formed with small blood	5
Gross bleeding, >6 liquid stools or nocturnal diarrhea	10
Patient functioning, general well-being (Recall, 1 week)	
No limitation of activities, well	0
Occasional difficulties in maintaining age appropriate activities, below par	5
Frequent limitation of activities, very poor	10
Weight	
Weight gain or voluntary weight loss	0
Involuntary weight loss 1–9%	5
Weight loss >10%	10
Height	
<1 channel decrease (or height velocity >–SD)	0
>1 <2 channel decrease (or height velocity <–1SD >–2SD)	5
>2 channel decrease (or height velocity <–2SD)	10
Abdomen	
No tenderness, no mass	0
Tenderness, or mass without tenderness	5
Tenderness, involuntary guarding, definite mass	10
Peri-rectal disease	
None, asymptomatic tags	0
1–2 indolent fistula, scant drainage, tenderness of abscess	5
Active fistula, drainage, tenderness or abscess	10

Extra-intestinal manifestations
Fever >38.5 × 3 d in week, arthritis, uveitis, erythema nodosum, or pyoderma gangrenosum

	Points
None	0
One	5
Two	10

Hematocrit

<10 y	11–14 (male)	11–19 (female)	15–19 (male)	Points
>33	>35	>34	>37	0
28-33	30–34	29–33	32–36	2.5
<28	<30	<29	<32	5

ESR (mm/hr)	Points
< 20	0
20–50	2.5
>50	5
Albumin (g/L)	
>35	0
31–34	5
<30	10

Source: Hyems JS, Ferry GD, Mardel FS, et al. Development and Validation of a Pediatric Grohn's Disease Activity Index. J Pediatr Gastroenterol Nurt. 1991;12:439–47

transferase (TPMT) genotype or phenotype to identify child at risk of myelosuppression.[36,37] However, the facility to measure TPMT is not available at many centers in low-and middle-income countries. Thus, regular monitoring of complete blood counts and liver function tests needs to be done as proxy markers for TPMT activity (2 weekly for the first 4 weeks, monthly thereafter) till metabolite levels become available. Pancreatitis is the most common hypersensitivity reaction which can occur in 3–4% of all cases. Thiopurines, in conjunction with biologicals, have also been shown to increase the risk of Non-Hodgkin lymphoma and Hepatosplenic T-cell lymphoma.[35]

Infliximab (IFX) in a dose of 5 mg/kg at 0, 2 and 6 weeks followed by 5 mg/kg 8 weekly for maintenance is the agent of choice in patients with persistently active or steroid-dependant UC, not controlled by 5-ASA or steroids. It can also be considered in steroid-refractory disease. The usage of Adalimumab (ADA) in pediatric UC is anecdotal and limited to case reports; however, it can be considered in Infliximab failure or intolerance, prior to colectomy.[38]

Surgery should only be considered in cases of treatment failure with all first line and second line agents. Surgery can also be considered in symptomatic children who are on multiple immunosuppressants and are steroid-dependant. The dose of immuno-suppressants and biologicals need to be optimized before referring an ambulatory case for surgery. Sometimes changing IFX to ADA can also prove useful. It can also be considered in cases of toxic megacolon. A two step procedure (colectomy and pouch formation with ileostomy as the first step followed by ileostomy closure) is the most commonly performed surgery. Sometimes a single step procedure (restorative proctocolectomy/ileo-anal pouch without ileostomy) can be performed in children who are not on high dose steroids. As with major surgeries, pre-operative clinical status (malnutrition,

hypoalbuminemia, steroids) influence post-operative disease outcomes.[2,39]

Crohn's Disease

For management of CD, it is helpful to cate-gorize children into mild, moderate and severe phenotypes based on disease location, extent and severity. In addition, issues like decreased bone mass and impaired growth velocity have to be factored into the treatment regimen.

Induction of Remission

Exclusive enteral nutrition (EEN) has been recommended by ESPGHAN as the modality of choice in inducing remission in children with luminal CD. While steroids have been conventionally used, EEN has the obvious advantage of lacking the toxicity of parenteral steroids. Few studies have shown higher remission rates with EEN as compared to steroids. EEN is to be given for 6–8 weeks.[40,41] Towards the end of the exclusive feeding period, reintroduction of regular diet should be started gradually over a period of several weeks. Factors influencing the use of EEN include the child's and parents' choice, palatability, compliance and cost. Both polymeric and elemental feeds are available in the Western market. Various guidelines have advocated the use of nasogastric tubes and even gastrostomy to meet the volume required for providing adequate caloric intake (120% of total caloric requirement/day). If EEN does not induce a clinical response in 2 weeks, alternative therapeutic strategies should be employed. EEN is of questionable significance in children with severe pancolitis, oral and perianal CD.[22]

Oral corticosteroids (prednisolone 1–2 mg/kg/d) can be used for inducing remission in children with moderate to severe luminal CD, especially if EEN is not available or not tolerated. Steroids are helpful in achieving quick clinical remission though only a small percentage of cases demonstrate mucosal healing on endoscopy.[42] Budesonide has been used in mild to moderate ileo-cecal CD to induce remission. The drug is known for its high topical activity and low systemic absorption, by virtue of its affinity to the intestinal glucocorticoid receptor.[43,44] The steroids are to be given at full dose for 2–4 weeks followed by gradual tapering over the next 8 weeks. There is no role of steroids in the maintenance therapy of pediatric CD.[45]

Metronidazole (10–20 mg/kg/day) and ciprofloxacin (20 mg/kg/day) are the two antibiotics utilized for perianal CD, especially of the fistulizing type. A meta-analysis showed that antibiotics are superior to placebo in active CD.[46] Metronidazole is thought to be more efficacious in children with colitis while Ciprofloxacin is preferred in those with ileitis. Azithromycin and rifaximin are the other antibiotics that have shown benefit during induction of remission in mild luminal CD.

Anti-TNF therapy with agents like infliximab (IFX) is recommended to induce remission in children with steroid refractory CD and children with active peri-anal fistulizing CD. It can also be considered in children with high risk of poor outcome (deep ulcerations on endoscopy, pan-enteric disease, advanced osteoporosis, marked growth failure, and poor response to adequate initial therapy). The induction dose is same as for patients with UC.[47]

Maintenance of Remission

Thiopurines (AZA/6MP) are the recommended agents for maintaining steroid-free remission in children with CD. Patients who received 6-MP after induction of remission are more likely to remain in remission, when compared with placebo.[48] These immunomodulators should be prescribed in full doses from the beginning as they require 8–14 weeks to achieve full efficacy.

Methotrexate can also be used as monotherapy for maintenance of remission in CD.[49] It can also be used as a second line drug in children with thiopurine failure.[50] MTX is prescribed in a dose of 15 mg/m^2 (max 25 mg) weekly as a subcutaneous injection. It can also be given intramuscularly and orally. The bioavailability of oral MTX is variable. Oral folic acid (5 mg) 24 hours after MTX administration is necessary. Nausea and vomiting are a frequent side effects, and can be tackled by giving pre-injection Ondansetron. Other side effects include hepatotoxicity, myelosuppression and pulmonary toxicity.[51] Thiopurines are the agent of choice in maintaining remission in patients post-surgery.

Biologicals (anti-TNF agents) are recommended for maintaining remission in children with chronic active luminal CD, especially those in whom remission was induced with IFX. Other categories include children with perianal CD, in combination with appropriate surgical intervention for fistulizing disease. Severe extra-intestinal manifestations like arthropathy and pyoderma gangrenosum also respond well to anti-TNF therapy. The maintenance dose is 5 mg/kg every 8 weeks. Higher doses of 10 mg/kg, or shorter intervals of dosing, i.e. 4-weekly intervals may be required in cases where drug response or drug levels are low.[47] The REACH study evaluated the safety and efficacy of IFX in children with CD who had moderate to severe disease activity. They concluded that those children who had IFX in their induction regimen were more likely to be in remission at week 54th when given maintenance IFX at 8 weekly intervals.[52] ADA is another biological, which can be used in a dose of 0.6 mg/kg (maximum 40 mg) every alternate week. Switch from one biological agent to another can be made in case of non-response to one agent. Patients with sustained response to biological agents can be considered for step-down therapy to immunomodulators, especially if they are treatment-naïve.[53] Combinations of thiopurines and biologicals have also been tried in children with CD. The benefit of lower antibody development against IFX and greater response has to be weighed against the possibility of lymphoma.[54] The development of antibodies to anti-TNF drugs is responsible for causing loss of drug efficacy, drug infusion reactions and delayed hypersensitivity reactions. Anti TNF therapy can be associated with severe life threatening infections like meningitis, sepsis, herpes and fungal infections. Immunization schedules should be completed prior to initiation of IFX therapy.[54]

Amino-salicylates can be used in very mild colonic disease in doses similar to UC.[55] There use in pediatric population is limited to information from only two clinical trials.[56,57] However, there is no evidence to suggest that they induce mucosal healing or be used as stand-alone therapy. Partial enteral nutrition cannot be used to induce remission. However, it can be used as maintenance therapy in patients with very mild disease or low risk of relapse. Omega-3 fatty acids and probiotics are not recommended for maintenance of remission.

The indications for surgery in CD include failure of medical therapy, growth failure despite maximal therapy, extraintestinal involvement (eyes and joints), and disease complications like obstruction, fistulae and perforation. The surgical paradigm in CD is to resect areas with macroscopic disease, that mainly is the ileocolonic area, with a right hemicolectomy. The use of strictureplasty and balloon dilatation of strictures is limited to adult literature[39] Perianal CD behaves like a distinct disease subtype and requires optimal use of biologicals, early and correct use of antibiotics and abscess drainage along with seton placement, if required.

Stopping/Stepping-down Therapy

There are no definite guidelines on when to stop therapy. Immunomodulators and anti-TNF therapy, if effective, should be continued for a prolonged period, and should not be stopped during critical growth phases, especially during or before adolescence. Drug de-escalation can be considered in children, who have been in prolonged steroid-free remission, especially those with complete mucosal healing. Surrogate markers like CRP, hemoglobin level, fecal calprotectin can also be used as adjuncts to de-escalate therapy. Complete stoppage of therapy is generally not advisable and often not possible, except in few patients with very mild/limited disease. Stepping down from combination therapy (anti-TNF + thiopurines) to IFX monotherapy should be done after mucosal healing is achieved.[35]

Step-up therapy has been conventionally used in CD. It involves giving steroids, 5-ASA agents, nutrition and antibiotics to ameliorate symptoms of the disease. The non-responders are then given immunomodulators and subsequently biologicals. This approach is gentler, with lesser side effects and avoids over-treatment of a low risk patient. On the other hand, failure to optimize conventional therapy can lead to serious side effects including surgery and the need for potentially toxic drugs at higher doses for a prolonged period of time. Top-down therapy involves the early use of immunosuppressants and biologicals in certain disease phenotypes with a known poor outcome (perianal CD) to induce remission.[58] Several recent studies have shown lesser relapses, lesser complications, less need for surgery and less use of steroids with this approach.[59,60] Top-down therapy offers the potential for altering the natural history of CD, and might help in changing treatment paradigms. This approach; however, is fraught with complications like increased risk of life-threatening infections, tuberculosis and herpes zoster re-activation. In addition, it imposes an economic burden on the family.

CONCLUSION

Pediatric IBD is a complex disease, which continues to evolve. Diagnostic and treatment strategies are based mainly on multicentric adult studies and pediatric series. Treatment paradigms are gradually shifting from the step-up approach to the step-down approach, with increasing experience of the severity of certain disease sub-types. With more-and-more work being done in the field of genetics, the genotype-phenotype combination may ultimately guide disease treatment.

REFERENCES

1. Carvalho RS, Abadom V, Dilworth HP, Thompson R, Oliva-Hemker M, Cuffari C. Indeterminate colitis: a significant subgroup of pediatric IBD. Inflamm Bowel Dis 2006;12:258–62.

2. Abraham BP, Mehta S, El-Serag HB. Natural history of pediatric-onset inflammatory bowel disease: a systematic review. J Clin Gastroenterol 2012;46:581–9.

3. Martin-de-Carpi J, Rodriguez A, Ramos E, Jimenez S, Martinez-Gomez MJ, Medina E, et al. Increasing incidence of pediatric inflammatory bowel disease in Spain (1996-2009): the SPIRIT Registry. Inflamm Bowel Dis 2013; 19:73–80.

4. Castro M, Papadatou B, Baldassare M, Balli F, Barabino A, Barbera C, et al. Inflammatory bowel disease in children and adolescents in Italy: data from the pediatric national IBD register (1996-2003). Inflamm Bowel Dis 2008; 14:1246–52.

5. Heyman MB, Kirschner BS, Gold BD, Ferry G, Baldassano R, Cohen SA, et al. Children with early-onset inflammatory bowel disease (IBD): analysis of a pediatric IBD consortium registry. J Pediatr 2005;146:35–40.

6. Sauer CG, Kugathasan S. Pediatric inflammatory bowel disease: highlighting pediatric differences in IBD. Med Clin North Am 2010;94:35–52.

7. Benchimol EI, Fortinsky KJ, Gozdyra P, Van den Heuvel M, Van Limbergen J, Griffiths AM. Epidemiology of pedia-tric inflammatory bowel disease: a systematic review of international trends. Inflamm Bowel Dis 2011;17:423–39.

8. Sathiyasekaran M, Raju BB, Shivbalan S, Rajarajan K. Pediatric Crohn's disease in South India. Indian Pediatr 2005;42:459–63.

9. Avinash B, Dutta AK, Chacko A. Pediatric inflammatory bowel disease in South India. Indian Pediatr 2009;46:639–40.

10. Sathiyasekaran M, Bavanandam S, Sankara-narayanan S, Mohan N, Geetha M, Wadhwa N, et al. A questionnaire survey of pediatric inflammatory bowel disease in India. Indian J Gastroenterol 2014;33:543–9.

11. Biank V, Broeckel U, Kugathasan S. Pediatric inflammatory bowel disease: clinical and molecular genetics. Inflamm Bowel Dis 2007;13: 1430–8.

12. Aujnarain A, Mack DR, Benchimol EI. The role of the environment in the development of pediatric inflammatory bowel disease. Curr Gastroenterol Rep 2013;15:326.

13. Timm S, Svanes C, Janson C, Sigsgaard T, Johannessen A, Gislason T, et al. Place of upbringing in early childhood as related to inflammatory bowel diseases in adulthood: a population-based cohort study in Northern Europe. Eur J Epidemiol 2014;29:429–37.

14. Aloi M, Cucchiara S. Extradigestive manifestations of IBD in pediatrics. Eur Rev Med Pharmacol Sci 2009;13:23–32.

15. Bousvaros A, Sylvester F, Kugathasan S, Szigethy E, Fiocchi C, Colletti R, et al. Challenges in pediatric inflammatory bowel disease. Inflamm Bowel Dis 2006;12:885–913.

16. Kwon YH, Kim YJ. Pre-diagnostic clinical presentations and medical history prior to the diagnosis of inflammatory bowel disease in children. Pediatr Gastroenterol Hepatol Nutr 2013;16: 178–84.

17. Davis MK, Andres JM, Jolley CD, Novak DA, Haafiz AB, Gonzalez-Peralta RP. Antibodies to Escherichia coli outer membrane porin C in the absence of anti-Saccharomyces cerevisiae antibodies and anti-neutrophil cytoplasmic antibodies are an unreliable marker of Crohn disease and ulcerative colitis. J Pediatr Gastroenterol Nutr 2007; 45:409–13.

18. Davis MK, Valentine JF, Weinstein DA, Polyak S. Antibodies to CBir1 are associated with glycogen storage disease type Ib. J Pediatr Gastroenterol Nutr 2010;51:14–8.

19. Aomatsu T, Yoden A, Matsumoto K, Kimura E, Inoue K, Andoh A, et al. Fecal calprotectin is a useful marker for disease activity in pediatric patients with inflammatory bowel disease. Dig Dis Sci 2011;56:2372–7.

20. Chang MH, Chou JW, Chen SM, Tsai MC, Sun YS, Lin CC, et al. Faecal calprotectin as a novel biomarker for differentiating between inflammatory bowel disease and irritable bowel syndrome. Mol Med Rep 2014;10:522–6.

21. Levine A, Koletzko S, Turner D, Escher JC, Cucchiara S, de Ridder L, et al. ESPGHAN revised porto criteria for the diagnosis of inflammatory bowel disease in children and adolescents. J Pediatr Gastroenterol Nutr 2014;58:795–806.

22. Ruemmele FM, Veres G, Kolho KL, Griffiths A, Levine A, Escher JC, et al. Consensus guidelines of ECCO/ESPGHAN on the medical management of pediatric Crohn's disease. J Crohns Colitis 2014;8:1179–207.

23. Turner D, Griffiths AM. Esophageal, gastric, and duodenal manifestations of IBD and the role of

upper endoscopy in IBD diagnosis. Curr Gastro-enterol Rep 2009;11:234–7.

24. Eszter Muller K, Laszlo Lakatos P, Papp M, Veres G. Incidence and paris classification of pediatric inflammatory bowel disease. Gastroenterol Res Pract 2014;2014:904307.

25. Alliet P, Desimpelaere J, Hauser B, Janssens E, Khamis J, Lewin M, et al. MR enterography in children with Crohn disease: results from the Belgian pediatric Crohn registry (Belcro). Acta Gastroenterol Belg 2013;76:45–8.

26. Gralnek IM, Cohen SA, Ephrath H, Napier A, Gobin T, Sherrod O, et al. Small bowel capsule endoscopy impacts diagnosis and management of pediatric inflammatory bowel disease: a prospective study. Dig Dis Sci 2012;57:465–71.

27. Hudesman D, Mazurek J, Swaminath A. Capsule endoscopy in Crohn's disease: are we seeing any better? World J Gastroenterol 2014;20:13044–51.

28. Min SB, Le-Carlson M, Singh N, Nylund CM, Gebbia J, Haas K, et al. Video capsule endoscopy impacts decision making in pediatric IBD: a single tertiary care center experience. Inflamm Bowel Dis 2013;19:2139–45.

29. North American Society for Pediatric Gastro-enterology Hepatology and Nutrition, Crohn's and Colitis Foundation of America, Bousvaros A, Antonioli DA, Colletti RB, et al. Differentiating ulcerative colitis from Crohn disease in children and young adults: report of a working group of the North American Society for Pediatric Gastro-enterology, Hepatology, and Nutrition and the Crohn's and Colitis Foundation of America. J Pediatr Gastroenterol Nutr 2007;44:653–74.

30. Frush DP, Goske MJ. Image Gently: toward optimizing the practice of pediatric CT through resources and dialogue. Pediatr Radiol 2015; 45:471–5.

31. Weng MT, Wei SC, Lin CC, Tsang YM, Shun CT, Wang JY, et al. Seminar Report From the 2014 Taiwan Society of Inflammatory Bowel Disease (TSIBD) Spring Forum (May 24th, 2014): Crohn's disease versus intestinal tuberculosis infection. Intest Res 2015;13:6–10.

32. Makharia GK, Srivastava S, Das P, Goswami P, Singh U, Tripathi M, et al. Clinical, endoscopic, and histological differentiations between Crohn's disease and intestinal tuberculosis. Am J Gastro-enterol 2010;105:642–51.

33. Turner D, Hyams J, Markowitz J, Lerer T, Mack DR, Evans J, et al. Appraisal of the pediatric ulcerative colitis activity index (PUCAI). Inflamm Bowel Dis 2009;15:1218–23.

34. Turner D, Travis SP, Griffiths AM, Ruemmele FM, Levine A, Benchimol EI, et al. Consensus for managing acute severe ulcerative colitis in children: a systematic review and joint statement from ECCO, ESPGHAN, and the Porto IBD Working Group of ESPGHAN. Am J Gastroen-terol 2011;106:574–88.

35. Aloi M, Nuti F, Stronati L, Cucchiara S. Advances in the medical management of paediatric IBD. Nat Rev Gastroenterol Hepatol 2014;11:99–108.

36. Weinshilboum RM, Sladek SL. Mercaptopurine pharmacogenetics: monogenic inheritance of erythrocyte thiopurine methyltransferase activity. Am J Hum Genet 1980;32:651–62.

37. Dubinsky MC, Lamothe S, Yang HY, Targan SR, Sinnett D, Theoret Y, et al. Pharmacogenomics and metabolite measurement for 6-mercapto-purine therapy in inflammatory bowel disease. Gastroenterology 2000;118:705–13.

38. Yang LS, Alex G, Catto-Smith AG. The use of biologic agents in pediatric inflammatory bowel disease. Curr Opin Pediatr 2012;24:609–14.

39. Baillie CT, Smith JA. Surgical strategies in paediatric inflammatory bowel disease. World J Gastroenterol 2015;21:6101–16.

40. Berni Canani R, Terrin G, Borrelli O, Romano MT, Manguso F, Coruzzo A, et al. Short- and long-term therapeutic efficacy of nutritional therapy and corticosteroids in paediatric Crohn's disease. Dig Liver Dis 2006;38:381-7.

41. Whitten KE, Rogers P, Ooi CY, Day AS. International survey of enteral nutrition protocols used in children with Crohn's disease. J Dig Dis 2012;13:107–12.

42. Bousvaros A. Mucosal healing in children with Crohn's disease: appropriate therapeutic goal or medical overkill? Inflamm Bowel Dis 2004;10: 481–3.

43. Escher JC, European Collaborative Research Group on Budesonide in Paediatric IBD. Budeso-nide versus prednisolone for the treatment of active Crohn's disease in children: a randomized, double-blind, controlled, multi-centre trial. Eur J Gastroenterol Hepatol 2004;16:47–54.

44. Levine A, Weizman Z, Broide E, Shamir R, Shaoul R, Pacht A, et al. A comparison of budesonide and prednisone for the treatment of active pediatric Crohn disease. J Pediatr Gastroenterol Nutr 2003; 36:248–52.

45. Dimakou K, Pachoula I, Panayotou I, Stefanaki K, Orfanou I, Lagona E, et al. Pediatric inflammatory bowel disease in Greece: 30-years experience of a single center. Ann Gastroenterol 2015;28:81–6.

46. Khan KJ, Ullman TA, Ford AC, Abreu MT, Abadir A, Marshall JK, et al. Antibiotic therapy in inflammatory bowel disease: a systematic review and meta-analysis. Am J Gastroenterol 2011;106: 661–73.

47. Olbjorn C, Nakstad B, Smastuen MC, Thiis-Evensen E, Vatn MH, Perminow G. Early anti-TNF treatment in pediatric Crohn's disease. Predictors of clinical outcome in a population-based cohort of newly diagnosed patients. Scand J Gastroenterol 2014;49:1425–31.

48. Markowitz J, Grancher K, Kohn N, Lesser M, Daum F. A multicenter trial of 6-mercaptopurine and prednisone in children with newly diagnosed Crohn's disease. Gastroenterology. 2000; 119:895–902.

49. Uhlen S, Belbouab R, Narebski K, Goulet O, Schmitz J, Cezard JP, et al. Efficacy of methotrexate in pediatric Crohn's disease: a French multicenter study. Inflamm Bowel Dis 2006;12: 1053–7.

50. Turner D, Grossman AB, Rosh J, Kugathasan S, Gilman AR, Baldassano R, et al. Methotrexate following unsuccessful thiopurine therapy in pediatric Crohn's disease. Am J Gastroenterol 2007;102:2804–12.

51. Sunseri W, Hyams JS, Lerer T, Mack DR, Griffiths AM, Otley AR, et al. Retrospective cohort study of methotrexate use in the treatment of pediatric Crohn's disease. Inflamm Bowel Dis. 2014;20: 1341–5.

52. Hyams J, Crandall W, Kugathasan S, Griffiths A, Olson A, Johanns J, et al. Induction and maintenance infliximab therapy for the treatment of moderate-to-severe Crohn's disease in children. Gastroenterology 2007;132:863–73. Hepatol. 2014; 26:458–65.

53. Assa A, Hartman C, Weiss B, Broide E, Rosenbach Y, Zevit N, et al. Long-term outcome of tumor necrosis factor alpha antagonist's treatment in pediatric Crohn's disease. J Crohns Colitis 2013;7:369–76.

54. Ford AC, Kane SV, Khan KJ, Achkar JP, Talley NJ, Marshall JK, et al. Efficacy of 5-aminosalicylates in Crohn's disease: systematic review and meta-analysis. Am J Gastroenterol 2011;106:617–29.

55. Griffiths A, Koletzko S, Sylvester F, Marcon M, Sherman P. Slow-release 5-aminosalicylic acid therapy in children with small intestinal Crohn's disease. J Pediatr Gastroenterol Nutr 1993;17: 186–92.

56. Cezard JP, Munck A, Mouterde O, Morali A, Lenaerts C, Lachaux A, et al. Prevention of relapse by mesalazine (Pentasa) in pediatric Crohn's disease: A multicenter, double-blind, randomized, placebo-controlled trial. Gastroenterol Clin Biol 2009;33:31–40.

57. Lin MV, Blonski W, Lichtenstein GR. What is the optimal therapy for Crohn's disease: step-up or top-down? Expert Rev Gastroenterol Hepatol 2010;4:167–80.

58. Kim MJ, Lee JS, Lee JH, Kim JY, Choe YH. Infliximab therapy in children with Crohn's disease: A one-year evaluation of efficacy comparing 'top-down' and 'step-up' strategies. Acta Paediatr 2011;100:451–5.

59. Krupoves A, Mack DR, Seidman EG, Deslandres C, Bucionis V, Amre DK. Immediate and long-term outcomes of corticosteroid therapy in pediatric Crohn's disease patients. Inflamm Bowel Dis. 2011;17:954–62.

60. Mayberry JF, Lobo A, Ford AC, Thomas A. NICE clinical guideline (CG152): The management of Crohn's disease in adults, children and young people. Aliment Pharmacol Ther 2013;37:195–203.

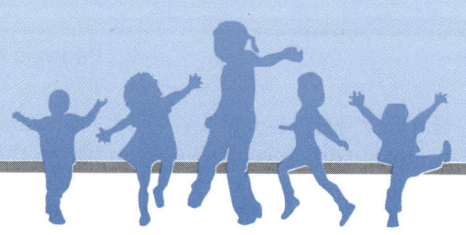

Clinical Effects of Prebiotics in Pediatric Population

Rok Orel, Lea Vodušek Reberšak

Prebiotics are non-digestible components of food that in a selective manner trigger the expansion of microbes in the gut with valuable effects for host health.[1] International Scientific Association for Probiotics and Prebiotics (ISAPP) postulated that prebiotics must fulfil three norms as: (i) escape digestion by human digestive enzymes in the upper gastrointestinal tract (GIT); (ii) be fermented by intestinal microorganisms; and (iii) selectively stimulate the growth and activity of those intestinal microorganisms that are associated with health and well-being of the presenter.[2]

All these demands are completed by non-digestible oligosaccharides that consist of three to ten sugar molecules, and are naturally present in fruits, vegetables, cereals, milk, etc., or can be industrially produced.[1,3,4] They represent an excellent meal for the resident society of saccharolytic bacteria in our gut. Main end-products of their fermentation are short-chain fatty acids (SCFAs). Different bacteria prefer one energy source over the other.[5] Consequently, diet becomes a powerful tool in directing gut microbial population.[6,7] That is in fact the foundation of prebiotic concept as we have the influence to supply favourite 'fuel' to specific microorganisms recognized as promoters of good health.

At the moment, animal and human studies favor the use of galacto-oligosaccharides (GOS), inulin, and fructo-oligosaccharides (FOS). In addition, to imitate the human milk oligosaccharides (HMO) a mixture of short-chain GOS and long-chain FOS was developed. According to the Commission Directive on infant formulae and follow-on formulae in European Union, fructo-oligosaccharides and galacto-oligosaccharides may be added to infant formulae, nonetheless their proportion must not exceed 0.8 g/100 mL in a combination of 90% oligogalactosyl-lactose and 10% high molecular weight oligofructosyl-saccharose.[8]

Nutritional and health benefits of prebiotics are gripping attention among consumers, food and pharmaceutical industry, and health professionals.[9,10] Some experts even established them to be superior to probiotics as they are cheaper to produce, more affordable for mass consumers, trust worthier compared to consuming live bacteria, and less susceptible to environmental stresses; nevertheless, probiotics cannot function in the absence of prebiotics.[11]

Special attention should therefore be focused on interpreting studies and conclusions as financial drive is enormous, whereas clinical evidence is often sparse.

For this review, we collected data through search of the MEDLINE, PubMed, UpToDate, Cochrane Database of Systemic Reviews and the Cochrane Controlled Trials Register database as well as through references from relevant articles. Duplicates were discarded. A search strategy was used based on combination of MeSH terms: 'prebiotics' and 'pediatrics'. The last search was conducted September 5th, 2015. 459 full-text articles were analyzed by two of the authors. A descriptive and explanatory qualitative approach was chosen for the content analysis.

MECHANISMS OF ACTION

Indirect effects of prebiotics arise through stimulation of health-promoting microbial taxa, such as Bifidobacterium and Bacteroides,[12–14] which block intestinal pathogens, improve intestinal barrier function and orchestrate immune pathways. There is even some evidence of gut microbiota influencing brain function over microbiota-gut-brain axis.[15]

Direct effects are due to the action of SCFAs. They are largely produced in colon where they act locally; however, some of them reach high concentration in the bloodstream carrying them across the body and allowing them to interact in extra-intestinal reactions.[16] The main SCFAs formed are acetate, propionate and butyrate. Their primary task is the energy supply for intestinal epithelial cells, though they also play a role in gene expression, gut motility and barrier function, metabolite absorption, lipid metabolism, appetite control, insulin resistance, gut-liver axis regulation, and regulation of the immune system, resulting in prevention of infection, diarrhea, constipation and allergies.[17]

CLINICAL USES IN CHILDREN

Infantile Colic

In a randomized non-blinded trial, published almost ten years ago, 96 formula-fed infants under 4 months of age with colic received a partially hydrolyzed whey protein formula containing FOS and GOS. They experienced a greater reduction of crying episodes after 7 and 14 days compared with those assigned to a standard formula and simethicone.[18] However, whether the effect is due to partially hydrolysed protein, the prebiotics, or both, is not clear. Pärtty, et al.[19] studied preterm infants randomized to receive a mixture of GOS and polydextrose (1:1), probiotics or placebo during first 2 months of life, and followed-up for 1 year. In both pre- and probiotic groups, significantly less frequent crying was observed compared with the placebo group (19% vs 19% vs 47%, respectively; P=0.02). On the other hand, a systematic review and meta-analysis including 12 prebiotic studies found no impact of prebiotics on the incidence of colic, regurgitation, crying, restlessness or vomiting.[20] Nonetheless, adding prebiotics to infant formula for full-term infants was reviewed. Although, further confirmatory studies are needed, no adverse effects of prebiotics were found during this review.

Constipation (Table 16.1)

Majority of clinical studies concerning the effects of supplementation of infant formulas with prebiotics confirmed increase in frequency of defecation and/or softer consistency of stools, similar to that of breast-fed infants.[21–31] Current analysis of stool characteristics of infants receiving short-chain GOS (scGOS) and long-chain FOS (lcFOS) in ratio 9:1 showed that effects on stool consistency were more often found to be significant than effects on stool frequency.[32] Bongers, et al.[33] published the only therapeutic randomized controlled trial (RCT) using prebiotic formula for functional constipation in 2007. The consumption of a high concentration sn-2 palmitic acid, scGOS/lcFOS 8 g/L and partially hydrolyzed whey protein formula resulted in a strong tendency of softer stools in constipated infants, but not in a difference in defecation frequency. In a randomized, double-blind, prospective study,[25] it was shown that prebiotics can soften stools and increase stool frequency even in toddlers.[25]

TABLE 16.1: Summary of randomized controled trial evaluating prebiotics in infantile case and constipation

Prebiotic study	Inclusion criteria, n	Treatment used in study groups	Treatment duration	Reported outcome
Infantile Colic				
Savino, *et al.*[18] 2006	Formula-fed infants, aged <4 months with infantile colic *n*=99	PG: partially hydrolysed formula with FOS and GOS CG: standard formula and simethicone (6 mg/kg 2×/d)	2 weeks	Reduction of crying episodes in infants with colic after 7 and 14 days in PG.
Pärtty, *et al.*[19] 2013	Gestational age 32–36 weeks and birth weight >1500 g *n*=63	PG: mixture of GOS and PDX (ratio 1:1) 600 mg/d day 1–30 and 1200 mg/d day 31–60 CG: standard formula	First 2 months of life and follow up for 1 year	Significantly less excessive criers in PG.
Constipation				
Holscher, *et al.*[21] 2012	Full-term formula-fed infants *n*=139	PG: a partially hydrolyzed whey formula with GOS & FOS (9:1) 4 g/L CG: a partially hydrolyzed whey formula BG	6 weeks	Prebiotic formula was well tolerated. Increased abundance, proportion of bifidobacteria, and reduced fecal pH in PG.
Williams, *et al.*[22] 2014	Healthy term infants *n*=180	PG 1: GOS 4 g/L PG 2: GOS 8 g/L CG: standard formula	First 4 months of life	PG 1 was well-tolerated in terms of stool consistency. Significantly higher percentage of watery stools in PG 2 group. No increase in stool frequency in PGs.
Scalabrin, *et al.*[23] 2012	Term infants *n*=230	PG: PDX & GOS (1:1) 4 g/L CG: standard formula BG	60 days	PDX & GOS produced soft stools and a bifidogenic effect closer to breast milk.
Ashley, *et al.*[24] 2012	Healthy 12- to 16-day old infants *n*=419	PG 1: PDX & GOS (1:1) 4 g/L PG 2: GOS 4 g/L CG: cow's milk—based infnat formula	From 14 to 120 days of age	Softer stooling pattern similar to that reported in breastfed infants in both PGs. No group differences in growth rate.

Contd...

TABLE 16.1: Summary of randomized controled trial evaluating prebiotics in infantile case and constipation *(Contd...)*

Prebiotic study	Inclusion criteria, n	Treatment used in study groups	Treatment duration	Reported outcome
Ribeiro, et al.[25] 2011	Healthy 9- to 48-months old children n=129	PG: PDX & GOS 2 g/d CG: cow's milk—based follow-on formula	108 days	More frequent and softer stools in PG.
Veereman-Wauters, et al.[26] 2011	Healthy neonates n=110	PG 1: oligofructose & FOS (1:1) 0.8 g/dL PG 2:GOS & FOS (9:1) 0.8 g/dL CG: standard formula BG	First month of life	Stool consistency and bacterial composition of infants in both PGs were closer to the breastfed pattern.
Westerbeek, et al.[27] 2011	Preterm infants n=113	PG: scGOS & lcFOS and AOS CG: maltodextrin	Between days 3 and 30	Prebiotic mixture decreases stool viscosity and stool pH with a trend towards increaased stool frequency.
Vivatvakin, et al.[28] 2010	Healthy term infants n=144	PG: a whey-predominant formula containing long-chain polyunsaturated fatty acids and GOS & FOS CG: case in-predominant formula BG	From 30 days to 4 months of age	Softer stools, stool microbiota, gastric and intestinal transit times were closer to that of the breastfed group. No group differences in growth rate.
Bisceglia, et al.[29] 2009	Healthy newborns n=76	PG: scGOS/lcFOS (9:1) 0.8 g/100 mL CG:standard formula	28 days	A larger number of stools in PG.
Bongers, et al.[33] 2007	Otherwise healthy constipated term infants aged 3–20 weeks n=38	PG: scGOS/lcFOS (9:1) 0.8 g/100 mL, high concentration of *sn-2* palmitic acid and partially hydrolyzed whey protein CG: standard formula	Period 1 (3 weeks in PG) and crossed-over to period 2 (CG)	A strong tendency of softer stools but no difference in defecation frequency in PG.

n=number of participants, PG-prebiotic group, CG-Control group, BG-breast-fed comparison group, FOS-fructo-oligosaccharides, GOS-galacto-oligosaccharides, scGOS-short chain GOS, lcFOS-long chain FOS, AOS-acidic oligosaccharides, PDX-polydextrose

A more recent study,[34] indicated a significant rush of motilin following prebiotic supplementation. Motilin being a peptide, produced by endocrine M cells, largely presents especially in duodenum and jejunum. Its essential role is to clean undigested food from the gut by controlling inter-digestive migrating contractions.[34] All together suggesting an association with improved gastric emptying, better tolerance to food and improved digestion in general.[35]

Changes in defecation patterns in pediatric population due to prebiotic supplementation mostly result in improvement of abdominal comfort and reduction of prevalence of functional constipation. Since constipation affects one third of children usually before the age of five[36–38] but often persists beyond puberty, these observations are relevant for preventive or curative treatment of this very common functional disorder.[39] Yet, to establish specific doses in avoiding diarrhea, more studies are awaited.

Absorption of Minerals (Table 16.2)

Acidic environment in colon increases solubility of certain minerals.[40] Bioavailability of calcium when consuming prebiotic ingredients has been well-studied. Animal studies verified the positive correlation; efficiency in humans is nevertheless not consistent. Abrams, et al.[41] found significantly enhanced calcium absorption and bone mineralization in adolescents after receiving inulin-type fructans daily for a year. On the contrary, no significant effect of prebiotics was observed on calcium absorption or other markers of bone mineralisation in infants.[42] Recent observations show that prebiotic oligosaccharides enhance iron absorption in deficient rats.[43] Clearly, further human trials are needed, but this seems to be encouraging information, given the prevalence of iron-deficiency in children.

Weight-gain (Table 16.2)

At the Summer Meeting of the Nutrition Society in 2010, it was announced that an overview of studies investigating effects of oral SCFA on appetite regulation did not reveal a positive connection. The experts concluded that sensory characteristics are those influencing our choice of which food we eat and the quantity of it rather than a physiological effect of SCFA.[44] In children, especially in the first months of life when milk is the basic nutrition, there are some encouraging results. For instance, Mugambi, et al.[20] conducted a meta-analysis that summarized positive context of prebiotics in infant formulas and increased weight gain; there was no impact on length or head circumference gain. Whether this is the result of intensified energy harvests by intestinal bacteria and/or increased absorption by enterocytes is not yet clear. It is very likely that the outcome is dose-dependent.[14] Interestingly, these results are to some extent antagonistic with the inverse correlation between fibre intake and obesity known in adults as well as in adolescents.[22,45,46] In fact, dietary fibre reduces the risk of childhood obesity by up to 21%.[47] Furthermore, Dasopoulou, et al.[35] found that supplementation of infant formula with scGOS/lcFOS resulted in significantly lower mean cholesterol values compared with preterm neonates fed with standard formula.

Diarrhea (Table 16.2)

An open-label RCT published six years ago,[48] included more than 300 healthy infants, age 1–2 months. The group receiving a GOS/FOS mix had a significantly lower number of gastrointestinal infections and antibiotic use per year.[48] Still, when Duggan, et al.[49] studied a group of 282 infants 6–12 months of age, there was no difference in diarrheal prevalence or the mean duration of diarrhea between those receiving an infant cereal enriched with oligofructose with and without prebiotics.[49]

Destruction of microbial population in GIT has the power to start the so called antibiotic-

TABLE 16.2: Summary of randomized controlled trial evaluating efficacy of prebiotics in nutrient absorption, weight gain and diarrhea

Prebiotic study	Inclusion criteria, n	Treatment used in study groups	Treatment duration	Reported outcome
Absorption of minerals				
Abrams, et al.[41] 2005	9 and 13 years of age a BMI between the 5th and 95th percentiles for age and sex n=98	PG: mixed short and long degree of polymerization insulin-type, 8 g/d CG: maltodextrin	8 weeks and 1 year	Calcium absorption was significantly greater in the PG at 8 weeks and at 1 year.
Hicks, et al.[42] 2012	Term infants to 10 weeks of age with birth weight ≥2500 g n=74	PG: GOS & PDX (1:1) 4 g/L CG: cow milk-based formula BG	A minimum of 14 days	No significant effect of prebiotics on calcium absorption or other markers of bone mineral metabolism.
Weight gain				
Dasopoulou, et al.[35] 2015	Healthy formula-fed preterms n=167	PG: scGOS & lcFOS, 0.8 g/100 mL CG: preterm formula	16 days	Mean cholesterol and low density lipo-protein (LDL) increased significantly in the CG. Mean weight increased in the CG. Significant surtge of motilin in PG.
Diarrhea				
Bruzzese, et al.[48] 2009	Healthy infants aged 1–2 months n=342	PG: GOS & FOS formula CG: standard formula	1 year	The incidence of gastroenteritis lower in the PG.
Duggan, et al.[49] 2003	Healthy infants aged 6–12 months n=251	PG: cereal with oligofructose 0.55 g/15 g cereal CG: non-supplemented	6 months	Prebiotic cereal was not associated with any change in diarrhea prevalence.
Brunser, et al.[50] 2006	Healthy infants aged 1–2 years n=140	PG: insulin and oligofructose, 4.5 g/L CG: standard formula	3 weeks after they had ended amoxicillin therapy for respiratory infects	No significant difference in the fre-quency of AAD.

Contd...

TABLE 16.2: Summary of randomized controlled trial evaluating efficacy of prebiotics in nutrient obsorption, weight gain and diarrhea (Contd...)

Prebiotic study	Inclusion criteria, n	Treatment used in study groups	Treatment duration	Reported outcome
ESPGHAN[51] 2012	6 months to 11 years old children with oral and/or intravenous	PG: insulin and FOS age-dependent doses (max. 5 g/day) CG: maltodextrin	For as long as they were taking antimicrobial drugs	No effect regarding AAD.
Hoekstra, et al.[52] 2004	1 month to 3 years old children with acute diarrhea n=144	PG: ORS with prebiotic mixture (soy polysaccharides 25%, alpha-cellulose 9%, gum arabic 19%, FOS 18.5%, insulin 21.5%, resistant starch 7%) CG: non-supplemented ORS	During mild to moderate dehydration	No significant difference between participants concerning mean 48-h stool qantity, need for intravenous rehydration, duration of symptoms and hospitalization
Vaisman, et al.[53] consistency 2010	9 to 24 months old children with acute diarrhea n=119	PG: 80% lcFOS & scGOS and 20% AOS 2 g, 3x/d CG: maltodextrin	12 days	Importantly increased stool but not total of daily stools number.
Passariello, et al.[54] 2011	3 months to 3 years old children with acute diarrhea n=60	PG: ORS with FOS and xilooligosaccharides-both 0.35 g/L CG: non-supplemented ORS	During dehydration	Higher rate of diarrhea resolution at 72 hours, greater ORS intake during first 24 hours and reduced number of missed working days by parents.
Alam, et al.[55] 2000	4 to 18 months old infant with watery non-choleric diarrhea of <48 hours of duration n=150	PG: ORS with partially hydrolyzed guar gum CG: non-supplemented ORS	During dehydration	Important reduction of total duration of acute diarrhea in PG.

n=number of participants, BMI-Body mass index, PG-prebiotic group, CG-Control group, BG-breast-fed comparison group, FOS-fructo-oligosaccharides, GOS-galacto-oligosaccharides, scGOS-short chain GOS, lcFOS-long chain FOS, AOS-acidic oligosaccharides, PDX-polydextrose

associated diarrhea. Preventive intervention by giving prebiotics after or along with antibiotic treatment has so far not been properly evaluated. A RCT published in 2006 by Brunser, *et al.*[50] showed no significant difference in the frequency of antibiotic-induced diarrhea between two groups, aged 1-2 years. The first group received inulin and oligofructose (total of 4.5 g/L) containing milk formula for 3 weeks after they had ended amoxicillin therapy for respiratory infection. The second group received prebiotic-free milk formula.[50] Another trial was organized by the ESPGHAN Working Group on Pro- and Pre-biotics. In this multi-centre trial, children with oral and/or intravenous antibiotic therapy covering common infections were treated with inulin and FOS in age-dependent doses (max 5 g/day) for as long as they were taking antimicrobial drugs. These children were below 11 years old and tolerated the mixture well; nonetheless, it had no effect regarding antibiotic-associated diarrhea. The study was stopped before time because of slow recruitment and the working group concluded that overall prevalence of diarrhea was not high and caution must be taken when judging the results. However, there is a need for further research with different prebiotics.[51]

Administration of prebiotic compounds via oral rehydration solution (ORS) is under investigation. A decade ago, Hoekstra, *et al.*[52] also completed a multi-centre European double-blind randomized placebo controlled study on behalf of the ESPGHAN (European Society for Paediatric Gastroenterology, Hepatology, and Nutrition) Working Group on intestinal infection. The subject was ORS containing a mixture of prebiotics (soy polysaccharides 25%, alpha-cellulose 9%, gum arabic 19%, FOS 18.5%, inulin 21.5%, resistant starch 7%) in the acute diarrhea treatment. Children aged 1 month to 3 years with acute diarrhea resulting in mild-to-moderate dehydration were given either supplemented or non-supplemented ORS.[52] There was no significant difference between participants of the two groups in mean 48-h stool quantity, duration of symptoms and hospitalization.[52] No significant influence on clinical course of acute gastroenteritis was also reported by Israeli analysts. A mixture of 80% lcFOS/scGOS and 20% AOS in a three 2-g sachets per day significantly increased stool consistency (P=0.048) but not total of daily stools number (P=0.66) in 9- to 24-month-old children.[53] A recent randomized controlled trial in Italian children showed significant efficiency when FOS and xylo-oligosaccharides–both 0.35 g/L were consumed along with hypotonic ORS. Children aged 3 months to 3 years in prebiotic group drunk more ORS in the first 24 hours (P<0.001), diarrhea was over after 72 hours in a greater percentage (P=0.01) and their parents missed fewer working days compared to placebo "team" of parents (P<0.001).[54] An older double-blind, placebo controlled RCT including boys from Bangladesh enrolled a group of 150 male children, aged 4 to 18 months that looked for medical help because of watery non-cholera diarrhea of less than 48 hours of duration. Adding partially hydro-lyzed guar gum to oral rehydration solution resulted in important reduction of total extent of acute gastroenteritis.[55]

Respiratory Infections (Table 16.3)

It would be simple, safe and economical if prebiotics would help to prevent respiratory infections. There are some supportive results revealed by Luoto and colleagues in a recent RCT. Ninety-four preterm infants were randomized to receive PDX/GOS 1:1 (600 mg/24h day 1 to 30, 1200 mg/24h day 31 to 60), probiotic (Lactobacillus rhamnosus GG (LGG); 1×109 colony-forming units/24h day 1 to 30, 2×109 colony-forming units/24h day 31 to 60) or placebo for 60 days, starting on the third day of life. Follow-up visits were dated five times in the adjacent year. Significantly lower incidence of respiratory tract infections (RTI) was confirmed in the prebiotic group (P<0.001) as well as in the probiotic group (P=0.022). Specifically, Rhinovirus being etiological cause

TABLE 16.3: Summary of randomized controlled trial evaluating efficacy of prebiotics in respiratory infections and atopic eczema

Prebiotic study	Inclusion criteria, n	Treatment used in study groups	Treatment duration	Reported outcome
Respiratory infections				
Luoto, et al[56] 2014	Gastational age 32–36 weeks n=94	PG: PDX & GOS (1:1), 600 mg/d day 1 to 30, 1200 mg/d day 31 to 60 CG: standard formula	60 days, starting on the third day of life and follow-up for 1 year	Significantly lower incidence of RTI in the PG, no difference among participants in severity and duration of RTI.
Niele, et al[57] 2013	Preterm infants (gestational age <32 week and/or birth weight <1500 g) n=113	PG: prebiotic mixture 80% scGOS & lcFOS + 20% AOS, maximum of 1,5 g/kg/day CG: standard formula	Between days 3 and 30 of life	No difference in the incidence of RTI.
Atopic eczema				
Grüber, et al[58] 2010	Healthy term infants with low atopy risk before the age of 8 weeks n=1130	PG: formula containing GOS & FOS (9:1) 6.8 g/L plus AOS 1.2 g/L CG: standard formula BG	1 year follow-up	The cumulative incidence of atopic eczema in the PG was in the low range of the breastfed group.
Niele, et al[57] 2013	Preterm infants (gestational age <32 weeks and/or birth weight <1500 g) n=113	PG: prebiotic mixture 80% scGOS & FOS + 20% AOS, maximum of 1,5 g/kg/day CG: standard formula	Between days 3 and 30 of life	No difference in prevalence of atopic eczema.
Ziegler, et al[31] 2007	Healthy, formula-fed, term infants n=226	PG 1: PDX & GOS 4 g/L PG 2: PDX & GOS and lactulose: 8 g/L CG: standard formula	Up to 120 days of age	PGs had a statistically important risk for developing eczema.
Moro, et al[59] 2006	Infants at high risk for atopy n=259	PG: extensively hydrolyzed formula with prebiotics scGOS & lcFOS 8 g/L CG: maltodextrine	First 6 months of life	A beneficial effect of prebiotics on the development of atopic dermatitis.
Arslanoglu, et al[60] 2008	Infants at high risk for atopy n=152	PG: extensively hydrolyzed formula with prebiotics scGOS/lcFOS 8 g/L CG: maltodextrine	Follow-up until second birthday	Cumulative incidence of atopic dermatitis significantly lower in PG.
Arslanoglu, et al[61] 2012	Infants at high risk for atopy n=92	PG: extensively hydrolyzed formula with prebiotics scGOS & lsFOS 8 g/L significantly lower in the PG. CG: maltodextrine	Follow-up until fifth birthday	The prevalence and the persistence of any allergic symptoms were

n=number of participants, PG=prebiotic group, CG-Control group, BG-breast-fed comparison group, FOS-fructo-oligosaccharides, GOS-galacto-oligosaccharides, scGOS-short chain GOS, lcFOS-long chain FOS, AOS-acidic oligosaccharides, PDX-polydextrose, RTI-respiratory tract infections

of 80% of contemplated RTIs, occurred less frequently in both non-placebo groups (prebiotic group: P=0.003; probiotic group: P=0.051). There was; however, no difference among participants in severity and duration of RTI.[56] On the contrary, a study published in 2012 found no difference in the incidence of infections of respiratory and gastrointestinal system in preterm neonates supplemented with a prebiotic mixture (80% scGOS/lcFOS + 20% AOS, maximum of 1,5 g/kg/day) between days 3 and 30 of life compared to placebo.[57]

To summarize, evidence to date is often contradictory but in general does not uphold the role of prebiotics in prevention or treatment of infectious diseases. However, supplementation of prebiotic compounds in infant formulas, as early as preterm period of life, and in ORS seems to be the most useful.

Eczema (Table 16.3)

Grüber and his team performed an international double-blind placebo-controlled trial in 832 low atopy-risk infants.[58] They were assigned either to the formula containing 6.8 g/L GOS/FOS (9:1) plus AOS 1.2 g/L, or standard formula. Results were compared to 300 breast-fed infants. At one year follow-up, the prebiotic group had almost comparable incidence of eczema to breastfed babies (5.7 vs 7.3%, vs controls 9.7%). However, a similarly designed but more recent study found no difference in prevalence of atopic eczema and bronchial hyper-reactivity when GOS/FOS plus acidic oligosaccharides (4:1) mixture was added to milk formula in a lower dose (1.5 g/kg/day) in 92 preterm, low birth weight infants.[57] On the other hand, Ziegler, et al.[31] found that unselected term infants fed with chosen blends of prebiotics (polydextrose and GOS: 4 g/L vs polydextrose and GOS and lactulose: 8 g/L vs control) have a statistically important elevated risk for developing eczema (18% vs 4% vs 7%).

When concerning infants with family history of allergic disease, the representative series of studies must be the three completed by Moro and Arslanoglu together with their colleagues. They began in 2006 with a pool of 259 children assigned to extensively hydrolyzed infant formula with or without prebiotics (scGOS/lcFOS 8 g/L) them during the first six month of life. In the intervention group, 9.8% developed atopic dermatitis, and 23.1% in the placebo group (P<0.05).[59] Blinded, follow-up continued until second birthday, 107 participants dropped out. Cumulative incidences of atopic dermatitis, recurrent wheezing and allergic urticaria were higher in the control group (27.9; 20.6 and 10.3 %, respectively) compared to the prebiotic group (13.6; 7.6, and 1.5%) (P<0.05).[60] After 5 years, with 92 children remaining in the study, both the prevalence and the persistence of any allergic symptoms were significantly lower in the supplemented (30.9% and 4.8%, respectively) than in the non-supplemented group (66% and 26%, respectively) (P<0.01). The differences for rhino conjunctivitis (2.4 vs 14%) and atopic dermatitis (19.1 vs 38%) (P<0.05) were significant but not for persistent wheezing (4.8 vs 14%).[61]

There are still many questions about not only the etiology, immunology and genetics, but also about the role of prebiotic substances in prevention and/or treatment of allergic diseases. Evidence is still very sketchy; however, it seems that early supplementation, at least in predisposed population, might be of benefit.

SUMMARY

Regarding the mechanisms of action, prebiotics seem to be very appealing in prevention and treatment of many clinical conditions as in contrast to probiotics they may have more extensive influence on overall bacterial community in the gut, both regarding its composition and functioning. However, in contrast to probiotics the number of published methodologically adequate clinical trials on the efficacy of prebiotics, especially RCTs, supported with exact type and dose information, is rather sparse, especially beyond the age of infancy. The strongest evidence on beneficial effects of prebiotics in children exists in relation to the fight against constipation, poor weight-gain in preterm infants and eczema in atopic children. The reasonableness of using prebiotics in some other diseases, including infantile colic, absorption of minerals and infectious diseases is still under investigation. It must be highlighted; however, that the safety profile of prebiotic use is excellent as no adverse effects were found in this review.

In conclusion, due to their strong potential to influence gut microbiota composition and function, as well as the extremely low risk of their use for serious adverse effects, prebiotics seem to be more than a promising tool for supporting health, prevention and treatment of many pathologic conditions in the intestine and beyond it. However, further large clinical studies are required using commercially available products to help health care providers and users in making an appropriate decision concerning the correct use of prebiotics in these conditions.

REFERENCES

1. Roberfroid M, Gibson GR, Hoyles L, McCartney AL, Rastall R, Rowland I, et al. Prebiotic effects: metabolic and health benefits. Br J Nutr 2010; 104:S1-S63.

2. First ISAPP Annual Meeting Report. Available from: http://isappscience.org/annual-meeting-reports/ Accessed May 1, 2016.

3. Goldsmith JR, Sartor RB. The role of diet on intestinal microbiota metabolism: Downstream impacts on host immune function and health, and therapeutic implications. J Gastroenterol 2014;49: 785–98.

4. Weijers CAGM, Franssen MCR, Visser GM. Glycosyltransferase-catalyzed synthesis of bioactive oligosaccharides. Biotechnol Adv 2008; 26:436–56.

5. Morris C, Morris GA. The effect of inulin and fructo-oligosaccharide supplementation on the textural, rheological and sensory properties of bread and their role in weight management: A review. Food Chem 2012;133:237–48.

6. Gibson GR, Probert HM, Loo JV, Rastall RA, Roberfroid MB. Dietary modulation of the human colonic microbiota: updating the concept of prebiotics. Nutr Res Rev 2004;17:259–75.

7. Scott KP, Gratz SW, Sheridan PO, Flint HJ, Duncan SH. The influence of diet on the gut microbiota. Pharmacol Res 2013;69:52–60.

8. Commission Directive 2006/141/EC of 22 Dec 2006 on infant formulae and follow-on formulae and amending Directive 1999/21/EC. Available from: http://eurlex. europa.eu/legal-content/EN/TXT/?uri=OJ:L: 2006:401:TOC. Accessed January 24, 2016.

9. Lamsal BP. Production, health aspects and potential food uses of dairy prebiotic galacto-oligosaccharides. J Sci Food Agric 2012;92:2020–8.

10. Kothari D, Patel S, Goyal A. Therapeutic spectrum of nondigestible oligosaccharides: overview of current state and prospect. J Food Sci 2014;79: R1491–8.

11. Homayoni Rad A, Akbarzadeh F, Mehrabany EV. Which are more important: prebiotics or probiotics? Nutrition 2012;28:1196–7.

12. Everard A, Lazarevic V, Derrien M, Girard M, Muccioli GG, Neyrinck AM, et al. Responses of gut microbiota and glucose and lipid metabolism to prebiotics in genetic obese and diet-induced leptin-resistant mice. Diabetes 2011;60:2775–86.

13. Neyrinck AM, Possemiers S, Druart C, Van de Wiele T, De Backer F, Cani PD, et al. Prebiotic effect of wheat arabinoxylan related to the increase in bifidobacteria, Roseburia and Bacteroides/Prevotella in diet-induced obese mice. PLoS One 2011;6:e20944.

14. Parnell JA, Peimer RA. Prebiotic fibres dose-dependently increase satiety hormones and alter Bacteroidetes and Firmicutes in lean and obese ICR:LA-cp rats. Br J Nutr 2012;107:601–13.

15. Wasilewski A, Zielińska M, Storr M, Fichna J. Beneficial effects of probiotics, prebiotics, synbiotics, and psychobiotics in inflammatory bowel disease. Inflamm Bowel Dis 2015;21:1674–82.

16. Marcobal A, Sonnenburg JL. Human milk oligosaccharide consumption by intestinal microbiota. Clin Microbiol Infect 2012;18:12–5.

17. Jakobsdottir G, Nyman M, Fåk F. Designing future prebiotic fiber to target metabolic syndrome. Nutrition 2014;30:497–502.

18. Savino F, Palumeri E, Castagno E, Cresi F, Dalmasso P, Cavallo F, et al. Reduction of crying episodes owing to infantile colic: A randomized

controlled study on the efficacy of a new infant formula. Eur J Clin Nutr 2006;60:1304–10.

19. Pärtty A, Luoto R, Kalliomäki M, Salminen S, Isolauri E. Effects of early prebiotic and probiotic supplementation on development of gut microbiota and fussing and crying in preterm infants: a randomized, double-blind, placebo-controlled trial. J Pediatr 2013;163:1272–7.e1-2.

20. Mugambi MN, Musekiwa A, Lombard M, Young T, Blaauw R. Synbiotics, probiotics or prebiotics in infant formula for full term infants: a systematic review. Nutr J 2012;11:81.

21. Holscher HD, Faust KL, Czerkies LA, Litov R, Ziegler EE, Lessin H, et al. Effects of prebiotic-containing infant formula on gastrointestinal tolerance and fecal microbiota in a randomized controlled trial. J Parenter Enteral Nutr. 2012;36: 95S-105S.

22. Williams T, Choe Y, Price P, Katz G, Suarez F, Paule C, et al. Tolerance of forumals containing prebiotics in healthy, term infants. J Pediatr Gastroenterol Nutr 2014;59:653–8.

23. Scalabrin DM, Mitmesser SH, Welling GW, Harris CL, Marunycz JD, Walker DC, et al. New prebiotic blend of polydextrose and galacto-oligosaccharides has a bifidogenic effect in young infants. J Pediatr Gastroenterol Nutr 2012;54: 343–52.

24. Ashley C, Johnston WH, Harris CL, Stolz SI, Wampler JL, Berseth CL. Growth and tolerance of infants fed formula supplemented with poly-dextrose (PDX) and/or galactooligosaccharides (GOS): double-blind, rando-mized, controlled trial. Nutr J 2012;11:38.

25. Ribeiro TC, Costa-Ribeiro H Jr, Almeida PS, Pontes MV, Leite ME, Filadelfo LR, et al. Stool pattern changes in toddlers consuming a follow-on formula supplemented with polydextrose and galactooligosaccharides. J Pediatr Gastroenterol Nutr 2012;54:288–90.

26. Veereman-Wauters G, Staelens S, Van de Broek H, Plaskie K, Wesling F, Roger LC, et al. Physiological and bifidogenic effects of prebiotic supplements in infant formulae. J Pediatr Gastroenterol Nutr 2011;52:763–71.

27. Westerbeek EA, Hensgens RL, Mihatsch WA, Boehm G, Lafeber HN, van Elburg RM. The effect of neutral and acidic oligosaccharides on stool viscosity, stool frequency and stool pH in preterm infants. Acta Paediatr 2011;100:1426–31.

28. Vivatvakin B, Mahayosnond A, Theamboonlers A, Steenhout PG, Conus NJ. Effect of a whey-predominant starter formula containing LCPUFAs

and oligosaccharides (FOS/GOS) on gastrointestinal comfort in infants. Asia Pac J Clin Nutr 2010;19:473–80.

29. Bisceglia M, Indrio F, Riezzo G, Poerio V, Corapi U, Raimondi F. The effect of prebiotics in the management of neonatal hyperbilirubinaemia. Acta Paediatr 2009; 98:1579–81.

30. Rao S, Srinivasjois R, Patole S. Prebiotic supplementation in full-term neonates: a systematic review of randomized controlled trials. Arch Pediatr Adolesc Med 2009;163:755–64.

31. Ziegler E, Vanderhoof JA, Petschow B, Mitmesser SH, Stolz SI, Harris CL, et al. Term infants fed formula supplemented with selected blends of prebiotics grow normally and have soft stools similar to those reported for breast-fed infants. J Pediatr Gastroenterol Nutr 2007;44:359–64.

32. Scholtens PA, Goossens DA, Staiano A. Stool characteristics of infants receiving short-chain galacto-oligosaccharides andlong-chain fructo-oligosaccharides: a review. World J Gastroenterol 2014;20:13446–52.

33. Bongers ME, de Lorijn F, Reitsma JB, Groeneweg M, Taminiau JA, Benninga MA. The clinical effect of a new infant formula in term infants with constipation: a double-blind, randomized crossover trial. Nutr J 2007;6:8.

34. Szurszewski JH. A migrating electric complex of canine small intestine. Am J Physiol 1969;217: 1757-63.

35. Dasopoulou M, Briana DD, Boutsikou T, Karakasidou E, Roma E, Costalos C, et al. Motilin and gastrin secretion and lipid profile in preterm neonates following prebiotics supplementation: a double-blind randomized controlled study. J Parenter Enteral Nutr 2015;39:359–68.

36. Issenman RM, Hewson S, Pirhonen D, Taylor W, Tirosh A. Are chronic digestive complaints the result of abnormal dietary patterns? Diet and digestive complaints in children at 22 and 40 months of age. Am J Dis Child 1987;141:679–82.

37. Ip KS, Lee WT, Chan JS, Young BW. A community-based study of the prevalence of constipation in young children and the role of dietary fibre. Hong Kong Med J 2005;11:431–6.

38. Hyman PE, Milla PJ, Benninga MA, Davidson GP, Fleisher DF, Taminiau J. Childhood functional gastrointestinal disorders: neonate/toddler. Gastroenterology 2006;130:1519–26.

39. Van Ginkel R, Reitsma JB, Büller HA, van Wijk MP, Taminiau JA, Benninga MA. Childhood constipation: longitudinal follow-up beyond puberty. Gastro-enterology 2003;125:357–363.

40. Sabater-Molina M, Larqué E, Torrella F, Zamora S. Dietary fructooligosaccharides and potential benefits on health. J Physiol Biochem 2009;65: 315–28.

41. Abrams SA, Griffin IJ, Hawthorne KM, Liang L, Gunn SK, Darlington G, *et al.* A combination of prebiotic short- and long-chain inulin-type fructans enhances calcium absorption and bone mineralization in young adolescents. Am J Clin Nutr 2005;82:471–6.

42. Hicks PD, Hawthorne KM, Berseth CL, Marunycz JD, Heubi JE, Abrams SA. Total calcium absorption is similar from infant formulas with and without prebiotics and exceeds that in human milk-fed infants. BMC Pediatr 2012; 12:118.

43. Laparra JM, Díez-Municio M, Herrero M, Moreno FJ. Structural differences of prebiotic oligosaccharides influence their capability to enhance iron absorption in deficient rats. Food Funct 2014;5: 2430–7.

44. Darzi J, Frost GS, Robertson MD. Do SCFA have a role in appetite regulation? Proc Nutr Soc. 2011;70:119–28.

45. Carlson JJ, Eisenmann JC, Norman GJ, Ortiz KA, Young PC. Dietary fiber and nutrient density are inversely associated with the metabolic syndrome in US adolescents. J Am Diet Assoc 2011; 111:1688–95.

46. Liu S, Willett WC, Manson JE, Hu FB, Rosner B, Colditz G. Relation between changes in intakes of dietary fiber and grain products and changes in weight and development of obesity among middle-aged women. Am J Clin Nutr 2003;78: 920–7.

47. Brauchla M, Juan W, Story J, Kranz S. Sources of Dietary Fiber and the Association of Fiber Intake with Childhood Obesity Risk (in 2–18 year olds) and Diabetes Risk of Adolescents 12–18 year olds: NHANES 2003–2006. Nutr Metab 2012; 2012:736258.

48. Bruzzese E, Volpicelli M, Squeglia V, Bruzzese D, Salvini F, Bisceglia M, *et al.* A formula containing galacto- and fructo-oligosaccharides prevents intestinal and extra-intestinal infections: An observational study. Clin Nutr 2009;28:156–61.

49. Duggan C, Penny ME, Hibberd P, Gil A, Huapaya A, Cooper A, *et al.* Oligofructose-supplemented infant cereal: 2 randomized, blinded, community-basedtrials in Peruvian infants. Am J Clin Nutr. 2003;77:937–42.

50. Brunser O, Gotteland M, Cruchet S, Figueroa G, Garrido D, Steenhout P. Effect of a milk formula with prebiotics on the intestinal microbiota of infants after anantibiotic treatment. Pediatr Res 2006;59:451–6.

51. ESPGHAN Working Group on Probiotics and Prebiotics, Szajewska H, Weizman Z, Abu-Zekry M, Kekez AJ, Braegger CP, Kolacek S, Micetic-Turk D, Ruszczyñski M, Vukavic T. Inulin and fructo-oligosaccharides for the prevention of antibiotic-associated diarrhea in children: report by the ESPGHAN Working Group on Probiotics and Prebiotics. J Pediatr Gastroenterol Nutr 2012; 54:828–9.

52. Hoekstra JH, Szajewska H, Zikri MA, Micetic-Turk D, Weizman Z, Papadopoulou A, *et al.* Oral rehydration solution containing a mixture of non-digestible carbohydrates in the treatment of acute diarrhea: a multicenter randomized placebo controlled study on behalf of the ESPGHAN working group on intestinal infections. J Pediatr Gastroenterol Nutr 2004;39:239–45.

53. Vaisman N, Press J, Leibovitz E, Boehm G, Barak V. Short-term effect of prebiotics administration on stool characteristics and serumcytokines dynamics in very young children with acute diarrhea. Nutrients 2010;2:683–92.

54. Passariello A, Terrin G, De Marco G, Cecere G, Ruotolo S, Marino A, *et al.* Efficacy of a new hypotonic oral rehydration solution containing zinc and prebioticsin the treatment of childhood acute diarrhea: a randomized controlled trial. J Pediatr 2011;158:288–92.

55. Alam NH, Meier R, Schneider H, Sarker SA, Bardhan PK, Mahalanabis D, *et al.* Partially hydrolyzed guar gum-supplemented oral rehydration solution in thetreatment of acute diarrhea in children. J Pediatr Gastroenterol Nutr 2000; 31:503–7.

56. Luoto R, Ruuskanen O, Waris M, Kalliomäki M, Salminen S, Isolauri E. Prebiotic and probiotic supplementation prevents rhinovirus infections in preterm infants: a randomized, placebo-controlled trial. J Allergy Clin Immunol 2014;133: 405–13.

57. Niele N, van Zwol A, Westerbeek EA, Lafeber HN, van Elburg RM. Effect of non-human neutral and acidic oligosaccharides on allergic and infectious diseases in preterm infants. Eur J Pediatr 2013;172:317–23.

58. Grüber C, van Stuijvenberg M, Mosca F, Moro G, Chirico G, Braegger CP, *et al.* MIPS 1 Working Group. Reduced occurrence of early atopic

dermatitis because of immunoactive prebiotic-samong low-atopy-risk infants. J Allergy Clin Immunol 2010;126:791–7.

59. Moro G, Arslanoglu S, Stahl B, Jelinek J, Wahn U, Boehm G. A mixture of prebiotic oligosaccharides reduces the incidence of atopic dermatitis during the first six months of age. Arch Dis Child 2006;91:814–9.

60. Arslanoglu S, Moro GE, Schmitt J, Tandoi L, Rizzardi S, Boehm G. Early dietary inter-vention with a mixture of prebiotic oligosac-charides reduces the incidence of allergic mani-festations and infections during the first two years of life. J Nutr 2008;138:1091–5.

61. Arslanoglu S, Moro GE, Boehm G, Wienz F, Stahl B, Bertino E. Early neutral prebiotic oligosaccharide supplementation reduces the incidence of some allergic manifestations in the first 5 years of life. J Biol Regul Homeost Agents 2012;26:49–59.

Introduction of Inactivated Poliovirus Vaccine in National Immunization Program and Polio Endgame Strategy

Vipin M Vashishtha, Jaydeep Choudhary, Sangeeta Yadav, Jeeson C Unni, Pramod Jog, Sachidanand S Kamath, Anupam Sachdeva, Sanjay Srirampur, Baldev Prajapati, Bakul J Parekh

In January 2013, the Global Polio Eradication Initiative (GPEI) launched the Polio Eradication and Endgame Strategic Plan 2013–2018, which was developed with an approach to tackle both wild and vaccine virus eradication in parallel rather than sequential manner.[1] In the November 2013 meeting, the Strategic Advisory Group of Experts (SAGE) on immunization recommended a global, coordinated withdrawal of the type 2 component of trivalent oral polio vaccine (tOPV) from immunization programmes by April 2016. For countries which use only tOPV in their routine infant immunization programmes, this will require switching from tOPV to bOPV (containing only types 1 and 3) for that purpose.[2] Prior to this switch, SAGE recommends that all countries introduce at least one dose of inactivated poliovirus vaccine (IPV) into their infant immunization schedules as a risk mitigation measure by providing immunity in case a type 2 poliovirus re-emerges or is reintroduced.[2] Initially, the plan stresses the need to introduce IPV at least 6 months in advance to the proposed switch date in order to provide adequate time to enhance population immunity against type 2.[1] SAGE recommends that one dose of IPV should be administered at or after 14 weeks of age through routine immunization (RI), in addition to the 3–4 doses of OPV. The group also offers flexibility to countries to consider alternative schedules (e.g. earlier IPV administration) based on local conditions; for example, documented risk of vaccine-associated paralytic poliomyelitis (VAPP) prior to 4 months of age.[2]

Three main risks are identified following type 2 poliovirus removal. These include immediate time-limited risk of circulating vaccine-derived poliovirus type 2 (cVDPV2) emergence; medium- and long-term risks of type 2 poliovirus re-introduction from a vaccine manufacturing site, research facility, diagnostic laboratory or a bioterrorism event; and spread of virus from rare immune-deficient individuals who are chronically infected with OPV2.[3] All these risks have the potential to cause substantial polio outbreaks or even re-establishment of polio virus transmission in polio-free regions.

GOVERNMENT OF INDIA INITIATIVES

Following SAGE recommendations and GPEI directives, the Government of India (GoI) has taken following decisions regarding polio immunization during implementation of endgame strategies in India:

- Introduction of at least single dose of intramuscular IPV (IM-IPV) administration at

14 weeks or first contact afterwards in the RI along with 3rd dose of DTP in 6 states viz. Bihar, Uttar Pradesh, Madhya Pradesh, Gujarat, Punjab and Assam;[4]

- Nationally coordinated switch from tOPV to bOPV all over the country on 25th April 2016 associated with cessation of use, withdrawal, destruction and validation of all available tOPV stocks from all over the country.[5]
- Introduction of fractional dose (0.1 mL) intradermal IPV (ID-fIPV) at 6 and 14 weeks in Orissa, Andhra Pradesh, Telangana, Tamil Nadu, Kerala, Karnataka, Maharashtra and Puducherry from April, 2016.[6] This change in approach from single-dose intramuscular IPV to fractional-dose intradermal IPV is mainly due to scarcity of IPV.

PERSPECTIVES OF ADVISORY COMMITTEE OF VACCINES AND IMMUNIZATION PRACTICES (ACVIP) OF INDIAN ACADEMY OF PAEDIATRICS (IAP)

Role of IPV in Raising Population Immunity Against Type 2 Poliovirus Before the 'Switch'

The GPEI has recommended introduction of IPV in RI well-before (i.e. 6 months prior) to the proposed 'switch' in order to raise population immunity against type 2.[1] The committee has reviewed the practical aspects of this decision and concludes that the impact of IPV would not be significant in raising population immunity against type 2 virus before the 'switch'. There are many states that have not yet introduced IPV in their immunization schedules. On the other hand, there is no data regarding the coverage of single dose of IPV from the Indian states that have already introduced the vaccine. The 'population immunity' is a product of IPV immunogenicity and coverage. Hence, the immunity provided by tOPV, through RI and supplementary immunization activities (SIAs) would ultimately determine the population immunity against type 2 poliovirus prior to proposed global switch to bOPV from tOPV. The

committee believes that a high performance round with tOPV would have benefitted more than IPV introduction to raise population immunity against type 2 before the switch. In recent trials, tOPV is found to be more immunogenic than IPV against type 2 poliovirus.[7]

Single Dose of Intramuscular IPV at 14 Weeks: Will it be Effective?

The ACVIP has also reviewed the decision to administer a single dose of IM-IPV at 14 weeks. It believes that the combined schedule of bOPV and IPV shall provide adequate protection against type 1 and 3 polioviruses; however, it is the protection against type 2 polioviruses, especially for the children born post-switch that should be the major concern. A single dose of IPV at 14 weeks may not provide adequate seroconversion, especially against type 2 in the vaccinees. The committee reiterates its earlier recommendation that at least two doses of IPV—given at or after 8 weeks of age with 8 week interval—are mandatory to provide adequate seroprotection to all the three serotypes of poliovirus.[8] A recent systematic review conducted on immunogenicity and effectiveness of 1 or 2 doses of IPV vaccine has also reaffirmed ACVIP's above recommendations. The review concludes that routine immunization with two full or fractional doses of IPV given after 10 weeks of age is likely to protect >80% of recipients against all types of polioviruses.[9] According to this review, one and two full doses of intramuscular IPV seroconverted 41% and 80% subjects, respectively, against serotype 2.[9] The GPEI's decision of introducing a single dose of IPV is based on a Cuban study[10] in which 63% of subjects seroconverted to a single dose when given at 4 months of age and among those who did not seroconvert (37%), 98% had a priming response to a subsequent dose of IPV.[10] However, there are certain issues that deserve attention. First, there is no incontrovertible proof of reasonably good seroconversion of single dose of IPV at 14 weeks. In the Cuban trial, the first dose of IPV was given at

4 months, not at 14 weeks. It is not yet clear whether immunological priming after a single dose of IPV is protective against paralytic disease. Another risk would be leaving children 'unprotected' against type 2 for first 3–4 months of life. Further, the coverage attained with 14-week IPV dose would be considerably less than at 6 weeks, considering the current 'drop-out' rates of DTP 3. A recent study from Bangladesh[7] revealed promising degree of priming with an early (6 week) dose of IPV. The cumulative effect of one dose given at 6 weeks (seroconversion and priming) was seen in 90.2% of subjects.[7] The committee opines that decisions having far reaching impact on global health should have broader evidence base; solely relying on few studies may prove perilous.

Intradermal Fractional Doses of IPV at 6 and 14 Weeks: IAP ACVIP's Viewpoint

The ACVIP has not yet approved the use of intradermal fractional-dose IPV (ID-fIPV) for office-practice. However, in wake of recent developments, the committee has reviewed all the available recent studies on immunogenicity and priming of ID-fIPV[7,10–14] (Table 17.1). Most of these studies have reported lower immunogenicity of a one-fifth (i.e. 0.1 mL) ID-fIPV dose compared with full dose (i.e. 0.5 mL) IM-IPV. Also, the geometric mean titers (GMTs) of poliovirus-specific serum neutralizing antibodies were found significantly lower than full dose IM-IPV.[7,10–14] Seroconversion appears to be dependent on the age at administration of the first dose and the interval between the doses. However, despite limited seroconversion with first dose, a considerable priming responses were observed even after one dose of ID-fIPV given at different ages.[7,10] In all of these studies, barring one,[11] different types of needle-free devices (jet injectors or micro-needle based devices) were utilized to deliver ID dose of IPV. In the Indian study conducted in Vellore,[11] needle and syringes were used to deliver ID-fIPV. In this study, the seroconversion against type 2 poliovirus after 4 weeks of 2nd dose at 14 weeks was 70%.[11]

The recent recommendation of GPEI/GoI to use fractional dose IPV by ID route is based on the trial done in Bangladesh.[7] In this study, ID-fIPV failed the non-inferiority test (i.e. with a non-inferiority margin of 10% in seroconversion) when compared with full dose IM-IPV for all serotypes for seroconversion and priming observed with 1 or 2 doses. The seroconversion at 18 weeks following two doses of fIPV at 6 and 14 weeks was 80.9% whereas the corresponding rate for IM-IPV was 91%.[7] Further, the GoI intends to use standard BCG needle and syringe for intradermal administration of ID-fIPV whereas in the Bangladesh study, a microneedle based device (MicronJet 600) was used.[7] It would have been more appropriate to consider Vellore study[11] while recommending two-dose ID-fIPV schedule for eight states as in this study, needle and syringes instead of needle-free devices were used as GoI is now planning to utilize in field.

THE CURRENT SCENARIO AND THE NEW OBJECTIVES OF IAP-ACVIP RECOMMENDATIONS

With the introduction of single dose of intramuscular IPV in RI of six Indian states from November 2015, and GoI's proposed introduction of two doses of ID-fIPV in rest of the country from April 2016, there is a lot of confusion amongst pediatricians/IAP members regarding the exact IPV schedule for primary immunization. The scarcity of IPV, particularly in private market, has further aggravated the confusion. The IAP-ACVIP is recommending three doses of IPV, given intramuscularly at 6, 10, and 14 weeks or two doses at 8 and 16 weeks of age for primary immunization in its schedule.[8]

The main objective of GoI's initiatives (described above) is to enhance population immunity against type 2 poliovirus just prior to proposed switch from t-OPV to b-OPV in April 2016 so that the risks associated with the complete removal of type 2 vaccine virus can be mitigated. The decision to employ only a single dose of IPV and two doses of intra-

TABLE 17.1: Seroconversion after two intradermal fractional (1/5th) dose of inactivated poliovirus vaccine (ID-fIPV)

Reference	Place	Schedule (age at doses)	Age at which SC by serotype*	Mode of delivery (of ID-fIPV)	No. of participants	SC by serotype* (%)					
						(After 1st dose)			(After 2nd dose)		
						P1	P2	P3	P1	P2	P3
Nirmal, et al.[11]	India	6, 14 wk	18 wk	Needle and syringe	30	–	–	–	90	70	97
Resik, et al.[12]	Cuba	6, 10 wk	10 and 14 wk	Biojector 2000	187	5	19	7	27	55	43
Mohammed, et al.[13]	Oman	2 m, 4 m	4 and 6 m	Biojector 2000	186	10	17	9	70	72	72
Estívariz, et al.[14]	India	6–9 m	4 wk later	PharmaJet	Variable#	100#	59	36	–	–	–
Resik, et al.[10]	Cuba	4 m, 8 m	8 and 9 m	Biojector 2000	157	17	47	15	94	98	93
Anand, et al.[7]	Bangladesh	6, 14 wk	14 and 18 wk	MicronJet 600	155	13	19	14	88	81	89

SC: Seroconversion; ID-fIPV: Intradermal fractional dose IPV; *Definition of seroconversion: 4-fold increase in serum neutralising antibodies over expected titre based on 28–30 day half-life of maternal antibodies, or a change from undetectable to detectable antibodies; **In this study conducted in Moradabad, India, the enrolled subjects had already received multiple doses of OPV; #A single dose of fIPV was given to 6–9 m old children. The above figure shows seroconversion of seronegative children. In type 1 group, only 1 child was seronegative; in type 2 and type 3 groups, 41 and 78 children were seronegative, respectively. In children who were type-1 seropositive, an increase of more than four times in antibody titre was detected 56% (9/16) subjects 28 days after they were given intradermal IPV.

dermal IPV is only an interim arrangement owing mainly to the limited supply and availability of IPV. On the other hand, the main aim of existing IAP-ACVIP guidelines on polio immunization[8] is to provide almost 100% protection against VAPP along with the best possible humoral and mucosal protection against polioviruses to an individual child in office practice setting. Considering the recent initiatives taken by the GoI as described above, the ACVIP will have to add another objective, i.e. to provide protection against type 2 poliovirus to naive children born post-switch. IPV would be the only source of providing immunity against type 2 poliovirus to children after April 2016. Therefore, the focus would be protection against VAPP along with provision of protection against type 2 poliovirus by maximizing type 2 population immunity. Since the threat of cVDPV type 2 emergence would be greatest, at least for one year following tOPV to bOPV switch, the latter objective would need to override the former for the time being.

REFERENCES

1. Global Polio Eradication Initiative. Polio Eradication & Endgame Strategic Plan 2013–2018. WHO/POLIO/13.02. Available from: http://www.polioeradication.org/Portals/0/Document/Resources/StrategyWork/PEESP_EN_US.pdf 2013. Accessed on April 5, 2016.

2. Meeting of the Strategic Advisory Group of Experts on immunization, November 2013–Conclusions and recommendations. Wkly Epidemiol Rec 2014;89:1–20.

3. World Health Organization, Background and Technical Rationale for Introduction of One dose of Inactivated Polio Vaccine (IPV) in Routine Immunization Schedule, October 2015. Available from:http://www.who.int/immunization/diseases/poliomyelitis/inactivated_polio_vaccine/ipv-technical-manual-aug2014.pdf. Accessed April 05, 2016.

4. Prasad R. A vaccine boost to India's polio fight. The Hindu, November 29, 2015. Available from: http://www.thehindu.com/opinion/op-ed/a-vaccine-boost-to-indias-polio-fight/article7927744.ece Accessed December 26, 2015.

5. Ministry of Health and Family Welfare, Government of India. Minutes of the meeting for tOPV to bOPV switch. Available from: http://emedinews.in/2016/jan/Final-Minutes-of-meeting-on-tOPV-to-bOPV-Switch-in-India.pdf. Accessed December 26, 2015.

6. Deliberations at Mini-India Expert Advisory Group (IEAG) on Polio Eradication held on 26th February, 2016, New Delhi. Available from: www.who.int/immunization/sage/meetings/2016/april/3-Conclusions-recommendations_mini_IEAG_26_Feb2016_NewDelhi.pdf. Accessed July 26, 2016.

7. Anand A, Zaman K, Estívariz CF, Yunus M, Gary HE, Weldon WC, et al. Early priming with inactivated poliovirus vaccine (IPV) and intradermal fractional dose IPV administered by a microneedle device: A randomized controlled trial. Vaccine 2015;33:6816–22.

8. Indian Academy of Pediatrics Committee on Immunization (IAPCOI). Consensus recommendations on immunization and IAP immunization timetable 2012. Indian Pediatr 2012;49:549–64.

9. Grassly NC. Immunogenicity and effectiveness of routine immunization with 1 or 2 doses of inactivated poliovirus vaccine: systematic review and meta-analysis. J Infect Dis 2014;210 (Suppl 1): S439–46.

10. Resik S, Tejeda A, Sutter RW, Diaz M, Sarmiento L, Alemañi N, et al. Priming after a fractional dose of inactivated poliovirus vaccine. N Engl J Med 2013;368:416–24.

11. Nirmal S, Cherian T, Samuel BU, Rajasingh J, Raghupathy P, John TJ. Immune response of infants to fractional doses of intradermally administered inactivated poliovirus vaccine. Vaccine 1998;16:928–31.

12. Resik S, Tejeda A, Lago PM, Diaz M, Carmenates A, Sarmiento L, et al. Randomized controlled clinical trial of fractional doses of inactivated poliovirus vaccine administered intradermally by needle-free device in Cuba. J Infect Dis 2010;201: 1344–52.

13. Mohammed AJ, Al Awaidy S, Bawikar S, Kurup PJ, Elamir E, Shaban MM, et al. Fractional doses of inactivated poliovirus vaccine in Oman. N Engl J Med 2010;362:2351–9.

14. Estívariz CF, Jafari H, Sutter RW, John TJ, Jain V, Agarwal A, et al. Immunogenicity of supplemental doses of poliovirus vaccine for children aged 6–9 months in Moradabad, India: A community-based, randomised controlled trial. Lancet Infect Dis 2012;12:128–35.

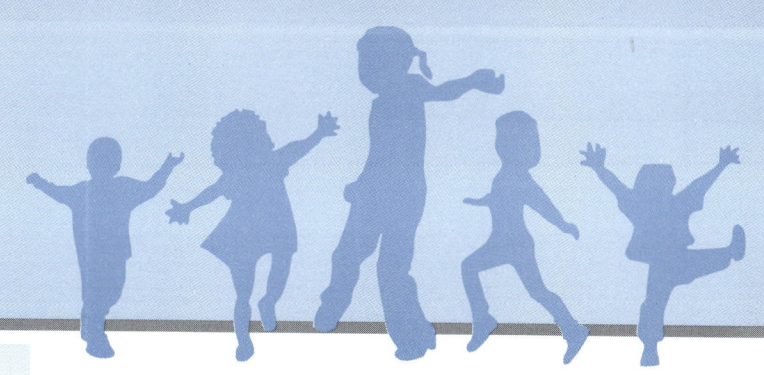

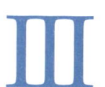

IAP-ACVIP Recommended Immunization Schedule (2018–19) and Update on Immunization*

S Balasubramanian, Abhay Shah, Harish K Pemde, Pallab Chatterjee, S Shivananda, Vijay Kumar Guduru, Santosh Soans, Digant Shastri, Remesh Kumar

The Indian Academy of Pediatrics (IAP) Advisory Committee on Vaccines and Immunization Practices (ACVIP) has recently reviewed and updated the recommended immunization schedule for children aged 0 through 18 years based on recent evidence for the vaccines licensed in India. The process of preparing the new recommendations consisted of review of data and literature, consultative meetings twice (4th and 5th August 2018 at Mangalore, and 22nd and 23rd September 2018 at Chennai), taking the opinion of various National Experts and arriving at a consensus and drafting the recommendations while taking into consideration the existing National immunization schedule and policies of the government. All decisions were taken unanimously and voting was not required for any issue. The recommendations in brief along with supporting evidence from relevant literature are presented in this article. The detailed information will be presented later in IAP Guidebook on Immunization. While using these guidelines, pediatricians are free to use their discretion in a particular situation within the suggested framework.

The current IAP ACVIP recommendations for the 2018–19 IAP Immunization Timetable are presented in Table 18.1 and Fig. 18.1, and this also include some alterations from the earlier recommended schedule.[1]

HEPATITIS B VACCINE

The burden of chronic hepatitis B virus infection is substantial as the coverage of the birth-dose (estimated as 39% globally) is still low. World Health Organization (WHO) Position paper 2017 states that hepatitis B vaccine (HBV) should be administered as a birth dose, preferably within 24 hours (timely birth dose).[2] This dose may only be delayed if the mother is known to be hepatitis-B surface antigen (HBsAg) negative at the time of delivery. When the HBsAg report of the mother is not known or reported incorrectly, or in case of infants born to HBsAg positive mothers, this dose becomes a very important safety net.[3]

Four doses of hepatitis B vaccine may be administered for programmatic reasons (e.g. 3 doses of hepatitis B-containing combination vaccine or monovalent HBV after a single monovalent dose at birth.[2]

---

*Indian Academy of Pediatrics (IAP)-Advisory Committee on vaccines and Immunization Practices (ACVIP) Recommended Immunization Schedule (2018–19) and Update on Immunization for Children Aged 0 Through 18 Years

TABLE 18.1: Key updates and major changes in recommendations for IAP immunization timetable, 2018–2019

Hepatitis B vaccine
- One dose of hepatitis B vaccine within 24 hours of birth.
- In case of use of a combination vaccines a total of four doses of hepatitis B vaccine are justified.

DTwP, DTaP and combination vaccines
- DTwP or DTaP can be offered in primary series.

Polio vaccines
- Ideally IPV should replace OPV as early as possible.
- Three doses of intramuscular IPV in primary series is the best option.
- Two doses of intramuscular IPV instead of three for primary series if started at 8 weeks, with an interval of 8 weeks between two doses is an alternative.
- In case IPV is not available or feasible, the child should be offered three doses of bOPV. In such cases, the child should be referred for two fractional doses of IPV at a Government facility at 6 and 14 weeks or at least one dose of intramuscular IPV, either standalone or as a combination vaccine, at 14 weeks of age.

Rotavirus vaccine
- In case of Rotavirus vaccine, RV1 can be used in 6, 10 weeks schedule.

Influenza vaccine
- Inactivated influenza vaccine (either trivalent or quadrivalent) is recommended routinely to all children below 5 years of age starting from 6 months of age annually (2–4 weeks before influenza season).

Measles-containing vaccines
- Measles-containing vaccine (MMR/MR) should be administered after 9 months of age.
- MR vaccine as part of the national campaign is to be administered irrespective of previous vaccination.

Typhoid vaccines
- Single dose of any of Typhoid conjugate vaccine (TCV 25 mg) is recommended from 6 months onwards and can be administered with MMR also.
- Booster dose of Typhoid conjugate vaccine not recommended in subsequent years.

Rabies vaccines
- ACVIP IAP endorses administration of a 4-dose schedule of Rabies vaccine recommended by WHO 2018 for Post-exposure prophylaxis.
- ACVIP also endorses administration of Rabies monoclonal antibody as an alternative to Rabies immunoglobulin for category-III bites.

ACVIP: Advisory Committee on Vaccines and Immunization Practices; IAP: Indian Academy of Pediatrics; IPV: Injectable polio vaccine; OPV: Oral polio vaccine; bOPV: bivalent oral polio vaccine; MR: Measles-Rubella vaccine; MMR: Measles-Mumps-Rubella vaccine

DIPTHERIA, TETANUS AND PERTUSSIS VACCINES (DTWP AND DTAP)

Long-term efficacy over 10 years has been observed to be superior with whole cell pertussis vaccine (wP).[4] Recent outbreaks of pertussis in various developed countries have sparked a debate on the effectiveness of acellular pertussis (aP) vaccines. However, none of these countries are planning to revert back to whole-cell pertussis vaccines as that can result in an increase in the prevalence of the disease due to poor acceptance of a vaccine that is much more reactogenic.[5] Though the reasons for this resurgence are complex and vary from place to place, the lesser duration of protection and decreased impact on transmission of the disease by acellular pertussis vaccines appears to be crucial.[6] Waning of immunity has been reported with whole cell and acellular vaccines over a period of time. Current evidence suggests that the efficacy of

	Birth	6 wk	10 wk	14 wk	6 m	9 m	12 m	13 m	15 m	16–18 m	2–3 yr	4–6 yr	9–14 yr	15–18 yr
BCG	BCG													
Hepatitis B	HB 1	HB 2	HB 3	HB*4										
Polio	OPV 0	IPV** 1	IPV** 2	IPV** 3						IPV*** B1				
DTwP/DTaP		DTP 1	DTP 2	DTP 3						DTP B1		DTP B2		
HiB		HiB 1	HiB 2	HiB 3						HiB B1				
Pneumococcal		PCV 1	PCV 2	PCV 3					PCV B1				PCV	
Rotavirus		Rota 1	Rota 2	Rota 3****										
MMR						MMR 1			MMR 2			MMR3/MMRV		
Varicella									Varicella 1			Varicella 2		
Hepatitis A							Hep A1			Hep A2*****				
Typhoid					TCV#									
Influenza							Influenza (yearly)******							
Meningococcal						MCV 1	MCV 2				MCV			
JE							JE 1	JE 2						
Tdap													Tdap	Td
HPV##													HPV 1 and 2	HPV 1,2,3
Cholera									Cholera 1 and 2					
	Range of recommended age for all children								Range of recommended age for catch-up immunization					
	Range of recommended age for high-risk children/area								Not recommended					

*Fourth dose of hepatitis B permissible for combination vaccines only

**In case IPV is not available or feasible, the child should be offered bOPV (3 doses). In such cases, give two fractional doses of IPV at 6 wk and 14 wk

***b–OPV, if IPV booster (standalone or combination not feasible

****Third dose not required for RV1. Catch-up to 1 year of age UIP schedule

*****Live attenuated Hepatitis A vaccine: single dose only

******Begin influenza vaccination after 6 months of age, about 2–4 weeks before season; give 2 doses at the interval of 4 weeks during first year and then single does yearly till 5 years of age

TCV= Typhoid conjugate vaccine; ## HPV= Human papilloma virus

Meningococcal vaccine (MCV): 9 months through 23 months: 2 doses, at least 3 months apart; 2 years through 55 years; single dose only

Japanese Encephalitis (JE): For individuals living in endemic areas and for travelers to JE endemic area provided their expected stay is for a minimum period of 4 weeks

HPV: Two doses at 6 months interval 9–14 years age; 3 doses (at 0,1–2 and 6 months) 15 years or older and immunocompromised

Cholera vaccine: Two doses 2 weeks apart for >1 year old; for individuals living in high endemic area and traveling to areas where risk to transmission is very high

Fig. 18.1: IAP-ACVIP Recommended immunization schedule for children aged 0–18 years (2018–19)

both aP and wP vaccines in preventing pertussis in the first year is equivalent. After the first year, the immunity wanes more rapidly with the aP vaccines and the impact on transmission by aP vaccines is also inferior to wP vaccines.[7–9] WHO clearly mentions that countries currently using the wP vaccine in their national programs should continue the same for the primary series,[10,11] while those using the aP vaccine should continue the same and consider additional boosters and strategies like immunization of mothers in case of pertussis resurgence.[10] The duration of protection for both the aP and wP vaccines after the three primary doses and a booster dose at least after a year varies from 6–12 years.[11] A German study reported acellular pertussis vaccine being quite efficacious (88.7%) (95% CI, 76.6% to 94.6%).[12]

Number of Components

In a couple of systematic reviews, it was concluded that multi-component acellular pertussis vaccines are more efficacious than the single- or two-component vaccines.[13,14] However, effectiveness studies of long-term usage of two-component acellular pertussis vaccines in Sweden[15] and Japan,[16] and the mono-component vaccine in Denmark showed high effectiveness in prevention of pertussis. Thus the higher efficacy for the multi-component vaccine as demonstrated in the trials should be cautiously interpreted, and at present the evidence is insufficient to conclude categorically that the effectiveness of the aP vaccines is related to the number of components alone.[10]

IAP-ACVIP Recommendation on Pertussis-Containing Vaccines

The primary series should be completed with three doses of either wP or aP vaccines, irrespective of the number of components. wP vaccine is definitely superior to aP vaccine in terms of immunogenicity and duration of protection but more reactogenic. In view of parental anxiety and concerns for its reacto-

genicity, aP vaccine can also be administered even in the primary series. The primary aim is to increase the vaccination coverage with either of the vaccines.

POLIO VACCINES

The elimination of circulating wild poliovirus from our country and the decline worldwide in the number of cases is the proof of efficacy of Oral polio vaccine (OPV). At the beginning of 2013, 126 countries using OPV exclusively, decided to introduce Injectable polio vaccine (IPV), at least one dose, in their National Immunization Schedule. This was part of WHO's Endgame Plan to withdraw type-2 polio virus and prepare for 'the switch' from trivalent OPV (tOPV) to bivalent OPV (bOPV) in April 2016.[17,18] However, IPV introduction in these countries has increased the global IPV demand, to over 200 million in 2016 from 80 million in 2013.[17,18] The attempt to meet the global requirements for IPV by rapidly increasing the IPV production has led to multiple challenges, resulting in a shortage worldwide. Intradermal IPV administration with fractional doses of IPV (fIPV) (0.1 mL or one-fifth of a full dose) offers potential cost reduction and allows immunization of a larger number of persons with a given vaccine supply.[19] Two fractional doses administered *via* the intradermal (ID) route offer higher immunogenicity compared to one full intramuscular (IM) dose of IPV.[20–23] As a result, a two-dose fIPV schedule has been strongly recommended to countries that are endemic and the those with high risk of importation of wild polio virus.[24]

Private medical practitioners have irregular and inadequate access to standalone IPV, and are thus compelled to administer combination vaccines, and thus are not able to follow the Indian government schedule, which consists of fIPV and standalone IPV. It is not feasible for pediatricians in private settings to refer all children to government facilities for the same. In addition, the recent controversy of the contamination of OPV with type-2 Poliovirus has resulted in the awareness of vaccine-derived paralytic poliomyelitis (VDPP) amongst public. In this background, there is a need to recommend a regimen containing IPV as combination vaccine in the private settings.

IAP-ACVIP Recommendations

- Birth dose of OPV is a must.
- Extra doses of OPV on all Supplementary immunization activities should continue.
- No child should leave the health facility without polio immunization (IPV or OPV), if indicated by the schedule.
- bOPV should be continued in place of IPV, only if IPV is not feasible, with a minimum of 3 doses at 6,10,14 weeks of age.
- Minimum age of administration of IPV is 6 weeks with the best option being 3 doses of IM IPV in 6–10–14 weeks schedule. This can be as a combination vaccine, in view of non-availability of standalone IM IPV.
- Two doses of IM IPV, instead of 3 doses can be administered provided the primary series is started at 8 weeks with the minimum interval between them being 8 weeks.
- In case IPV is not available or feasible, the child should be offered 3 doses of bOPV in a 6–10–14 weeks schedule. In such cases, the child should be advised to receive two fractional doses of IPV at a Government facility at 6 and 14 weeks of age or at least one dose of IM IPV either standalone or as a part of combination vaccine at 14 weeks.

ROTAVIRUS VACCINES

A review of studies from 38 populations found that all rotavirus gastroenteritis events (RVGE) occurred in 1%, 3%, 6%, 8%, 10%, 22% and 32% children by age 6, 9, 13, 15, 17, 26 and 32 weeks, respectively. Mortality was mostly related to RVGE events occurring before 32 weeks of age.[25] The highest risk of mortality was noted in the children having earliest exposure to rotavirus, living in poor rural households, and having lowest level of vaccine coverage.[26] It is ideal if immunization schedule is completed early in developing countries where natural infection might occur early.[27]

Infants in developing countries may be at risk of developing RVGE at an earlier age than those in developed countries. They also tend to have a higher risk of mortality coupled with the risk of lower vaccine coverage. No observational study has compared different ages at first dose. A schedule of two doses at 10 and 14 weeks may result in incomplete course of vaccination, especially in developing countries because of restriction of upper age limit for rotavirus vaccine administration. Such children would remain immunologically susceptible to get rotavirus infection. Early administration of the first dose of rotavirus vaccine as soon as possible after 6 weeks of age has been recommended by WHO recently.[27] Administration of RV1 or RV5 vaccine at 6 weeks has also been recommended and approved even in developed countries.[28]

Two randomized controlled trials reported data on severe rotavirus gastroenteritis with up to one year follow-up, and directly compared children who received the first dose of RV1 at age 6 weeks *vs* 10 to 11 weeks. No statistically significant difference in efficacy was found between these two schedules.[29] The South Africa and Malawi RV1 trial[30] reported similar efficacy of vaccination schedules beginning at 6 weeks or 10 to 11 weeks against severe RVGE during the second year follow-up using only the Malawi cohort. Indirect comparisons based on stratification of RV1 and RV5 trials using different schedules showed no impact on mortality for different ages at first dose.

Considering these factors, ACVIP recommends RV1 in a schedule of 6 and 10 weeks. The recommendations for the schedule of other vaccines remain the same.

Currently the following live oral rotavirus vaccines are available in India: (i) Human monovalent live vaccine (RV1); (ii) Human bovine pentavalent live vaccine (RV5); (iii) Indian neonatal rotavirus live vaccine,

116 E; (iv) Bovine Rotavirus Vaccine–Pentavalent (BRV-PV). BRV-PV is a recently introduced pentavalent rotavirus vaccine that contains serotypes G1, G2, G3, G4, and G9 obtained from Bovine (UK) X Human Rotavirus Reassortant strains. It is a thermostable vaccine and can be stored below 24°C till the duration of the shelf life of 30 months. This vaccine remains stable for 36 months at temperature below 25°C, for 18 months between 37°C and 40°C, and a short-term exposure at 55°C.[31]

IAP-ACVIP Recommendation on Rotavirus Vaccines

Any of the available rotavirus vaccines may be routinely administered as per the manufacturer's recommendations. All the available vaccines have been demonstrated to be safe and immunogenic.

- Minimum age: 6 weeks for all available brands
- Only two doses of RV-1 are recommended at 6 and 10 weeks
- If any dose in series was RV-5 or RV-116E or vaccine product is unknown for any dose in the series, a total of three doses of RV vaccine should be administered.

Recommendations on the age limit for the first dose and the last dose (16 and 32 weeks) should continue in spite of recommendation for increase in the age limit as per recent NIP guidelines.

TYPHOID VACCINE

Considering the continuation of significant burden of typhoid fever, widespread prevalence of antibiotic-resistant strains of S. typhi and availability of favorable evidence on the efficacy, effectiveness, immunogenicity, safety, and cost-effectiveness of typhoid vaccines, WHO recommends use of typhoid vaccines in national programs for the control of typhoid fever.[32,33] Typhoid conjugate vaccine (TCV) is preferred at all ages as it has improved immunological properties, can be used in younger children, and is expected to provide longer duration of protection. A meta-analysis summarized that typhoid cases across the age groups; 14% to 29% in <5 years, 30% to 44% in 5–9 years and 28% to 52% in 10–14 years.[34] It has been observed that more than one-fourth of all cases occur in children aged below 4 years, with approximately 30% of cases in children aged below 2 years, and 10% in children aged below 1 year.[35] Based on this, WHO has recommended TCV for infants and children from 6 months of age as a 0.5 mL single dose,[36] and the same is endorsed by ACVIP.

Booster Doses/Revaccination

The need for revaccination with TCV is currently unclear.[36] The protection with TCV may last for up to 5 years after the administration of one dose, and natural boosting may occur in endemic areas.[37] The evidence concerning the need for booster vaccination is lacking currently. Until more data is generated or available, the ACVIP recommends only a single dose of TCV from 6 months onwards. If a child has received Typhoid polysachharide vaccine, it is recommended to offer one dose of TCV at least 4 weeks following the receipt of polysaccharide vaccine.

Currently, three products of TCV are licensed in India. Two of them contain 25 µg of purified Vi PS of S. typhi, and one of them containing 5 µg purified Vi PS of S. typhi. The WHO position paper in 2018 has remarked that the body of evidence for the 5 µg vaccine is very limited.

IAP-ACVIP Recommendation on Typhoid Vaccines

Primary Schedule

- A single dose of TCV 25 µg is recommended from the age of 6 months onwards routinely.
- An interval of at least 4 weeks is not mandatory between TCV and measles-containing vaccine when it is offered at age of 9 months or beyond.
- For a child who has received only Typhoid polysaccharide vaccine, a single dose of

TCV is recommended at least 4 weeks following the receipt of polysaccharide vaccine. Routine booster for TCV at 2 years is not recommended as of now.

MEASLES, MUMPS AND RUBELLA (MMR/MR) VACCINES

Standalone measles vaccine is now not available for regular use. Measles-containing vaccine (MMR/MR) should be administered after 9 months of age (270 days). MR (Measles-Rubella) vaccine is currently not available in the private sector. Hence in view of morbidity following mumps infection, it has been recommended that MMR is administered instead of MR at 9 months, 15 months, and 4–6 years,[38] or as two doses at 12 to 15 months of age with the second dose between 4 to 6 years of age.[39] Additional dose of MR vaccine during MR campaign for children 9 months to 15 years, irrespective of previous vaccination status is to be administered, keeping in mind the need to support national programs.

INFLUENZA VACCINE

A meta-analysis and systematic review evaluating studies published between 1995 to 2010 estimated that children under 5 years of age had 90 million (95% CI 49–162 million) new influenza episodes, 20 million (95% CI 13–32 million) cases of acute lower respiratory infections (ALRI) where influenza was associated, and 1 million (95% CI 1–2 million) cases of severe ALRI (associated with influenza). This resulted in 28,000–111,500 deaths attributed to influenza, with 99% of them from developing countries.[40] Another study estimated that globally 160,000–450,000 children below 5 years of age die in hospitals each year due to all-cause ALRI.[41]

A systematic literature review described that during the peak rainy season, influenza accounted for 20–42% of monthly acute medical illness hospitalizations in India.[42] This suggests that influenza is a substantial contributor to severe respiratory illness and hospitalization. The findings from the studies also show that influenza circulation and influenza-associated hospitalization are major public health concerns in India. There is poor uptake of the influenza vaccine in India. IAP position paper on influenza in 2013 stated the while it may not be practical to recommend routine influenza vaccination to everyone in India, the vaccination for high-risk groups such as the elderly, children below 5 years, medical practitioners and pregnant women should be seriously considered.[43] Influenza incidence in children below 5 years of age from developing countries is three times higher than those from developed countries, with a 15-fold higher case-fatality.[41]

Health utilization surveys conducted in two rural sites (Ballabgarh, Haryana and Vadu, Maharashtra) in 2010–2012 reported adjusted all-age incidence rates of influenza-associated hospitalization as 3.8–5.4 per 10,000 in Ballabgarh and 20.3–51.6 per 10,000 in Vadu.[44] The age-specific influenza-associated hospitalization rates varied from year to year. In 2010, these rates were highest among persons aged <1 year, in 2011 among patients >59 years of age, and in 2012 in children 1–4 years in Ballabhgarh. Whereas in Vadu, in 2010, these rates were highest among persons aged 1–4 years, in 2011 in children <1 year, and in 2012 in children 5–14 years. Influenza viruses were found throughout the year and the peaks coincided with peaks in rain fall at both the sites.

The Influenza Serotype-B is reported almost round the year in India. A multi-site influenza study in India found that 27.8% isolates were Influenza A (H1N1) virus, 29.8% were type A (H3N2), and 42.3% isolates were type B.[45] A global influenza study found that during seasons, out of all influenza B isolates, Victoria and Yamagata lineages predominated or co-circulated (>20% of total detections), and this accounted for 64% and 36% of seasons respectively. The vaccine virus mismatch was found in 25% of the seasons.[46]

With the available data, there is enough reason to believe that the magnitude of the problem is much higher in developing countries (including India) vis-a-vis developed countries. India lies within the northern hemisphere. Some parts of the country experience a distinct tropical environment because of its location close to the equator. These areas have a southern hemisphere seasonality with almost round-the-year circulation of influenza viruses peaking during monsoon. Northern parts of India experience another peak during winters similar to northern hemisphere pattern. There is continuous influenza activity across the nation, with seasonal peaks during monsoon and winter, and an ever increasing number of influenza-like illnesses affecting a large number of children who can transmit the disease to their peers and adult counterparts.

In view of influenza activity round the year with seasonal peaks, high morbidity and mortality in high-risk groups, including children below 5 years, paucity of facilities for laboratory diagnosis, high transmission rate, substantial socioeconomic burden, limitations of oseltamivir, availability of moderately efficacious vaccine, it would be justifiable to use Influenza vaccine routinely in the high-risk group of children below age of 5 years.

Vaccine Strains

FDA recommended the following combinations for 2018–19 influenza vaccines.
- Trivalent vaccines-to have (i) an A/Michigan/45/2015 (H1N1)pdm09-like virus, (ii) an A/Singapore/INFIMH-16-0019/2016 (H3N2)-like virus; and (iii) a B/Colorado/06/2017-like virus (Victoria lineage).
- Quadrivalent vaccines to contain the above three, and a B/Phuket/3073/2013-like virus (Yamagata lineage).[47]

IAP-ACVIP Recommendations

ACVIP recommends that quadrivalent/trivalent inactivated influenza vaccine should be routinely offered annually to all children between 6 months to 5 years of age. The latest available influenza vaccine can be adminisred after 6 months of age, 2–4 weeks prior to the influenza season: two doses at the interval of one month in the first year, and one dose annually before the influenza season up to 5 years of age.

RABIES VACCINE

Recent data indicate that duration and number of doses for post-exposure prophylaxis (PEP) and pre-exposure prophylaxis (PrEP) regimens can be shortened. ACVIP endorses the new schedule suggested by WHO in 2018.[48]

Pre-exposure prophylaxis (Pre-EP) is recommended in the following two situations.
- Children exposed to pets in home.
- Children identified to have a higher risk of being bitten by dogs.

WHO recommends a "1-site vaccine administration on days 0 and 7 for intramuscular administration".[48]

For post-exposure prophylaxis, recently the WHO[48] has recommended a new 4-dose schedule of either of the following: (i) 1-site intramuscular administration of vaccine on days 0, 3, 7 and between day 14–28, or (ii) 2-sites intramuscular administration on days 0 and 1-site on days 7, 21 (intramuscular).

Rabies Human Monoclonal Antibody (RHMAB)

Access to Rabies immunoglobulin (RIG) is limited resulting in high rabies mortality. RHMAB is a completely human IgG1 monoclonal antibody that binds to the ectodomain of the G glycoprotein produced by recombinant technology. It has been demonstrated to neutralize 25 different isolates of wild-type or street isolates of rabies virus. A recent study found that it is not inferior to Human rabies immunoglobulin (HRIG) in producing rabies virus neutralizing antibody in 200 subjects with WHO category-III suspected rabies exposures. The study subjects received either RMHAB or HRIG (1:1 ratio) in wounds, and intramuscularly wherever necessary, on day-0. All these patients also received five doses of rabies vaccine intramuscularly on 0, 3, 7, 14 and 28 days.[49]

This newly introduced monoclonal antibody has emerged as a safe and potent alternative to rabies immunoglobulin. The WHO position paper on Rabies in 2018 has also suggested encouragement of use of this product, if available, instead of RIG. The comparative advantages include easy availability, standardized production quality, possibly greater effectiveness, no requirement of animals in its production, and less adverse events.

In view of the irregular availability and high cost of Rabies immunoglobin (RIG), ACVIP endorses the use of RHMAB as an alternative to RIG – human or equine – along with rabies vaccines in all category-III bites. RHMAB is licensed in India (as Rabisheild, Serum Institute of India; 40 IU/mL) since 2017. The recommended dose is 3.33 IU/kg body weight, preferably at the time of the first vaccine dose. However, this may also be administered up to the 7th day after the first dose of vaccine is given. If the calculated dose is insufficient (to infiltrate all the wounds), it should be diluted in sterile normal saline to get a volume that is enough to be infiltrated around all the wounds.

REFERENCES

1. Vashishtha VM, Choudhury P, Kalra A, Bose A, Thacker N, Yewale VN, et al. Indian Academy of Pediatrics (IAP) recommended immunization schedule for children aged 0 through 18 years–India, 2014 and updates on immunization. Indian Pediatr 2014;51:785–800.

2. Hepatitis B vaccines: WHO position paper – No 27, 2017, World Health Organization. Weekly epidemiological record. No 27, 2017;92:369–92.

3. Elizabeth D. Barnett, Give first dose of HepB vaccine within 24 hours of birth: American Academy of Pediatrics August 28, 2017. Available from: http://www.aappublications.org/news/2017/08/28/HepB082817. Accessed Nov 6, 2018.

4. Cherry JD. Pertussis and Immunizations: Facts, Myths, and Misconceptions. Available from: http://aap-ca.org/pertussis-and-immunizations-facts-myths-and-misconceptions. Accessed November 6, 2018.

5. Munoz FM. Safer pertussis vaccines for children: Trading efficacy for safety. Pediatrics 2018;142: e20181036.

6. Jackson DW, Rohani P. Perplexities of pertussis: Recent global epidemiological trends and their potential causes. Epidemiol Infect 2013;16:1–13.

7. Winter K, Harriman K, Zipprich J, Schechter R, Talarico J, Watt J, et al. California pertussis epidemic, 2010. J Pediatr 2012;161:1091–6.

8. Centers for Disease Control and Prevention (CDC). Pertussis epidemic—Washington, 2012. Morb Mortal Wkly Rep 2012;61:517–22.

9. Pertussis vaccines: WHO Position Paper – August 2015 No. 35. World Health Organization. Weekly Epidemiological Record 2015;90:433–60.

10. World Health Organization. Pertussis Vaccine Evidence to Recommendations (WHO). Available from: http://www.who.int/immunization/position_papers/Pertussis GradeTable3.pdf. Accessed November 6, 2018.

11. WHO Position paper on Pertusis Vaccine, 2005. World Health Organization. Weekly Epidemiological Record 2005;4:29–40.

12. Schmitt HJ, von König CH, Neiss A, Bogaerts H, Bock HL, Schulte-Wissermann H, et al. Efficacy of acellular pertussis vaccine in early childhood after household exposure. JAMA 1996;275:37–41.

13. Jefferson T, Rudin M, DiPietrantonj C. Systematic review of the effects of pertussis vaccines in children. Vaccine 2003;21:2003–14.

14. Carlsson R, Trollfors B. Control of pertussis-lessons learnt from a 10-year surveillance programme in Sweden. Vaccine 2009;27:5709–18.

15. Okada K, Ohashi Y, Matsuo F, Uno S, Soh M, Nishima S. Effectiveness of an acellular pertussis vaccine in Japanese children during a non-epidemic period: a matched case-control study. Epidem Infection 2009;137:124–30.

16. World Health Organization. WHO SAGE Pertussis Working Group. Background Paper. SAGE April 2014. Available from: http://www.who.int/immunization/sage/ meetings/2014/april/1_Pertussis_background_FINAL4_web.pdf? ua=. Accessed November 15, 2018.

17. World Health Organization. Use of Fractional Dose IPV in Routine Immunization Programmes: Considerations for Decision-making. Available

from: http://www.who. int/immunization/diseases/poliomyelitis/endgame_objective2/inactivated_polio_vaccine/fIPV_considerations_for_decision-making_April2017.pdf?ua=1. Accessed November 6, 2018.

18. Indian Academy of Pediatrics (IAP) Advisory committee on vaccines and Immunization Practices (ACVIP), Vasishtha VM, Choudhary J, Yadav S, Unni JC, Jog P, Kamath SS, *et al*. Introduction of inactivated poliovirus vaccine in National Immunization Program and polio endgame strategy. Indian Pediatr 2016; 53(Suppl.1):S65–9.

19. Bahl S, Verma H, Bhatnagar P, Haldar P, Satapathy A, Arun Kumar KN, *et al*. Fractional-dose inactivated poliovirus vaccine immunization campaign — Telangana State, India, June 2016. MMWR 2016;65:859–63.

20. Resik S, Tejeda A, Mach O, Fonseca M, Diaz M, Alemany N, *et al*. Immune responses after fractional doses of inactivated poliovirus vaccine using newly developed intradermal jet injectors: A randomized controlled trial in Cuba. Vaccine 2015;33:307–13.

21. Clarke E, Saidu Y, Adetifa JU, Adigweme I, Hydara MB, Bashorun AO, *et al*. Safety and immunogenicity of inactivated poliovirus vaccine when given with measles-rubella combined vaccine and yellow fever vaccine and when given *via* different administration routes: A phase 4, randomised, non-inferiority trial in The Gambia. Lancet Glob Health 2016;4:e534–47.

22. Troy SB, Kouiavskaia D, Siik J, Kochba E, Beydoun H, Mirochnitchenko O, *et al*. Comparison of the immunogenicity of various booster doses of inactivated polio vaccine delivered intradermally versus intramuscularly to HIV-infected adults. J Infect Dis 2015;15:1969–76.

23. Saleem AF, Mach O, Yousafzai MT, Khan A, Weldon WC, Oberste MS, *et al*. Needle adapters for intradermal administration of fractional dose of inactivated poliovirus vaccine: Evaluation of immunogenicity and programmatic feasibility in Pakistan. Vaccine 2017;35:3209–14.

24. Polio vaccines: WHO Position Paper, March 2016. World Health Organization. Weekly Epidemiological Record 2016;91:145–68.

25. World Health Organization. Detailed Review Paper on Rotavirus Vaccines (presented to the WHO Strategic Advisory Group of Experts (SAGE) on Immunization in April 2009). Geneva, World Health Organization, 2009. Available

from: http://www.who.int/immunization/sage/3_Detailed_Review_Paper_on_Rota_Vaccines_ 17_3_2009.pdf. Accessed November 08, 2018.

26. Phua KB, Lim FS, Lau YL, Nelson EA, Huang LM, Quak SH, *et al*. Rotavirus vaccine RIX4414 efficacy sustained during the third year of life: A randomized clinical trial in an Asian population. Vaccine 2012;30:4552–7.

27. Rotavirus vaccines WHO Position Paper–January 2013. Weekly Epidemiological Record 2013;88:49–64.

28. Rotavirus. In: Hamborsky J, Kroger A, Wolfe S, (Eds). Centers for Disease Control and Prevention. Epidemiology and Prevention of Vaccine-preventable Diseases. 13th ed. Washington DC: Public Health Foundation, 2015. Available from:https://www.cdc.gov/vaccines/pubs/ pinkbook/downloads/rota.pdf. Accessed November 15, 2018.

29. World Health Organization. Rotavirus Report, February 2012. Rotavirus Vaccines Schedules: A Systematic Review of Safety and Efficacy from Randomized Controlled Trials and Observational Studies of Childhood Schedules Using RV1 and RV5 Vaccines. Available from: http://www.who.int/immunization/sage/meetings/2012/april/Soares_K_et_al_SAGE_April_rotavirus.pdf. Accessed November 08, 2018.

30. World Health Organization. Grading of Scientific Evidence – Tables 1–4: Does RV1and RV5 induce protection against rotavirus morbidity and mortality in young children both in low and high mortality settings? Available from: http://www.who.int/immunization/position_papers/rotavirus_ grad_rv1_rv5_protection. Accessed November 8, 2018.

31. Naik SP, Zade JK, Sabale RN, Pisal SS, Menon R, Bankar SG, *et al*. Stability of heat stable, live attenuated rotavirus vaccine (ROTASIIL®). Vaccine 2017;35:2962–9.

32. World Health Organization. Background Paper on Typhoid Vaccines for SAGE Meeting (October 2017). Available from: http://www.who.int/immunization/sage /meetings/ 2017/october/1_Typhoid_SAGE_background_paper_Final_v3B.pdf. Accessed November 08, 2018.

33. World Health Organization. Guidelines on The Quality, Safety and Efficacy of Typhoid Conjugate Vaccines, 2013. Available from: http://www.who.int/biologicals/areas/vaccines/TYPHOID_BS2215_doc_v1.14_WEB_ VERSION.pdf. Accessed July 12, 2016.

34. Britto C, Pollard AJ, Voysey M, Blohmke CJ. An appraisal of the clinical features of pediatric enteric fever: Systematic review and meta-analysis of the age-stratified disease occurrence. Clin Infect Dis 2017;64:1604–11.

35. World Health Organization. Background Paper to SAGE on Typhoid Policy Recommendations. 2017. Available from: http://www.who.int/immunization/sage/meetings/2017/october/1_Typhoid_SAGE_background_paper_Final_v3B.pdf?ua=1. Accessed November 08, 2018.

36. Typhoid vaccines: WHO Position Paper – March 2018. Weekly Epidemiological Record 2018;93: 153–72.

37. Voysey M, Pollard AJ. Sero-efficacy of Vi-poly-saccharide tetanus-toxoid typhoid conjugate vaccine (Typbar-TCV). Clin Infect Dis 2018;67: 18-24.

38. Vashishtha VM, Yewale VN, Bansal CP, Mehta PJ. Indian Academy of Pediatrics, Advisory Committee on Vaccines and Immunization Practices (ACVIP). IAP perspectives on measles and rubella elimination strategies. Indian Pediatr 2014;51:719–22.

39. Centers for Disease Control and Prevention. Measles, Mumps, and Rubella (MMR) Vaccination: What Everyone Should Know. Available from: https://www.cdc.gov/vaccines/vpd/mmr/public/index.html. Accessed November 18, 2018.

40. Nair H, Brooks WA, Katz M, Roca A, Berkley JA, Madhi SA, et al. Global burden of respiratory infections due to seasonal influenza in young children: A systematic review and meta-analysis. Lancet 2011;378:1917–30.

41. Rudan I, Theodoratou E, Zgaga L, Nair H, Chan KY, Tomlinson M, et al. Setting priorities for development of emerging interventions against childhood pneumonia, meningitis and influenza. J Glob Health 2012;2:10304.

42. Venkatesh M, Doarn CR, Steinhoff M, Yung J. Assessment of burden of seasonal influenza in India and consideration of vaccination policy. Glob J Med Pub Health 2016;5:1–10. Available from: http://www.gjmedph.com/uploads/R1-Vo5No5.pdf. Accessed November 18, 2018.

43. Vashishtha VM, Kalra A, Choudhury P. Influenza vaccination in India: Position Paper of Indian Academy of Pediatrics, 2013. Indian Pediatr 2013;50:867–74.

44. Hirve S, Krishnan A, Dawood FS, Lele P, Saha S, Rai S, et al. Incidence of influenza-associated hospitalization in rural communities in western and northern India, 2010–2012: A multi-site population-based study. J Infect 2015;70:160–70.

45. Chadha MS, Broor S, Gunasekaran P, Potdar VA, Krishnan A, Chawla-Sarkar M, et al. Multisite virological influenza surveillance in India: 2004-2008. Influenza Other Respir Viruses 2012;6: 196–203.

46. Caini S, Huang QS, Ciblak MA, Kusznierz G, Owen R, Wangchuk S, et al. Epidemiological and virological characteristics of influenza B: results of the Global Influenza B Study. Influen Other Respir Viruses 2015;9:3–12.

47. Grohskopf LA, Sokolow LZ, Broder KR, Walter EB, Fry AM, Jernigan DB. Prevention and control of seasonal influenza with vaccines: Recommendations of the Advisory Committee on Immunization Practices—United States, 2018–19. Influenza Season. MMWR Recomm Rep 2018;67:1–20.

48. World Health Organization. Rabies vaccines: WHO Position Paper, April 2018 Recommendations. Vaccine 2018;36:5500–3.

49. Gogtay NJ, Munshi R, Ashwath Narayana DH, Mahendra BJ, Kshirsagar V, Gunale B, et al. Comparison of a novel human rabies monoclonal antibody to human rabies immunoglobulin for postexposure prophylaxis: A phase 2/3, randomized, single-blind, noninferiority, controlled study. Clin Infect Dis 2018;66:387–95.

Revised IAP Growth Charts for Height, Weight and BMI for 5- to 18-year-old Indian Children

Vaman Khadilkar, Sangeeta Yadav, KK Agrawal, Suchit Tamboli, Monidipa Banerjee, Alice Cherian,
Jagdish P Goyal, Anuradha Khadilkar, V Kumaravel, V Mohan, D Narayanappa, I Ray, Vijay Yewale

In 2007, the Indian Academy of Pediatrics (IAP) growth monitoring guideline committee designed growth charts for Indian children from birth to 18 years of age.[1] The growth references used in these guidelines were based on the then available multicentric data that was collected in 1989 on affluent Indian children, which is now more than 20 years old.[2,3] The pattern of growth of a population changes with time and hence it is recommended that references should be updated regularly so that they reflect current growth patterns of children and are representative of secular trends.[4] As the current IAP growth reference curves are based on data collected more than 2 decades ago, they may not be suitable for use any more, especially in an economically upwardly mobile country like India, where major changes in nutrition status of children have been witnessed. Recent studies from India on overweight and obesity in children have shown that not only is there a rise in the incidence of overweight and obesity but adiposity rebound is seen at a younger age.[5] The pattern of growth in children has thus changed and hence we urgently need to update Indian growth charts.

In 2006, the World Health Organization (WHO) published the first growth standards as prescriptive charts for children under the age of 5 years to be used as a single uniform global standard; IAP and Government of India have adopted these standards for use in Indian children under 5 years of age. These standards are aspirational models which define how under-five children of the world should grow rather than how they actually grow. Many countries have since then changed their growth charts for under-five children as per the WHO Multicentre Growth Reference Study.[6]

For children between 5–18 years of age, WHO has stated that it would not be possible to have prescriptive growth standards because environmental variables in this age group cannot be controlled for; hence, charts by the WHO for 5–18 year old children are based on statistical reconstruction of 1977 National Centre for Health Statistics data and are called growth references and not standards.[7] However, growth patterns differ amongst different populations, especially in children above the age of 5 years, as nutritional, environmental and genetic factors, and timing of puberty seem to play a major role not only in the attainment of final height but also in the characteristics of the growth curve. Hence, it is necessary to have country-specific growth charts to monitor growth of children between 5–18 years.

There are several recent reports on growth data of affluent Indian children, multicentric as well as regional, that can potentially be used as reference data; however, there is no national consensus on which charts to use.[8] While these studies have made an attempt to address the issue of monitoring growth in Indian children; to date, no unified charts have been constructed. Further, childhood obesity is a growing problem in urban India and hence there is a worry about "normalizing" obese children if growth charts are prepared on these contemporary data sets. Since a lot of children around the world are showing a rising trend of increasing weight, no population is perfect on whom ideal weight charts can be constructed. Hence, a statistical approach has been suggested by experts, including the WHO.[6,9] WHO has described a method to eliminate unhealthy weights from populations by removing children who have weight to height z scores above +2 SD. This method eliminates children with unhealthy weights especially at the upper percentiles reducing the effect of obesity which is common in children of today, thus effectively dealing with the issue of "normalizing" obese children's weight.

Growth is an integral part of childhood and growth monitoring is critical for the assessment of health and disease in an individual child and the community as a whole. Since growth is an indicator of a child's health and nutrition, updated population-specific reference growth charts are needed.[10] Taken together, there is an urgent need to construct unified growth charts, adjusted for weight, for assessing the growth of contemporary Indian children from 5–18 years to be used together with the WHO standards (0–5 years). With this aim, the IAP Growth Chart Committee constructed revised IAP growth references for 5–18 year old Indian children based on collated national data from published studies from last 10 years, performed on apparently healthy 87022 children and adolescents. Comparisons of collated data with previous Indian and contemporary International studies are also presented.

METHODS

A growth chart committee was formed by the IAP in January 2014 to design new growth charts for Indian children older than 5 years so that they are based on contemporary data that represents the growth of modern-day Indian children. A consultative committee scrutinized the methodology, results and scientific content of the manuscript in November 2014 in Mumbai when data compilation, analysis and results became available. Studies performed on children's growth, nutritional assessment and anthropometry published in various Indexed journals in the last decade were indentified through internet based search engines *viz.* Google, Pubmed and Embase. The criteria used for selecting studies were as follows: Studies presenting anthropometric data on apparently healthy Indian children between the age of 5 to 18 (Flowchart. 19.1)

Flowchart. 19.1: Data acquisition and analysis

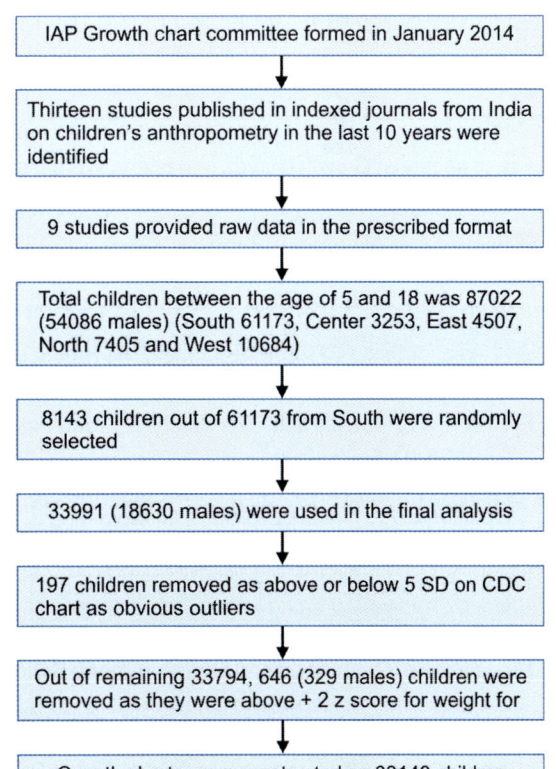

IAP Growth chart committee formed in January 2014

↓

Thirteen studies published in indexed journals from India on children's anthropometry in the last 10 years were identified

↓

9 studies provided raw data in the prescribed format

↓

Total children between the age of 5 and 18 was 87022 (54086 males) (South 61173, Center 3253, East 4507, North 7405 and West 10684)

↓

8143 children out of 61173 from South were randomly selected

↓

33991 (18630 males) were used in the final analysis

↓

197 children removed as above or below 5 SD on CDC chart as obvious outliers

↓

Out of remaining 33794, 646 (329 males) children were removed as they were above + 2 z score for weight for

↓

Growth charts were constructed on 33148 children

from the upper and middle socioeconomic classes were included where height, weight and age were available for every child. Studies performed on children of lower socioeconomic class (data on them may not represent the optimal growth potential of children due to under-nutrition) and where authors refused/could not share data were excluded.

Using these criteria, it was found that three studies were performed to construct growth percentiles,[11–13] one was primarily designed to construct waist circumference percentiles[14] but, height, weight and age were available for each child. Other studies were performed to assess incidence of underweight, over-weight and obesity in school-going children.[15–20] One study was primarily aimed at comparing available growth charts in India while studying anthropometry on normal Indian school-going children.[21] The committee contacted 13 study groups who had published their data in indexed journals from 2004 onwards and requested data from apparently healthy children from upper and middle socio-economic class. Out of 13 study groups that were contacted through electronic communication, phone calls and personal meetings, authors of nine studies were able to provide raw data on their study subjects (Table 19.1). Researchers were asked to provide raw data, including age, height, weight, socioeconomic class, region and gender in a pre-designed Microsoft excel template 2007. These raw data were then joined to form a single dataset. Total number of children from upper and middle class from 5 to 18 years was 87022 (54086 males). Data from fourteen cities (Agartala, Ahmadabad, Chandigarh, Chennai, Delhi, Hyderabad, Kochi, Kolkata, Madurai, Mumbai, Mysore, Pune, Raipur and Surat) were collated. To make the regional distribution more uniform, 8143 children out of 61173 from Southern India were randomly selected by generating random numbers in age-wise groups thus selecting approximately comparable number of children in each age group. Data from a total of 33991 (18630 males), were used in the final analysis. Using

TABLE 19.1: Published sources of raw data

Study title	Journal and year of publication	Total children
Cross-sectional Growth Curves for Height, Weight and Body Mass Index for Affluent Indian Children, 2007[11]	Indian Pediatrics 2009	18666
Mysore Childhood Obesity Study[16]	Indian Pediatrics 2009	43152
Determinants of Overweight and Obesity in Affluent Adolescent in Surat City, South Gujarat Region, India[17]	Indian Journal of Community Medicine 2011	5664
Body Mass Index Cut-offs for Screening for Childhood Overweight and Obesity in Indian Children[12]	Indian Pediatrics 2012	18666
Prevalence of Obesity and Overweight in Urban School Children in Kerala, India[18]	Indian Pediatrics 2012	1634
An anthropometric study on the children of Tripura: Nutritional and health coverage and redefining WHO percentile cut-off points[20]	International Journal of Scientific and Research Publications 2013	9498
Are the current Indian growth charts really representative? Analysis of anthropometric assessment of school children in a South Indian district[21]	Indian Journal of Endocrinology and Metabolism 2014	19668
Prevalence of Overweight and Obesity Among School Children and Adolescents in Chennai[19]	Indian Pediatrics 2014	18955
Waist Circumference Percentiles in 2–18 Year Old Indian Children[14]	American Journal of Pediatrics 2014	10842

CDC standards, children above and below 5 SD scores for height, weight and body mass index (BMI) were removed as obvious outliers.[22] Fourteen children were removed as height SD score was below –5.0 SD and 2 removed as height SD was above +5. Thirty-nine children were removed as weight SD scores were below –5 SD; no child was above +5 SD for weight. One hundred and forty-two children with BMI SD below –5SD were removed; no child had BMI SD above +5.

Method used to remove children with unhealthy weights: In case of cross sectional data WHO recommends removing observations that are above +2SD of the study population for weight for height as unhealthy overweight.[6] Weight for height z scores were computed using Cole's LMS method. Children who were above +2 SD scores were removed from analysis. A total of 646 children (329 males) were removed from analysis. We examined (using one way ANOVA) gender- and age group-wise regional differences, which showed that while there were significant differences in younger age groups amongst regions, there were no differences in height and weight SD scores post-puberty at 17 and 18 years between the five zones.

Cole's LMS method was then used to compute growth curves for height, weight and BMI using LMS method. LMS method constructs growth reference percentiles adjusted for skewness.[23] Each growth reference is summarized by three smooth curves plotted against age representing the median (M), the coefficient of variation (S) and the skewness (L) of the measurement distribution. For height and weight 3rd, 10th, 25th, 50th, 75th, 90th and 97th percentiles were generated. Body mass index (BMI) was calculated as weight in kg/height in meters square. For the BMI; however, using International Obesity Task Force (IOTF) approach 3rd, 5th, 10th, 25th, 50th, 23 adult equivalent (as overweight cut-off), and 27 adult equivalent (as obesity cut-off) percentiles were generated as per recent recommendations for

Asian Indian overweight and obesity cut offs.[24,25] The 3rd percentile was used to define thinness.[26]

RESULTS

Data on 33148 children were used in the construction of growth charts. Region wise distribution was 7227 (4514 boys, 2713 girls), 7835 (4263 boys, 3572 girls), 4408 (2131 boys, 2277 girls), 10474 (5473 boys, 5001 girls), 3204 (1789 boys, 1415 girls) from North, South, East, West and Central zones, respectively. Of the studies excluded, growth percentile data for comparison were available in only one study and the difference in median height in boys and girls at 18 years on comparison with current study results was <1 cm.[13]

Figure 19.2 shows the smoothed height and weight curves for Indian boys, using 3rd, 10th, 25th, 50th, 75th, 90th and 97th percentiles, respectively. Equivalent height and weight percentile values along with standard deviations are presented in Tables 19.2 and 19.3, respectively. Figure 19.3 shows the smoothed height and weight curves for Indian girls, using 3rd, 10th, 25th, 50th, 75th, 90th and 97th percentiles, respectively. Equivalent height and weight percentile values along with standard deviations are presented in Tables 19.4 and 19.5, respectively. Figure 19.4 shows the smoothed BMI percentile curves for boys showing 3rd, 5th, 10th, 25th, 50th, 23 adult equivalent (overweight) and 27 adult equivalent (obesity) percentiles. Equivalent values for BMI for boys along with SD are shown in Table 19.6. Figure 19.5 shows the smoothed BMI percentile curves for girls showing 3rd, 5th, 10th, 25th, 50th, 23 adult equivalent (overweight) and 27 adult equivalent (obesity) percentiles. Equivalent values for BMI for girls along with SD are shown in Table 19.7.

Tables 19.8 and 19.9 illustrate the comparison of height and weight in the current study with data from Saudi Arabia,[27] China,[28] IAP 2007,[1] CDC[29] and WHO.[7] The height percentiles of boys and girls from current

TABLE 19.2: Height (cm) centiles and standard deviation for boys

Age	3	10	25	50	75	90	97	SD
5.0	99.0	102.3	105.6	108.9	112.4	115.9	119.4	5.7
5.5	101.6	105.0	108.4	111.9	115.4	119.0	122.7	5.3
6.0	104.2	107.7	111.2	114.8	118.5	122.2	126.0	5.6
6.5	106.8	110.4	114.0	117.8	121.6	125.4	129.3	5.5
7.0	109.3	113.0	116.8	120.7	124.6	128.6	132.6	5.9
7.5	111.8	115.7	119.6	123.5	127.6	131.7	135.9	5.7
8.0	114.3	118.2	122.3	126.4	130.5	134.8	139.1	6.3
8.5	116.7	120.8	124.9	129.1	133.4	137.8	142.2	6.1
9.0	119.0	123.2	127.5	131.8	136.3	140.7	145.3	6.4
9.5	121.3	125.6	130.0	134.5	139.1	143.7	148.3	6.4
10.0	123.6	128.1	132.6	137.2	141.9	146.6	151.4	6.8
10.5	125.9	130.5	135.2	139.9	144.7	149.5	154.4	6.5
11.0	128.2	133.0	137.8	142.7	147.6	152.5	157.5	7.6
11.5	130.7	135.6	140.6	145.5	150.5	155.6	160.6	7.3
12.0	133.2	138.3	143.3	148.4	153.5	158.6	163.7	8.1
12.5	135.7	141.0	146.2	151.4	156.5	161.7	166.8	7.9
13.0	138.3	143.7	149.0	154.3	159.5	164.7	169.9	9.0
13.5	140.9	146.4	151.8	157.2	162.4	167.6	172.7	8.4
14.0	143.4	149.0	154.5	159.9	165.1	170.3	175.4	9.0
14.5	145.8	151.5	157.0	162.3	167.6	172.7	177.7	7.8
15.0	148.0	153.7	159.2	164.5	169.7	174.8	179.7	7.9
15.5	150.0	155.7	161.2	166.5	171.6	176.5	181.4	6.6
16.0	151.8	157.4	162.9	168.1	173.1	178.0	182.7	7.2
16.5	153.4	159.1	164.5	169.6	174.5	179.3	183.8	6.7
17.0	155.0	160.6	165.9	171.0	175.8	180.4	184.8	6.9
17.5	156.6	162.1	167.3	172.3	177.0	181.5	185.8	6.1
18.0	158.1	163.6	168.7	173.6	178.2	182.5	186.7	6.9

TABLE 19.3: Weight (kg) centiles and standard deviation for boys

Age	3	10	25	50	75	90	97	SD
5.0	13.2	14.3	15.6	17.1	19.0	21.3	24.2	3.2
5.5	13.8	15.0	16.5	18.2	20.3	22.9	26.1	2.9
6.0	14.5	15.8	17.4	19.3	21.7	24.6	28.3	3.6
6.5	15.3	16.8	18.6	20.7	23.3	26.6	30.8	3.8
7.0	16.0	17.6	19.6	21.9	24.9	28.6	33.4	4.2
7.5	16.7	18.5	20.7	23.3	26.6	30.8	36.2	4.9
8.0	17.5	19.5	21.9	24.8	28.5	33.2	39.4	5.7
8.5	18.3	20.5	23.2	26.4	30.5	35.7	42.6	6.5
9.0	19.1	21.5	24.3	27.9	32.3	38.0	45.5	6.3
9.5	19.9	22.4	25.6	29.4	34.3	40.5	48.6	7.0
10.0	20.7	23.5	26.9	31.1	36.3	43.0	51.8	7.9
10.5	21.6	24.6	28.3	32.8	38.5	45.8	55.2	8.3
11.0	22.6	25.9	29.8	34.7	40.9	48.7	58.7	8.9
11.5	23.8	27.3	31.6	36.9	43.5	51.8	62.5	9.3
12.0	24.9	28.7	33.3	39.0	46.0	54.8	66.1	10.0
12.5	26.1	30.2	35.1	41.2	48.6	57.8	69.5	10.6
13.0	27.5	31.8	37.0	43.3	51.1	60.7	72.6	11.3
13.5	29.0	33.6	39.1	45.7	53.8	63.6	75.6	11.4
14.0	30.7	35.5	41.3	48.2	56.4	66.3	78.3	12.1
14.5	32.6	37.7	43.7	50.8	59.1	69.1	80.9	11.6
15.0	34.5	39.8	45.9	53.1	61.6	71.5	83.1	12.1
15.5	36.1	41.6	47.9	55.2	63.6	73.4	84.7	11.2
16.0	37.5	43.1	49.5	56.8	65.2	74.8	85.8	12.2
16.5	38.7	44.4	50.9	58.2	66.6	76.1	86.8	12.6
17.0	39.8	45.6	52.1	59.5	67.8	77.1	87.5	12.3
17.5	40.8	46.7	53.2	60.6	68.7	77.8	88.0	12.3
18.0	41.8	47.7	54.3	61.6	69.7	78.6	88.4	11.3

study were almost at par with China and Saudi Arabia but were still lower than the CDC and WHO percentiles. Further, mean boys' height at the age of 18 year was found to be 2.8 cm higher than the mean as per the previous IAP growth charts, and the 97th percentile was also higher (186.7 cm *vs* 181.6 cm). In case of girls, the average height at the age of 18 year showed an increase of 0.8 cm from 157.0 to 157.8 while the 97th percentile showed an increase of 2.6 cm from 168.0 to 170.6, thus there was a secular trend in height which was more marked in boys. The upper weight percentiles in the current study are higher than IAP 2007 growth data for boys but comparable in girls, are lower than Saudi Arabia, China and CDC in case of

TABLE 19.4: Height (cm) centiles and standard deviation for girls

Age	3	10	25	50	75	90	97	SD
5.0	97.2	100.5	103.9	107.5	111.3	115.2	119.3	5.4
5.5	99.8	103.2	106.8	110.5	114.4	118.3	122.5	5.7
6.0	102.3	106.0	109.7	113.5	117.4	121.5	125.6	5.8
6.5	104.9	108.7	112.5	116.5	120.5	124.6	128.7	5.5
7.0	107.4	111.4	115.4	119.4	123.5	127.7	131.9	6.1
7.5	110.0	114.1	118.2	122.4	126.6	130.8	135.0	6.0
8.0	112.6	116.8	121.1	125.4	129.6	133.9	138.1	6.2
8.5	115.2	119.6	124.0	128.4	132.7	137.0	141.3	6.8
9.0	117.8	122.4	126.9	131.4	135.8	140.2	144.5	6.9
9.5	120.5	125.2	129.9	134.4	138.9	143.3	147.6	6.6
10.0	123.3	128.1	132.8	137.4	142.0	146.4	150.8	7.8
10.5	126.1	130.9	135.7	140.4	145.0	149.5	153.9	7.3
11.0	128.8	133.7	138.6	143.3	147.9	152.4	156.8	7.9
11.5	131.5	136.4	141.2	145.9	150.6	155.1	159.6	7.1
12.0	134.0	138.9	143.7	148.4	153.0	157.5	162.0	7.0
12.5	136.3	141.1	145.8	150.5	155.1	159.6	164.1	6.7
13.0	138.2	142.9	147.6	152.2	156.8	161.3	165.9	6.9
13.5	139.9	144.5	149.1	153.6	158.2	162.7	167.2	6.0
14.0	141.3	145.8	150.2	154.7	159.2	163.7	168.2	6.6
14.5	142.4	146.8	151.1	155.5	160.0	164.5	169.0	5.9
15.0	143.3	147.5	151.8	156.1	160.5	165.0	169.5	6.6
15.5	144.1	148.1	152.3	156.6	160.9	165.3	169.8	5.9
16.0	144.7	148.6	152.7	156.9	161.2	165.6	170.1	6.1
16.5	145.2	149.1	153.1	157.2	161.4	165.7	170.2	6.4
17.0	145.7	149.5	153.4	157.4	161.6	165.9	170.4	6.5
17.5	146.2	149.8	153.6	157.6	161.7	166.0	170.5	6.7
18.0	146.6	150.2	153.9	157.8	161.9	166.1	170.6	6.6

TABLE 19.5: Weight (kg) centiles and standard deviation for girls

Age	3	10	25	50	75	90	97	SD
5.0	12.3	13.4	14.8	16.4	18.5	21.3	25.0	2.5
5.5	13.0	14.3	15.7	17.6	19.9	22.9	27.0	3.5
6.0	13.7	15.1	16.7	18.7	21.3	24.6	29.1	3.4
6.5	14.4	15.9	17.7	19.9	22.7	26.3	31.2	4.1
7.0	15.1	16.8	18.7	21.2	24.2	28.2	33.4	4.4
7.5	15.9	17.7	19.9	22.5	25.9	30.1	35.7	4.8
8.0	16.7	18.7	21.1	24.0	27.6	32.2	38.1	5.2
8.5	17.5	19.7	22.3	25.5	29.5	34.4	40.7	6.4
9.0	18.5	20.9	23.7	27.2	31.5	36.7	43.4	6.4
9.5	19.5	22.1	25.3	29.0	33.6	39.3	46.3	6.9
10.0	20.7	23.5	26.9	31.0	36.0	42.0	49.4	7.7
10.5	22.0	25.1	28.8	33.2	38.4	44.8	52.6	8.3
11.0	23.3	26.7	30.7	35.4	41.0	47.7	55.9	8.5
11.5	24.8	28.4	32.6	37.6	43.6	50.6	59.1	9.1
12.0	26.2	30.0	34.5	39.8	46.0	53.4	62.1	9.0
12.5	27.6	31.6	36.3	41.8	48.2	55.8	64.8	9.7
13.0	28.9	33.1	37.9	43.6	50.2	57.9	67.1	9.4
13.5	30.2	34.4	39.4	45.1	51.8	59.7	69.0	9.8
14.0	31.3	35.6	40.6	46.4	53.2	61.1	70.4	9.6
14.5	32.3	36.6	41.7	47.5	54.3	62.2	71.4	9.4
15.0	33.1	37.5	42.5	48.4	55.1	62.9	72.1	9.6
15.5	34.0	38.3	43.3	49.1	55.8	63.5	72.5	8.7
16.0	34.7	39.1	44.0	49.7	56.3	64.0	72.8	8.7
16.5	35.5	39.8	44.7	50.3	56.9	64.4	73.1	9.2
17.0	36.2	40.5	45.3	50.9	57.3	64.7	73.3	8.8
17.5	36.9	41.1	46.0	51.5	57.8	65.0	73.4	9.5
18.0	37.6	41.8	46.6	52.0	58.2	65.3	73.5	10.2

boys and at par with Saudi Arabia and China but lower than CDC in case of girls.

DISCUSSION

We present here cross-sectional reference percentiles curves for height, weight and BMI based on data published on 5–18 year old apparently healthy Indian children from 14 Indian cities collected by nine research groups over the last decade. As compared to the previous IAP charts, boys and girls were taller at a younger age. At 18 years, average height of boys was 2.8 cm higher and the 97th percentile was 5 cm higher; for girls these figures were 0.8 cm and 2.6 cm. Thus, there

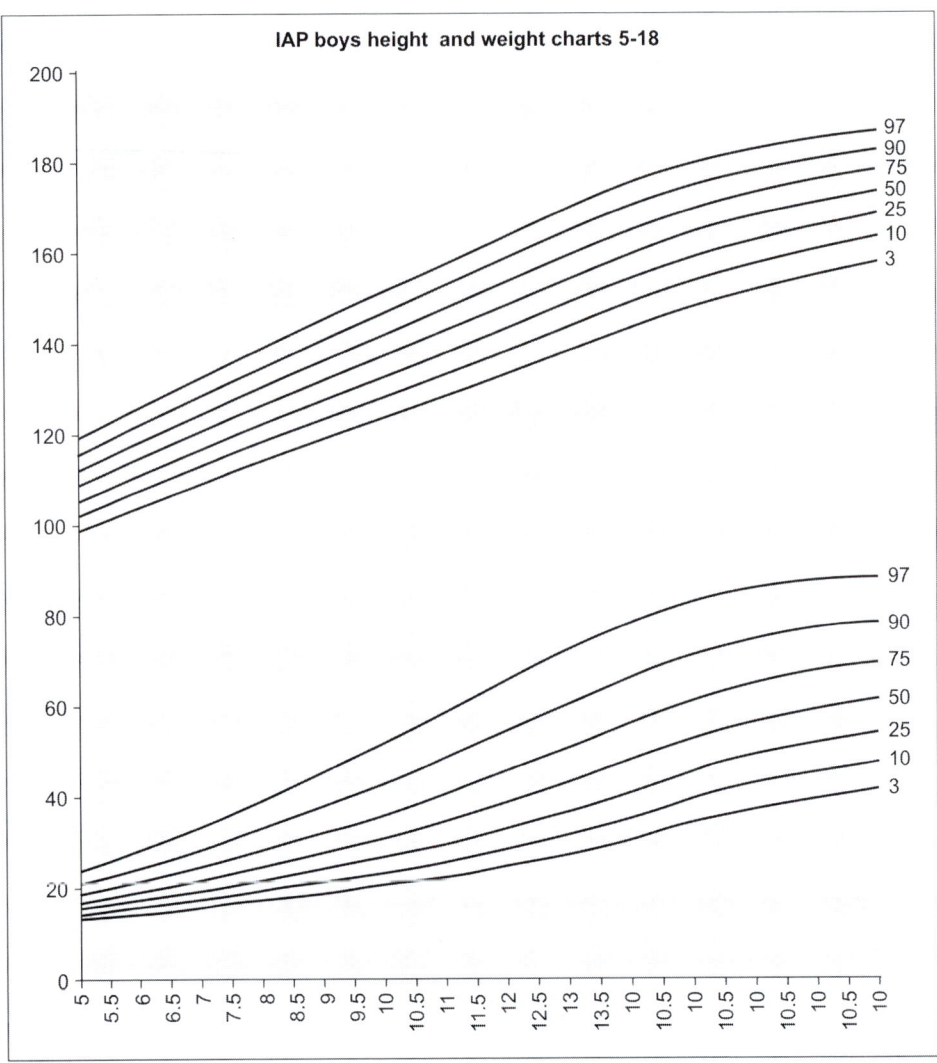

Fig. 19.2: Height and weight charts for boys

was a secular trend in height which underlines the importance of updating growth charts in a developing nation like India.

By adopting the approach as suggested by the WHO, it was possible to produce weight percentiles which were lower as compared to the recently published weight charts on affluent Indian children in 2011, thus reducing the impact of unhealthy weights on growth charts. At 5,10 and 18 years the 97th percentile was 5.3, 1.5 and 10.1 kg lower in comparison with the 2011 data, respectively, while the difference in the median at 5, 10, 18 years was 1.9, 1.9 and 4.7 kg, respectively in boys.[6,13] In girls, the equivalent values at 5, 10 and 18 years were 3.7, 3.3 and 6.6 kg at the 97th percentile, respectively and at 5, 10 and 18 years 2.1, 2.8 and 3.6 kg, respectively at the median. The same comparison with affluent Indian children data published in 2009 shows that in boys the difference in 97th percentile at 5, 10, 18 years was 1.9, 3 and

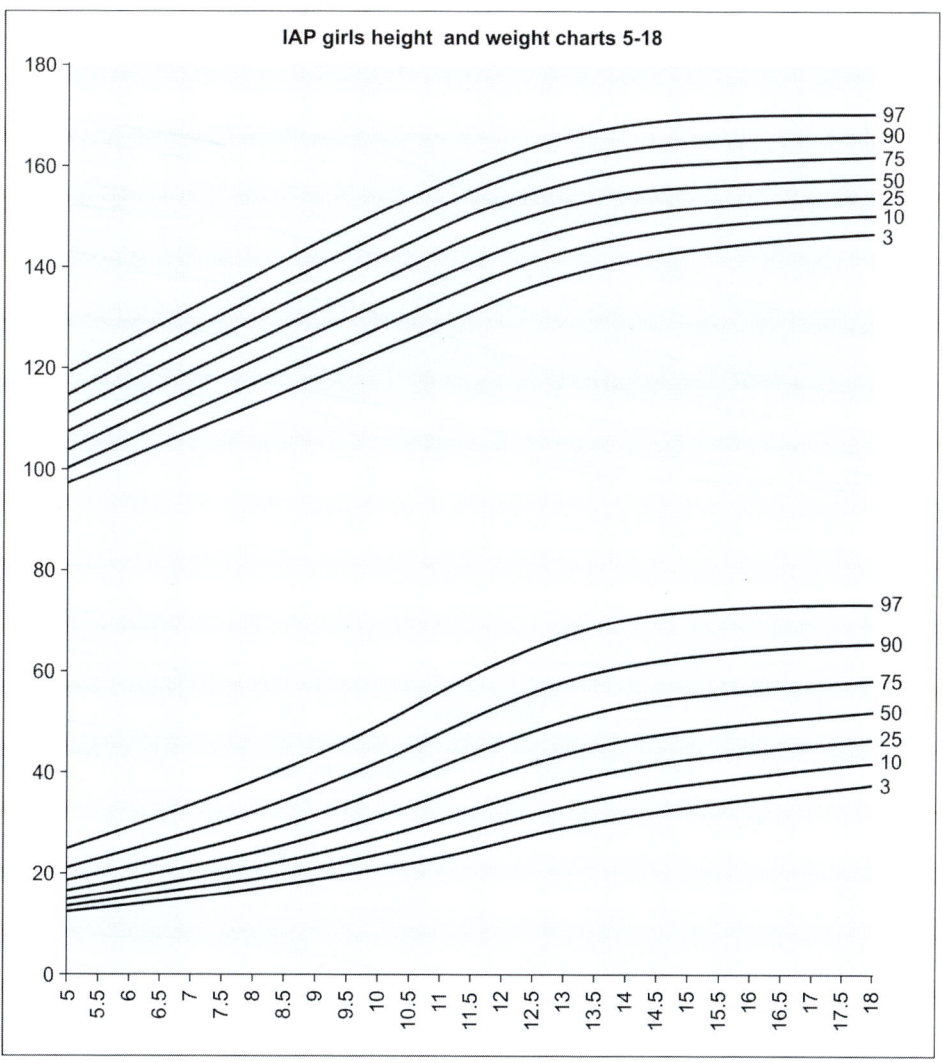

Fig. 19.3: Height and weight charts for girls

9.9 kg while the difference in the median was unremarkable. In girls, equivalent values at 5, 10 and 18 years were 0.3, 3.9 and 9.1 kgs at the 97th percentile while the difference in median was insignificant.[11] Thus the study reduced the impact of unhealthy weights on the weight charts.

BMI charts presented are based on the same method as IOTF.[24] The 23 and 27 adult equivalent cut offs lines (for risk of overweight and obesity, respectively) are more appro-priate for use in Asian children as Asians are known to have more adiposity and increased cardio-metabolic risk at a lower BMI.[25] The current study's 23 and 27 adult equivalent cut-offs are very close to IOTF's extended 23 and 27 cut-offs for both sexes, being slightly lower than the IOTF extended Asian cut-offs by about 0.5 in the 23rd equivalent line and by about 1 in the 27 equivalent line in boys. In case of girls the 23 and 27 equivalent lines are similar.[24]

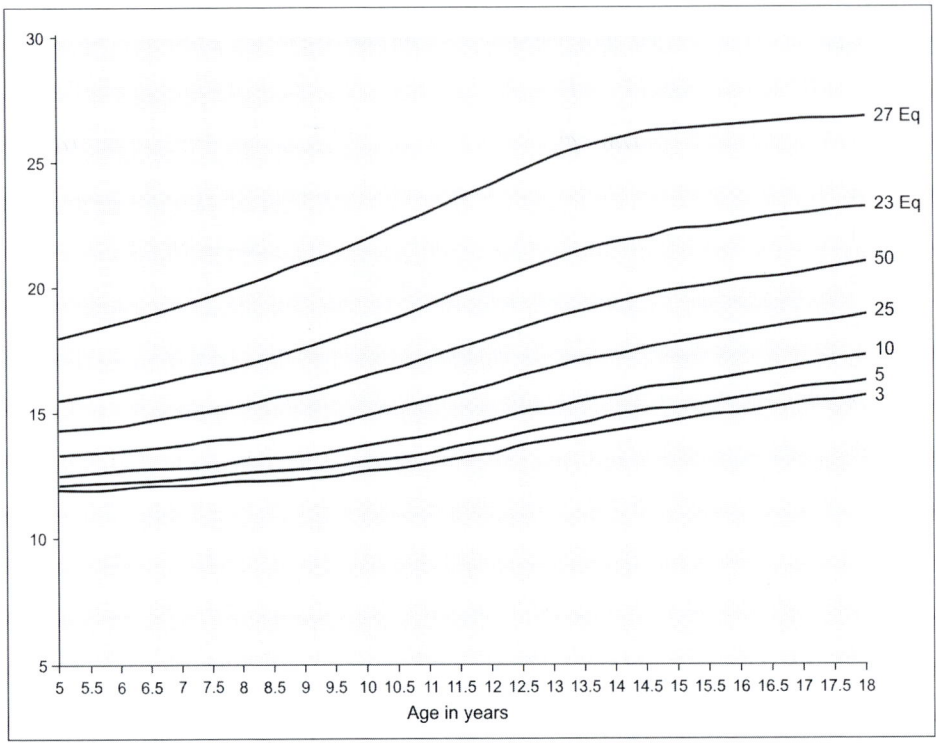

Fig. 19.4: Body mass index charts for boys

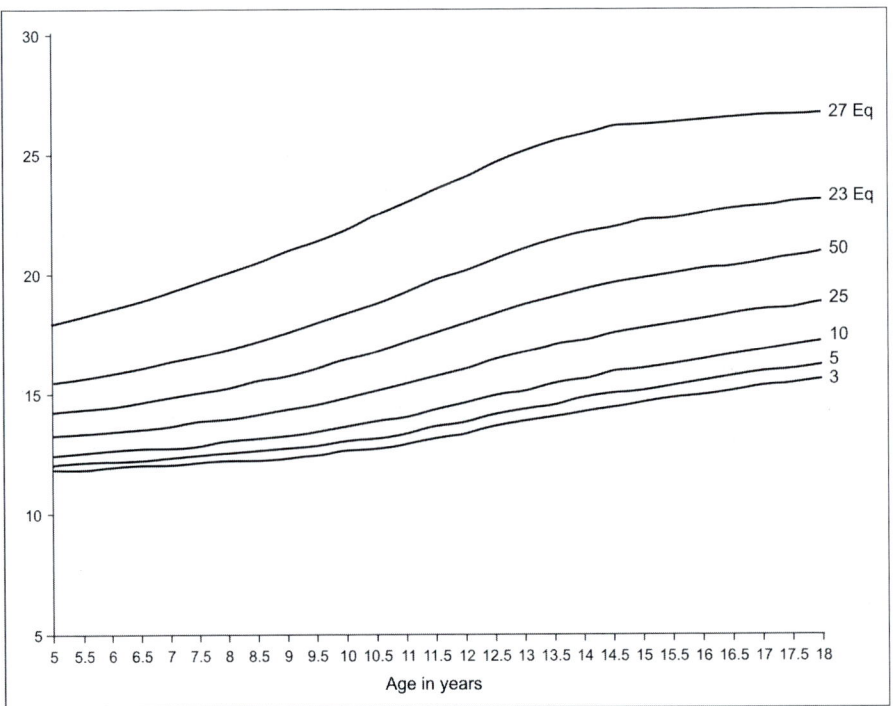

Fig. 219.5: Body mass index charts for girls

TABLE 19.6: Body mass index percentiles and standard deviations for boys

Age	3	5	10	25	50	23 Eq (75)	27 Eq (95)	SD
5.0	12.1	12.4	12.8	13.6	14.7	15.7	17.5	1.6
5.5	12.2	12.4	12.9	13.7	14.8	15.8	17.6	1.5
6.0	12.2	12.5	12.9	13.7	14.9	16.0	17.8	1.8
6.5	12.3	12.5	13.0	13.8	15.0	16.1	18.0	1.8
7.0	12.3	12.6	13.1	13.9	15.1	16.3	18.2	1.9
7.5	12.4	12.7	13.2	14.1	15.3	16.5	18.5	2.2
8.0	12.5	12.8	13.3	14.2	15.5	16.7	18.8	2.5
8.5	12.6	12.9	13.4	14.4	15.7	17.0	19.2	2.8
9.0	12.7	13.0	13.5	14.5	15.9	17.3	19.6	2.6
9.5	12.8	13.1	13.7	14.7	16.2	17.6	20.1	2.8
10.0	12.9	13.2	13.8	14.9	16.4	18.0	20.5	3.1
10.5	13.0	13.3	14.0	15.1	16.7	18.3	21.0	3.2
11.0	13.1	13.5	14.1	15.4	17.0	18.7	21.5	3.2
11.5	13.2	13.6	14.3	15.6	17.3	19.1	22.1	3.3
12.0	13.3	13.8	14.5	15.8	17.7	19.5	22.6	3.4
12.5	13.5	13.9	14.6	16.0	17.9	19.8	23.0	3.6
13.0	13.6	14.0	14.8	16.3	18.2	20.2	23.4	3.5
13.5	13.7	14.2	14.9	16.5	18.5	20.5	23.8	3.7
14.0	13.8	14.3	15.1	16.7	18.7	20.8	24.2	3.7
14.5	14.0	14.5	15.3	16.9	19.0	21.1	24.5	3.5
15.0	14.2	14.7	15.5	17.2	19.3	21.4	24.9	3.7
15.5	14.4	14.9	15.8	17.4	19.6	21.7	25.2	3.4
16.0	14.6	15.1	16.0	17.7	19.9	22.0	25.5	3.7
16.5	14.9	15.4	16.3	18.0	20.2	22.4	25.8	3.8
17.0	15.1	15.6	16.6	18.3	20.5	22.6	26.0	3.8
17.5	15.4	15.9	16.8	18.6	20.8	22.9	26.3	3.6
18.0	15.6	16.2	17.1	18.9	21.1	23.2	26.6	3.2

TABLE 19.7: Body mass index percentiles and standard deviations for girls

Age	3	5	10	25	50	23 Eq (75)	27 Eq (95)	SD
5.0	11.9	12.1	12.5	13.3	14.3	15.5	18.0	1.4
5.5	11.9	12.2	12.6	13.4	14.4	15.7	18.3	1.7
6.0	12.0	12.2	12.7	13.5	14.5	15.9	18.6	1.7
6.5	12.1	12.3	12.8	13.6	14.7	16.1	18.9	2.0
7.0	12.1	12.4	12.8	13.7	14.9	16.4	19.3	2.1
7.5	12.2	12.5	12.9	13.9	15.1	16.6	19.7	2.2
8.0	12.3	12.6	13.1	14.0	15.3	16.9	20.1	2.3
8.5	12.3	12.7	13.2	14.2	15.6	17.2	20.5	2.7
9.0	12.4	12.8	13.3	14.4	15.8	17.6	21.0	2.7
9.5	12.5	12.9	13.5	14.6	16.1	18.0	21.4	2.8
10.0	12.7	13.1	13.7	14.9	16.5	18.4	21.9	2.9
10.5	12.8	13.2	13.9	15.2	16.8	18.8	22.5	3.1
11.0	13.0	13.4	14.1	15.5	17.2	19.3	23.0	3.1
11.5	13.2	13.7	14.4	15.8	17.6	19.8	23.6	3.3
12.0	13.4	13.9	14.7	16.1	18.0	20.2	24.1	3.2
12.5	13.7	14.2	15.0	16.5	18.4	20.7	24.7	3.3
13.0	13.9	14.4	15.2	16.8	18.8	21.1	25.2	3.2
13.5	14.1	14.6	15.5	17.1	19.1	21.5	25.6	3.5
14.0	14.3	14.9	15.7	17.3	19.4	21.8	25.9	3.4
14.5	14.5	15.1	16.0	17.6	19.7	22.0	26.2	3.3
15.0	14.7	15.2	16.1	17.8	19.9	22.3	26.3	3.4
15.5	14.9	15.4	16.3	18.0	20.1	22.4	26.4	3.1
16.0	15.0	15.6	16.5	18.2	20.3	22.6	26.5	3.1
16.5	15.2	15.8	16.7	18.4	20.4	22.8	26.6	3.2
17.0	15.4	16.0	16.9	18.6	20.6	22.9	26.7	3.0
17.5	15.5	16.1	17.1	18.7	20.8	23.1	26.7	3.1
18.0	15.7	16.3	17.3	18.9	21.0	23.2	26.8	3.6

Comparing the final height and weight data with recent international studies from China, Saudi Arabia, WHO and CDC, it is clear that Indian children are growing almost at par with Chinese and Saudi Arabian children but are still shorter and lighter than their Caucasian counterparts[7,27–29] (Tables 19.7 and 19.8). Further, Indian children's stature seems to be comparable to Caucasian children until the onset of pubertal years, however, the growth spurt after puberty is attenuated in Indian children in both sexes, the effect being more

TABLE 19.8: Boys height and weight comparison at 18 years with IAP 2007 and international data

Parameter	Country/Study					
	Saudi (2007)	China (2009)	Current study	IAP (2007)	CDC (2000)	WHO (2007)
Height						
3rd	156	158	158	161.0	162.5	162.1
50th	169	170	173.6	169.8	176.2	176.1
97th	181	183	186.7	181.6	189.5	193.5
Weight						
3rd	41	47	41.8	47.6	51.7	–
50th	65	61	61.6	58.6	67.3	–
97th	103	85	88.4	83.6	97.2	–

TABLE 19.9: Girls height and weight comparison at 18 years with IAP 2007 and international data

Parameter	Country/Study					
	Saudi (2007)	China (2009)	Current study	IAP (2007)	CDC (2000)	WHO (2007)
Height						
3rd	144	147	146.6	148.3	150.9	150.6
50th	157	160	157.8	157.0	163.1	163.1
97th	170	171	170.6	168.0	175.3	175.5
Weight						
3rd	37	40	37.6	37.6	44.2	–
50th	56	51	52	48.4	52.9	–
97th	84	67	73.5	75.6	83.2	–

pronounced in girls. Thus, the average difference in height between Caucasian girls and Indian girls from 5 to 11 years of age is only about 1 cm; however this gap widens to 6 cm at 18 years. Similar figures in boys are 1 cm from the age of 5 to 12.5 years and 3.5 cm at 18 years. Interestingly, Chinese children also show a very similar growth pattern suggesting that this is possibly a characteristic of Asian children.[30] These finding are of particular relevance in interpreting target height and predicting final adult height based on prediction equations, thus stressing the need for ethnic specific growth charts.

Updating growth references and standards is necessary because with changing socioeconomic standards and demographic changes children's growth patterns also change and secular trends can be incorporated in the updated growth charts. This is particularly true in a developing country as nutrition transition influences growth patterns significantly and secular trends can be marked over a short time period.

The strengths of the growth charts presented here are that they are contemporary, have good national representation as they are prepared from 14 Indian cities from all five zones of IAP giving a true representation of current growth pattern of children across the country. The BMI charts give adult equivalent cut-offs which are more relevant for Asian children and the data have been corrected for unhealthy weights. A drawback of this study is that the study designs and measurement scales possibly used in the nine studies included are different; however, rigorous attention has been given to the methodology of all studies included here to minimize errors while data analysis was performed.

REFERENCES

1. Khadilkar VV, Khadilkar AV, Choudhury P, Agarwal KN, Ugra D, Shah NK. IAP growth monitoring guidelines for children from birth to 18 years. Indian Pediatr 2007;44:187–97.

2. Agarwal DK, Agarwal KN, Upadhyay SK, Mittal R, Prakash R, Rai S. Physical and sexual growth pattern of affluent Indian children from 5-18 years of age. Indian Pediatr 1992;29:1203–82.

3. Agarwal DK, Agarwal KN. Physical growth in Indian affluent children (Birth – 6 years). Indian Pediatr 1994;31:377–413.

4. Buckler JMH. Growth Disorders in Children. 1st ed. London: BMJ Publishing Group; 1994.

5. Khadilkar VV, Khadilkar AV, Cole TJ, Chiplonkar SA, Pandit D. Overweight and obesity prevalence and body mass index trends in Indian children. Int J Pediatr Obes 2011;6:e216–24.

6. WHO Child Growth Standards. Acta Pediatr Supplement 2006;450:5–101.

7. de Onis M, Onyango AW, Borghi E, Siyam A, Nishida C, Siekmann J. Development of a WHO growth reference for school-aged children and adolescents. Bull World Health Organ 2007;85: 660–7.

8. Khadilkar V, Phanse S. Growth charts from controversy to consensus. Indian J Endocrinol Metab 2012;16:S185–7.

9. Bhatia V. Growth charts, the secular trend and the growing concern of childhood obesity. Natl Med J India 2011;24:260–2.

10. Cameron N. The methods of auxological anthropometry. In: Falkner F, Tanner JM (eds). Human growth—A comprehensive treatise. Vol. III. 2nd ed. New York: Plenum Press 1986;3-46.

11. Khadilkar VV, Khadilkar AV, Cole TJ, Sayyad MG. Cross-sectional growth curves for height, weight and body mass index for affluent Indian children, 2007. Indian Pediatr 2009;46:477–89.

12. Khadilkar VV, Khadilkar AV, Borade AB, Chiplonkar SA. Body mass index cut-offs for screening for childhood overweight and obesity in Indian children. Indian Pediatr 2012;49:29–34.

13. Marwaha RK, Tandon N, Ganie MA, Kanwar R, Shivaprasad C, Sabharwal A, et al. Nationwide reference data for height, weight and body mass index of Indian schoolchildren. Natl Med J India 2011;24:269–77.

14. Khadilkar A, Ekbote V, Chiplonkar S, Khadilkar V, Kajale N, Kulkarni S, et al. Waist circumference

percentiles in 2–18 year old Indian children. J Pediatr 2014;164:1358–62.

15. Kaur S, Sachdev HP, Dwivedi SN, Lakshmy R, Kapil U. Prevalence of overweight and obesity amongst school children in Delhi, India. Asia Pac J Clin Nutr 2008;17:592–6.

16. Premanath M, Basavanagowdappa H, Shekar MA, Vikram SB, Narayanappa D. Mysore childhood obesity study. Indian Pediatr 2010;47: 171–3.

17. Goyal JP, Kumar N, Parmar I, Shah VB, Patel B. Determinants of overweight and obesity in affluent adolescent in Surat City, South Gujarat Region, India. Indian J Community Med. 2011;36: 296–300.

18. Cherian AT, Cherian SS, Subbiah S. Prevalence of obesity and overweight in urban school children in Kerala, India. Indian Pediatr 2012;49:475–7.

19. Jagadesan S, Harish R, Miranda P, Unnikrishnan R, Anjana RM, Mohan V. Prevalence of overweight and obesity among school children and adolescents in Chennai. Indian Pediatr 2014;51: 544–9.

20. Ray I, Amar K. An anthropometric study on the children of Tripura: Nutritional and health coverage and redefining WHO percentile cut-off points. Int J Sci Res Publi 2013;3:1–8.

21. Kumaravel V, Shriraam V, Anitharani M, Mahadevan S, Balamurugan AN, Sathiyasekaran BW. Are the current Indian growth charts really representative? Analysis of anthropometric assessment of school children in a South Indian district. Indian J Endocrinol Metab 2014;18:56–62.

22. Mansourian M, Marateb HR, Kelishadi R, Motlagh ME, Aminaee T, Taslimi M, et al. First growth curves based on the World Health Organization reference in a Nationally-representative sample of pediatric population in the Middle East and North Africa (MENA): the CASPIAN-III study. BMC Pediatr 2012;12:149.

23. Cole TJ, Green PJ. Smoothing reference centile curves: The LMS method and penalized likelihood. Stat Med 1992;11:1305–19.

24. Cole TJ, Lobstein T. Extended international (IOTF) body mass index cut-offs for thinness, overweight and obesity. Pediatr Obes 2012;7: 284–94.

25. WHO Expert Consultation. Appropriate body-mass index for Asian populations and its implications for policy and intervention strategies. Lancet 2004;10:157–63.

26. http://www.who.int/growthref/who2007_bmi_for_age/en/. Accessed November 13, 2014.

27. El-Mouzan MI, Al-Herbish AS, Al-Salloum AA, Qurachi MM, Al-Omar AA. Growth charts for Saudi children and adolescents. Saudi Med J 2007;28:1555–68.

28. Zong XN, Li H. Construction of a new growth references for China based on urban Chinese children: Comparison with the WHO growth standards. PLoS One 2013;8:e59569.

29. Kuczmarski RJ, Ogden CL, Guo SS, Grummer-Strawn LM, Flegal KM, Mei Z, et al. 2000 CDC Growth Charts for the United States: methods and development. Vital Health Stat. 11. 2002;246: 1–190.

30. Li H, Ji CY, Zong XN, Zhang YQ. Height and weight standardized growth charts for Chinese children and adolescents aged 0 to 18 years. Zhonghua Er Ke Za Zhi 2009;47:487–92.

Prevention and Treatment of Vitamin D and Calcium Deficiency in Children and Adolescents: IAP Guidelines

Anuradha Khadilkar, Vaman Khadilkar, Jagdish Chinnappa, Narendra Rathi, Rajesh Khadgawat, S Balasubramanian, Bakul Parekh, Pramod Jog

Vitamin D deficiency is increasingly being recognized the world over as also in India.[1–5] Reports from various parts of India and in all age groups from neonates to adolescents as well as pregnant and lactating mothers have reported vitamin D deficiency to the tune of 30–90%.[6–8] Further, habitually low calcium intakes are reported in children and adolescents from several studies all over India, especially those from lower socio-economic classes.[9,10] Given that vitamin D and calcium are both critical for musculoskeletal health in growing years, addressing the issues of their deficiency in the pediatric and adolescent population is critical.

Deficiency of vitamin D (with or without calcium deficiency) may result in rickets in an infant or adolescent or osteomalacia (abnormal mineralization of bone matrix) and muscle weakness in an older child/adolescent.[11] Vitamin D deficiency may also have a negative impact on the peak bone mass resulting in low bone mineral density in childhood, which may subsequently result in osteoporosis in adulthood.[12] Rickets in a neonate resulting from maternal vitamin D deficiency may result in hypocalcemic seizures and rarely cardiomyopathy.[13] There is lack of consensus amongst clinicians and scientists on the role of vitamin D supplementation in relation to extraskeletalal effects particularly in pediatrics; this Guideline therefore, does not deal with these effects of vitamin D.[14] Rickets resulting from deficiency of vitamin D and/or calcium deficiency may be prevented and treated with adequate intake of vitamin D and calcium.[15] However, children with vitamin D deficiency, without raised Parathormone (PTH) or signs of rickets are not at an increased risk of fractures.[16]

Less than 10% of vitamin D is derived from the diet while close to 90% is synthesized in the skin with sunlight exposure.[17] Socio-cultural practices, darker pigmentation, a diet low in calcium and high in phytates and oxalates which depletes vitamin D, absence of fortification with vitamin D, genetic factors such as increased 25(OH)D-24-hydroxylase, which degrades 25(OH)D to inactive metabolites, geographical location of various places in the country (India extends from 8 to 38 degrees north latitude) and environmental pollution are some reasons proposed for vitamin D deficiency in Indian children.[18–21] Together with these factors, changing lifestyles with sedentary behavior in children with indoor lifestyle (avoiding optimal hours of sun exposure between 10 AM to 3 PM, the best time to form Vitamin D in the skin) further reduce the sunlight exposure and thus increase the tendency for vitamin D deficiency.[21–23] Further, very few Indian foods are fortified with vitamin D, and that too, with small amounts.[23] Premature babies and children with renal, hepatic disorders, malabsorptive states, etc. are at special risk for metabolic bone disease.[24]

Given the plethora of literature on vitamin D deficiency, multiple guidelines suggested by various international bodies, lack of consensus about the ranges for deficiency and sufficiency, peculiarities of the Indian circumstances, evidence from India suggesting high prevalence of vitamin D and calcium deficiency in the pediatric population,[16,24–26] the practitioner may be confused regarding appropriate prevention and treatment of vitamin D and calcium deficiency. The Indian Academy of Pediatrics (IAP) therefore felt the need for a practice guideline for pediatricians for the prevention and treatment of vitamin D and calcium deficiency in children and adolescents. These guidelines do not include conditions causing non-nutritional rickets; e.g. renal disorders, disorders of the parathyroid hormone axis.

Methods

The 'Guideline for Vitamin D and Calcium in Children Committee' was formed by the IAP in September 2016. The consultative committee scrutinized the methodology, results and scientific content of the manuscript in November 2016 in Mumbai after data from an extensive search on prevalence of deficiency of vitamin D and calcium from India was performed. Guidelines on the deficiency of vitamin D and calcium with reference to deficiencies for children and adolescents published by various bodies in Indexed journals were identified through internet-based search engines *viz.* Google, PubMed and Embase.[16,24-27] Indian studies reporting the prevalence of vitamin D deficiency and intakes of calcium were also reviewed. Evidence from Indian studies and other previously published recommendations, which were pertinent to the

Indian circumstances, were collated for preparation of these guidelines. For vitamin D, the guidelines are based on the assumption of minimal sun exposure.[26]

DEFINITIONS

This is based on the serum concentrations of 25(OH)D. Although professional bodies recommend that the assessment should be performed by tandem mass spectrometry (TMS), most reports from India suggest that these are performed by enzyme-linked immunosorbent assay, chemiluminescence or radio-immuno assay. Very few centers have the facility for assessment of vitamin D with TMS. Although a fasting specimen is recommended, it is not required; further, diurnal variations are also not a major consideration.[28,29] Given the various methods and the variability in the values of vitamin D using different assays, reports for serum 25(OH)D should be interpreted with care, taking into account the laboratory and type of assay employed. Measurement of the active form of vitamin D, 1,25-dihydroxychole-calciferol for the assessment of vitamin D deficiency is not recommended.[25] Data suggest that 20 ng/mL (50 nmol/L) can be set as the serum 25(OH)D level that coincides with the level that would cover the needs of 97.5 percent of the population;[16,26] thus, vitamin D concentrations of >20 ng/mL (50 nmol/L) are considered as sufficient, between 12–20 ng/mL (30–50 nmol/L) as insufficient, and <12 ng/mL (<30 nmol/L) as deficient.[16]

Calcium deficiency is difficult to define as there is no specific biochemical marker for the reserves of calcium [like 25(OH)D for vitamin D]; therefore, these guidelines refer to dietary calcium deficiency.[30]

Although ensuring adequacy is important, there is also concern about excessive intake and administration of vitamin D, particularly on the basis of only low 25(OH)D concentrations. Toxicity is defined as vitamin D concentrations of 25(OH)D of >100 ng/mL

(250 nmol/L) with hypercalcemia, hypercalciuria and suppressed PTH concentrations.[31] Following inadvertent high doses of vitamin D, testing for serum levels of calcium and vitamin D are recommended, especially in children with symptoms of hypercalcemia such as irritability, constipation and polyuria.[32]

Hypercalcemia (that can result in vascular and soft tissue calcification, nephrocalcinosis, nephrolithiasis, etc.) occurs when serum calcium concentrations are above 10.5 mg/dL (reference to the laboratory values is also recommended).[33] Preferably, serum ionized calcium may be assessed as 1 gm% reduction in serum albumin will reduce total serum calcium by 0.8 mg%.[34]

Tolerable upper limit (i.e. the maximum level of total chronic daily intake of a nutrient from all sources judged to be unlikely to pose a risk of adverse health effects to humans) for intake of vitamin D and calcium during neonatal period, 1–12 months, 1–18 years are 1000 IU/day, 1000–1500 IU/day, 3000–4000 IU/day and 1000 mg/day, 1000–1500 mg/day, and 2500–3000 mg/day, respectively (Table 20.1).[16,25,33,35] Larger doses may be required for treatment of rickets; however, tolerable upper limits are not to be exceeded without supervision.

Screening for vitamin D deficiency: Routine screening of healthy children for vitamin D deficiency is not recommended.[16,25] However, screening may be performed for children, who are at risk of vitamin D deficiency, for determination of vitamin D concentrations and treatment.[25] Monitoring 25(OH)D levels in the population is not practical because of the need for drawing blood, high monetary cost of assessment, and also a low positive predictive value; and is thus reserved for high-risk groups.

Route of administration: Oral treatment is recommended; reports suggest that oral administration of vitamin D restores vitamin D concentrations more rapidly than by the intramuscular (IM) route.[16] This is especially important in the Indian context as injectable

	Vitamin D				Calcium		
Age	Prevention	*Tolerable upper limit	Treatment	#Treatment with large dose	Prevention	*Tolerable upper limit	Treatment
Premature neonates	400 IU/d	1000 IU/d	1000 IU/d	NA	Intake of 150 to 220 mg/kg/d	1000 mg/d	Maximum of 175–200 mg/kg/d
Neonates	400 IU/d	1000 IU/d	2000 IU/d$	NA	200 mg/d	1000 mg/d	500 mg/d
1–12 m	400 IU/d	1000–1500 IU/d	2000 IU/d$	60000 IU wkly for 6 wk (over 3 m of age)	250–500 mg/d	1000–1500 mg/d	500 mg/d
1–18 y	600 IU/d	3000 IU/d till 9 y, 4000 IU/d from 9–18 y	3000–6000 IU/d$	60000 IU wkly for 6 wk	600–800 mg/d 3000 mg/d	2500 mg/d till 8 y and for 9–18 y	600–800 mg/d
At-risk groups	400–1000 IU/d	as per age group	as per age group	as per age group	as per age group	as per age group	as per age group

TABLE 20.1: Recommendations for vitamin D and calcium deficiency–prevention and treatment

$For a minimum of 3 months after treatment, daily maintenance doses need to be given; *Tolerable Upper Limit—the maximum level of total chronic daily intake of a nutrient (from all sources) judged to be unlikely to pose a risk of adverse health effects to humans; #Oral route preferred

preparations of vitamin D are inadvertently used in very large doses for longer periods. The IM route with larger doses may only be considered when compliance or absorption from the gut is an issue. Further, vitamin D may be administered with a meal or on an empty stomach as absorption is independent of fed state.[25]

RECOMMENDATIONS

The recommendations for prevention and treatment of vitamin D and calcium deficiency for various age groups and for at-risk groups are provided in Table 20.1. Assessment of dietary intake of calcium to ensure that children are having adequate calcium for optimum bone health is required.

Prevention of Deficiency of Vitamin D and Deficiency of Calcium

Premature neonates: Calcium and phosphorus in breast milk do not meet the needs of rapidly growing premature infants who have missed some of the critical period of intrauterine bone growth; this puts them at a higher risk for metabolic bone disease.[36] Exposure to medications that alter mineral levels, immobilization, and long-term parenteral nutrition may further increase the risk of the premature baby for metabolic bone disease (MBD).[37,38] Routine measurement of serum 25(OH)D levels in premature infants is not recommended; however, in the presence of a likely impairment of 25-hydroxylation, such as might be present in an infant with cholestasis, measurement of serum 25(OH)D level may be considered.[26] Enteral calcium intake of about 150 to 220 mg/kg per day, phosphorous intake of 75–140 mg/kg/day and vitamin D intake of 400 IU/day is recommended.[37] Backstrom, *et al.* have found that an intake of 200 IU/kg of vitamin D in premature infants in first 6 weeks after birth lead to mean 25(OH)D concentrations of around 50 nmol/L.[38] It is however critical to avoid excessive administration of vitamin D that can lead to hypervitaminosis,

especially as various preparations with varying amount of vitamin D and calcium are available in India.

Neonates and infants up to 1 year of age: Although there is likelihood of a high prevalence of vitamin D deficiency in apparently healthy term neonates who are born to vitamin D deficient mothers, due to financial and logistic limitations in the Indian context, routine screening for vitamin D concentrations in this age group cannot be recommended. Breastmilk is not an adequate source of vitamin D;[39] 400 IU of vitamin D has been shown to maintain serum 25(OH)D concentrations at >50 nmol/L in breastfed infants.[40] Further, for formula-fed infants, the amount of formula milk to obtain 400 IU/day would be close to a liter, which a baby may not consume daily. Thus, for all newborns, 400 IU of vitamin D supplementation is recommended till one year of age; it is also recommended that supplementation be started in the first few days of life. It is critical to give careful instructions about the dosage and administration and to avoid excessive administration of vitamin D, which could lead to hypervitaminosis, particularly in infants.

There are no reports of full-term, vitamin D-replete infants developing calcium deficiency when exclusively fed human milk.[41] Also, calcium absorption is high in neonates to the tune of around 60% (facilitated by lactose from breast milk); hence, the adequate intake for calcium based on amounts of calcium in breast milk is 200 mg. In the first year of life, if dietary calcium intake is not adequate (250–500 mg), calcium supplementation is justified.[42,43]

Maternal concentrations of vitamin D determine the status of vitamin D of her fetus and newborn.[44] Thus, the neonate of a mother who has vitamin D deficiency is also likely to be vitamin D deficient. Hence, it is recommended that pregnant mothers receive 600 IU of vitamin D daily.[25] This supplementation is also to be continued during lactation. Breastmilk contains very little vitamin D, which is inadequate for the newborn who requires around 400 IU/day.[39] However, to increase content of breast milk vitamin D, very large doses are required to be given to lactating mothers. Thus, it is recommended that infants be supplemented with 400 IU daily and mothers continue to take 600 IU daily for their own vitamin D needs. Maternal dietary intake of calcium is not associated with breast milk content; however, it is recommended that mothers take 1200 mg of calcium, as advised by the ICMR.[17]

Children older than 1 year and adolescents: Vitamin D deficiency is likely to occur during rapid phases of growth as well as when there are physiological changes; Indian children are spending more and more time indoors and intake of milk and other calcium-containing foods is also low. As a result of this, as per reports, a very high percentage of children have vitamin D concentrations below 50 nmol/L. Hence, it is recommended that all children and adolescents be supplemented with 600 IU of vitamin D that is believed to maximize bone health.[2,25] Along with the vitamin D, it is recommended that adequate amounts of calcium, i.e. 600–800 mg/day should also be supplemented/derived from dietary sources; this may be obtained from 2–3 servings of milk and milk products/day (as per recommendations from the Indian Council of Medical Research).[17]

At-risk groups: In cases where there is an increased risk of deficiency of vitamin D such as in children with fat malabsorption, liver disease or renal insufficiency, transplant recipients, those on anti-seizure medications, children on treatment for malignancy, restricted sun exposure such as in children with physical disabilities, history of rickets, children with predisposition to osteoporosis such as in hypogonadism or Cushing's syndrome, etc., higher doses of vitamin D may be required to ensure adequate concentrations of vitamin D.[16,25,26] Thus, for at-risk infants,

400–1000 IU/day and from 1 year onwards, 600–1000 IU/day may be required to maintain 25(OH)D concentrations above 50 nmol/L.[25] Screening for vitamin D concentrations may be performed in this group of children and treatment with vitamin D advised accordingly. Repeat measurements of vitamin D at 3–6 monthly intervals may be performed as clinically indicated, especially if follow up radiological assessments show poor/inadequate healing of rickets. Adequate calcium intake as per the age group (Table 20.1) should also be ensured.

There is an inverse association of body fat with vitamin D concentrations; vitamin D being a fat soluble vitamin, is sequestrated in adipose tissue.[45] Thus, children who are obese may be given at least two to three times (between 400–1000 IU/day) more vitamin D for their age group to satisfy their body's vitamin D requirements.[25]

Treatment of Deficiency of Vitamin D and Deficiency of Calcium

For preterm infants with rickets/metabolic bone disease who are able to tolerate oral/enteral feeding, calcium intake of up to a maximum of to a maximum of 70–80 mg/kg/day of elemental calcium and 40–50 mg/kg/day elemental phosphorus is indicated.[37] Preterm infants with rickets are also provided the tolerable upper intake of 1000 IU/day of vitamin D [target serum 25(OH)D concentration of >20 ng/mL (50 nmol/L)].[27]

For the emergency treatment of hypocalcemia resulting in seizures in a neonate, calcium gluconate in a dose of 2 mL/kg as slow intravenous infusion and calcitriol [1–25(OH)2 D3] is recommended in a dose of 20–50 ng/kg/day. Also, vitamin D in a dose of 1000 IU/day is recommended.[46]

For neonates and infants till 1 year of age, daily 2000 IU of vitamin D with 500 mg of calcium for a 3-month period is recommended. At the end of 3 months, response to treatment should be reassessed and treatment continued, if required.[16] Response to treatment may be assessed on clinical biochemical and radiological parameters. If larger doses of vitamin D are to be given, then, 60,000 IU of vitamin D weekly for 6 weeks is recommended (only in infants older than 3 months of age).[16] After completion of this therapy with weekly doses, maintenance doses of 400 IU of vitamin D daily and 250–500 mg of calcium are necessary.

From one year onwards till 18 years of age, 3000–6000 IU/day of vitamin D along with calcium intake of 600–800 mg/day is recommended for a minimum of 3 months. For larger doses (oral preferred) 60,000 IU of vitamin D weekly for 6 weeks may be administered.[25] The maintenance doses of 600 IU/day of vitamin D and 600–800 mg of calcium need to be continued post therapy. Complete healing at 12 weeks has been observed in higher percentage of children with rickets who received combined therapy with vitamin D and calcium.[47] Calcitriol, the active form of vitamin D, should not be used for vitamin D deficiency rickets. Minimum treatment for vitamin D and calcium deficiency is advised for 3 months. If there are no radiological and biochemical signs of healing after 3 months, the patient may need to be investigated for non-nutritional rickets.[48]

Available Preparations

Vitamin D3 (cholecalciferol) has been reported to have greater efficacy in raising 25(OH)D concentrations, most supplements available thus contain D3. Reports suggest that there is variability in cholecalciferol content of commercial preparations available in the Indian pharmaceutical market; thus caution should be used when prescribing preparations of vitamin D.[49]

Most calcium supplements contain calcium carbonate, though preparations with gluconate and citrate are also available. Calcium carbonate contains the highest amount of elemental calcium (40%) compared to other preparations (gluconate, citrate). Thus, given the lower price and higher amount of elemental calcium, it should be the first choice.[50] Supplements containing calcium citrate may be taken with or without food. However, if the preparation contains calcium carbonate or any other form of calcium, it should be taken with food. All forms of calcium work better if taken in divided doses; however, compliance also needs to be considered. Very few preparations containing only calcium salts (without vitamin D) are available.

CONCLUSION

Considering the increased prevalence of vitamin D deficiency and the confusion about supplementation and treatment of vitamin D deficiency for various age groups, the IAP has put forth recommendations for prevention and treatment of vitamin D and calcium deficiency. The recommendations are in line with other international organizations. As a long term policy, fortifying everyday staple foods, which will be consumed by the at-risk segments of the population, with calcium and vitamin D is the solution to the problem. Till the time this can be implemented, supplementation of infants with 400 IU, and children and adolescents with 600 IU daily and higher doses for at-risk groups, with adequate calcium intake for prevention of deficiency is necessary. Adequate intake of calcium and continuing maintenance doses of vitamin D after treatment of rickets is warranted.

Disclaimer: The present guidelines are developed for the assistance of pediatricians in accordance with current scientific evidence and guidelines presented by major international bodies for preserving and promoting musculoskeletal health in children; however, many areas are still not clearly defined. Vitamin D has been reported to have many other important health benefits and when rigorous proof is available, guidelines will be suitably modified. These guidelines cannot establish a standard of care, and decisions about treatment should be based on the judgement of the pediatrician on a case-to-case basis.

REFERENCES

1. Mithal A, Wahl DA, Bonjour JP, Burckhardt P, Dawson-Hughes B, Eisman JA, et al. Global vitamin D status and determinants of hypovitaminosis D. Osteoporos Int. 2009;20:1807–20.

2. Puri S, Marwaha RK, Agarwal N, Tandon N, Agarwal R, Grewal K, et al. Vitamin D status of apparently healthy schoolgirls from two different socioeconomic strata in Delhi: relation to nutrition and lifestyle. Br J Nutr. 2008;99:876–82.

3. Garg MK, Marwaha RK, Khadgawat R, Ramot R, Obroi AK, Mehan N, et al. Efficacy of vitamin D loading doses on serum 25-hydroxy vitamin D levels in school going adolescents: an open label non-randomized prospective trial. J Pediatr Endocrinol Metab. 2013;26:515–23.

4. Ekbote VH, Khadilkar AV, Mughal MZ, Hanumante N, Sanwalka N, Khadilkar VV, et al. Sunlight exposure and development of rickets in Indian toddlers. Indian J Pediatr. 2010;77:61–5.

5. Rathi N, Rathi A. Vitamin D and child health in the 21st century. Indian Pediatr. 2011;48:619–25.

6. Kajale NA, Khadilkar VV, Mughal Z, Chiplonkar SA, Khadilkar AV. Changes in body composition of Indian lactating women: a longitudinal study. Asia Pac J Clin Nutr. 2016;25:556–62.

7. Sachan A, Gupta R, Das V, Agarwal A, Awasthi PK, Bhatia V. High prevalence of vitamin D deficiency among pregnant women and their newborns in northern India. Am J Clin Nutr. 2005;81:1060–4.

8. Balasubramanian S. Vitamin D deficiency in breastfed infants and the need for routine vitamin D supplementation. Indian J Med Res. 2011;133: 250–2.

9. Sanwalka NJ, Khadilkar AV, Mughal MZ, Sayyad MG, Khadilkar VV, Shirole SC, et al. A study of calcium intake and sources of calcium in adolescent boys and girls from two socioeconomic strata, in Pune, India. Asia Pac J Clin Nutr. 2010;19:324–9.

10. Harinarayan CV, Ramalakshmi T, Prasad UV, Sudhakar D, Srinivasarao PV, Sarma KV, et al. High prevalence of low dietary calcium, high phytate consumption and vitamin D deficiency in healthy south Indians. Am J Clin Nutr. 2007;85: 1062–7.

11. Lips P, van Schoor NM. The effect of vitamin D on bone and osteoporosis. Best Pract Res Clin Endocrinol Metab. 2011;25:585–91.

12. Golden NH, Abrams SA; Committee on Nutrition. Optimizing bone health in children and adolescents. Pediatrics. 2014;134:e1229–43.

13. Maiya S, Sullivan I, Allgrove J, Yates R, Malone M, Brain C, et al. Hypocalcaemia and vitamin D deficiency: an important, but preventable, cause of life-threatening infant heart failure. Heart. 2008;94:581–4.

14. Theodoratou E, Tzoulaki I, Zgaga L, Ioannidis JP. Vitamin D and multiple health outcomes: Umbrella review of systematic reviews and meta-analyses of observational studies and randomised trials. BMJ. 2014;348:g2035.

15. Thacher TD, Fischer PR, Strand MA, Pettifor JM. Nutritional rickets around the world: causes and future directions. Ann Trop Paediatr. 2006;26:1–16.

16. Munns CF, Shaw N, Kiely M, Specker BL, Thacher TD, Ozono K, et al. Global consensus recommendations on prevention and management of nutritional rickets. J Clin Endocrinol Metab. 2016;101:394–415.

17. Indian Council of Medical Research (ICMR), Nutrient Requirements and Recommended Dietary Allowances for Indians, a Report of the Expert Group of the Indian Council of Medical Research 2010. Hyderabad, India: National Institute of Nutrition; 2010.

18. Khadilkar AV. Vitamin D deficiency in Indian adolescents. Indian Pediatr. 2010; 47:755–6.

19. Harinarayan CV, Ramalakshmi T, Venkataprasad U. High prevalence of low dietary calcium and low vitamin D status in healthy south Indians. Asia Pac J Clin Nutr. 2004;13:359–64.

20. Awumey EM, Mitra DA, Hollis BW, Kumar R, Bell NH. Vitamin D metabolism is altered in Asian Indians in the southern United States: a clinical research center study. J Clin Endocrinol Metab. 1998;83:169–173.

21. Agarwal KS, Mughal MZ, Upadhyay P, Berry JL, Mawer EB, Puliyel JM. The impact of atmospheric pollution on vitamin D status of infants and toddlers in Delhi, India. Arch Dis Child. 2002; 87:111–3.

22. Meena P, Dabas A, Shet D, Malhotra RK, Madhu SV, Gupta P. Sunlight exposure and vitamin D status in breastfed infants. Indian Pediatr. 2017; 54:105–11.

23. Ritu G, Gupta A. Fortification of Foods with Vitamin D in India. Nutrients. 2014; 6:3601–23.

24. Nehra D, Carlson SJ, Fallon EM, Kalish B, Potemkin AK, Gura KM, et al. A.S.P.E.N. clinical

guidelines: Nutrition support of neonatal patients at risk for metabolic bone disease. J Parenter Enteral Nutr. 2013;37:570–98.

25. Holick MF, Binkley NC, Bischoff-Ferrari HA, Gordon CM, Hanley DA, Heaney RP, et al. Evaluation, treatment, and prevention of vitamin D deficiency: An Endocrine Society clinical practice guideline. J Clin Endocrinol Metab. 2011;96:1911–30.

26. A Catharine Ross; Institute of Medicine (US). Committee to Review Dietary Reference Intakes for vitamin D and Calcium. (2011). DRI, dietary reference intakes: calcium, vitamin D. Washington, DC: National Academies Press.

27. Wagner CL, Greer FR; American Academy of Pediatrics Section on Breastfeeding; American Academy of Pediatrics Committee on Nutrition. Prevention of rickets and vitamin D deficiency in infants, children, and adolescents. Pediatrics. 2008;122:1142–52.

28. Roth HJ, Schmidt-Gayk H, Weber H, Niederau C. Accuracy and clinical implications of seven 25-hydroxyvitamin D methods compared with liquid chromatography-tandem mass spectrometry as a reference. Ann Clin Biochem. 2008;45:153–9.

29. Laboratory Procedure Manual. 2015. Available from http://www.cdc.gov/nchs/data/nhanes/nhanes_05_06/VID_D_met_Vitamin_D.pdf. Accessed November 15, 2016.

30. Wang M, Yang X, Wang F, Li R, Ning H, Na L, et al. Calcium-deficiency assessment and biomarker identification by an integrated urinary metabonomics analysis. BMC Med. 2013;11:86.

31. Munns CF, Simm PJ, Rodda CP, Garnett SP, Zacharin MR, Ward LM, et al. Incidence of vitamin D deficiency rickets among Australian children: an Australian Paediatric Surveillance Unit study. Med J Aust. 2012;196:466–8.

32. Vogiatzi MG, Jacobson-Dickman E, DeBoer MD; Drugs, and Therapeutics Committee of the Pediatric Endocrine Society. Vitamin D supplementation and risk of toxicity in pediatrics: A review of current literature. J Clin Endocrinol Metab. 2014; 99:1132–41.

33. Institute of Medicine (US) Committee to Review Dietary Reference Intakes for Vitamin D and Calcium; Ross AC, Taylor CL, Yaktine AL, et al., editors. Dietary Reference Intakes for Calcium and Vitamin D. Washington (DC): National Academies Press (US); 2011. 6, Tolerable Upper Intake Levels: Calcium and Vitamin D. Available

from: https://www.ncbi.nlm.nih.gov/books/NBK56058/. Accessed November 26, 2017.

34. Calcium imbalances. In: Metheny NM. Fluid and Electrolyte Imbalances: Nursing considerations. 5th edition. USA: Jones & Bartlett Learning, LLC; 2015. 91–110.

35. Panel on Dietetic Products, Nutrition and Allergies. Scientific Opinion on the Tolerable Upper Intake Level of eicosapentaenoic acid (EPA), docosahexaenoic acid (DHA) and docosapentaenoic acid (DPA). EFSA J. 2012;10:2815.

36. Hosking DJ. Calcium homeostasis in pregnancy. Clin Endocrinol (Oxf). 1996;45: 1–6.

37. Abrams SA. Committee on Nutrition. Calcium and vitamin d requirements of enterally fed preterm infants. Pediatrics. 2013;131:e1676–83.

38. Backstrom MC, Maki R, Kuusela AL, Sievänen H, Koivisto AM, Ikonen RS, et al. Randomised controlled trial of vitamin D supplementation on bone density and bio-chemical indices in preterm infants. Arch Dis Child Fetal Neonatal Ed. 1999; 80:F161–F6.

39. Hollis BW, Wagner CL. Vitamin D requirements during lactation: High-dose maternal supplementation as therapy to prevent hypovitaminosis D for both the mother and the nursing infant. Am J Clin Nutr. 2004;80:1752S–8S.

40. Wagner CL, Hulsey TC, Fanning D, Ebeling M, Hollis BW. High-dose vitamin D3 supplementation in a cohort of breastfeeding mothers and their infants: a 6-month follow-up pilot study. Breastfeed Med. 2006;1:59–70.

41. Mimouni F, Campaigne B, Neylan M, Tsang RC. Bone mineralization in the first year of life in infants fed human milk, cow-milk formula, or soy-based formula. J Pediatr. 1993;122:348–54.

42. Fomon SJ, Nelson SE. Calcium, phosphorus, magnesium, and sulfur. In: Fomon SJ, editor. Nutrition of Normal Infants. Mosby-Year Book, Inc.; St. Louis, MO, USA: 1993. p. 192–218.

43. Widdowson EM. Absorption and excretion of fat, nitrogen, and minerals from "filled" milks by babies one week old. Lancet. 1965;2:1099–105.

44. Hollis BW, Pittard WB 3rd. Evaluation of the total feto-maternal vitamin D relationships at term: evidence for racial differences. J Clin Endocrinol Metab. 1984;59:652–7.

45. Wortsman J, Matsuoka LY, Chen TC, Lu Z, Holick MF. Decreased bioavailability of vitamin D in obesity. Am J Clin Nutr. 2000;72: 690–3.

46. Greenbaum LA. Rickets and Hypervitaminosis D. In: Kliegman RM, Stanton BF, Geme JW, Schor

NF, eds. Nelson Textbook of Paediatrics. 20th edition. Philadelphia (PA): Elsevier Health Sciences; 2015. p.331–40.

47. Aggarwal V, Seth A, Aneja S, Sharma B, Sonkar P, Singh S, *et al*. Role of calcium deficiency in development of nutritional rickets in Indian children: A case control study. J Clin Endocrinol Metab. 2012;97:3461–6.

48. Mughal MZ. Metabolic Bone Disorders. In: Desai MP, Menon P, Bhatia V, editors. Pediatric Endocrine Disorders. 3rd ed. Chennai: Orient Longman Private Ltd.; 2014. p.401–05.

49. Khadgawat R, Ramot R, Chacko KM, Marwaha RK. Disparity in cholecalciferol content of commercial preparations available in India. Indian J Endocr Metab. 2013;17:1100–3.

50. Heaney RP, Dowell MS, Bierman J, Hale CA, Bendich A. Absorbability and cost effectiveness in calcium supplementation. J Am Coll Nutr. 2001; 20:239–46.

Consensus Statement of the IAP on Newborn Hearing Screening

Abraham Paul, Chhaya Prasad, SS Kamath, Samir Dalwai, MKC Nair, Waheeda Pagarkar

Hearing impairment is one of the most critical sensory impairments with significant social and psychological consequences. Failure to detect children with congenital or acquired hearing loss may result in lifelong deficits in speech and language acquisition, poor academic performance and personal-social and behavior problems.[1,2] Deficits in speech and language lead to lack of stimulation, which adversely affects the structure of the synaptic junction. Lack of auditory stimulation leads to retrograde degeneration in the cell body and axon.[3]

Apart from the biological evidence, the data on congenital disabilities indicate that hearing loss has a substantially high incidence with congenital hearing loss affecting 30 per 10,000 children.[4] Significant hearing loss is the most common disorder, occurring in 1 to 2 newborns per 1000 in the general population, and 24 to 46% of newborns admitted to neonatal intensive care unit.[5,6] Vocabulary of a 3-year-old child with hearing impairment if remediated at birth is 300–700 words; if remediated at 6 months is 150–300 words and if remediated at 2 years is 0–50 words, respectively; as compared to vocabulary of a 3-year-old child with typical hearing which is 500–900 words.

In view of the above, standard guidelines for screening newborns for hearing loss are urgently needed. The meeting on formulation of National consensus guidelines on developmental disorders was organized by the Indian Academy of Pediatrics in Mumbai, on 18th and 19th December, 2015. The invited experts included Pediatricians, Developmental Pediatricians, Pediatric Neurologists and Clinical Psychologists. The participants framed guidelines after extensive discussions and review of literature. Thereafter, a committee was established to review and finalize the points discussed in the meeting.

Subsequent sections include the points of consensus on screening of newborn hearing.

RECOMMENDATIONS

Early Screening

Critical period for identification and remediation of hearing loss is before the age of 6 months. Since the pediatrician is the primary care provider for the child during the first few days of life, it is the sole responsibility of the pediatrician (or the primary physician) to evaluate the child for hearing loss (or ensure referral for the same). It has been observed that practice of neonatal screening has dramatically lowered the age of diagnosis of deafness from

1½–3 years to less than 6 months of age. Screening should ideally be 'universal', i.e. everybody is screened and at a minimum, screening should be 'targeted', i.e. 'high risk' babies are screened.

Causes of hearing loss are summarized in Box 21.1. These can be classified as: Conductive, Cochlear (i.e. Sensory: defect in the cochlea and Neural: defect in the 8th cranial/ auditory nerve), Retrocochlear (i.e. defect at the level of auditory nerve, brainstem auditory pathway or both) and Central (i.e. defect in the auditory area in cerebral cortex).

With respect to current guidelines, sensorineural hearing loss is most relevant and cochlear causes of sensorineural hearing loss are more common. Many risk factors for hearing loss have been identified and are listed in Box 21.2.

Congenital rubella syndrome, Usher syndrome and Jervell and Lange-Nielsen (JLN) syndrome have been noted to be associated with hearing loss; few other syndromes include Treacher-Collins syndrome, Apert syndrome, Alport syndrome, Neurofibromatosis syndrome, Achondroplasia, CHARGE syndrome, Brachio Oto Renal

---

BOX 21.2: Risk factors for hearing loss[7]

- Family history of hereditary childhood sensorineural hearing impairment
- Intrauterine infection (TORCH)
- Craniofacial anomalies
- Birth weight less than 1500 gram
- Hyperbilirubinemia at a serum level requiring exchange transfusion
- Ototoxic medications used in multiple courses, or in combination with loop diuretics.
- Bacterial meningitis
- APGAR scores 0–4 at 1 minute or 0–6 at 5 minute
- Mechanical ventilation for 5 days or longer
- Stigmata of other findings associated with a syndrome known to include sensorineural and/or conductive hearing loss.

---

syndrome, Chudley McCullough syndrome and Golden Har syndrome.[8]

Screening for Newborn Hearing Loss

In India, majority of hospitals do not conduct universal or high risk screening. In such a situation, a centralized facility catering to all hospitals in a city is a practical option. A two-stage screening protocol can be made, in which infants are screened first with otoacoustic emissions (OAE). Infants who fail the OAE are screened with auditory brainstem response (ABR). In this two tier screening program, the second tier being ABR (which is more expensive) is required only for a select few, making the program more practical and viable.

The Child Health Screening and Early Intervention Services Program (Rashtriya Bal Swasthya Karyakram) under National Rural Health Mission initiated by the Ministry of Health and Family Welfare of Government of India has included congenital deafness as one of the conditions to be included for early identification and remediation. It involves screening of infants and children under age 18 years by a mobile team and provision of appropriate treatment at District Early Intervention Centres (DEICs). This ambitious scheme is likely to streamline the management of hearing disabilities.[9]

BOX 21.1: Causes of hearing loss

- Causes in ear canal/Conductive (e.g., congenital atresia, wax, foreign body, trauma, external otitis, stenosis
- Causes in middle ear/Conductive (e.g., acute and chronic otitis media, perforation of tympanic membrane, congenital defects, trauma, malformations either hereditary or familial)
- Causes in the cochlea/Cochlear (e.g., ototoxic drugs, stay in neonatal intensive care unit due to jaundice or other causes, neonatal infections, head injury, noise); and
- Causes in auditory nerve/Retrocochlear (e.g., problems in cochlear nerve, auditory pathway or cortex like tumors, trauma, de myelination).
- Intrauterine infections (tetanus, toxoplasma, rubella, cytomegalovirus and herpes or TORCH group of infections) can be classified as cochlear or retrocochlear causes of Sensorineural hearing loss.

Otoacoustic emissions (OAEs) are quicker methods (as compared to electrophysiologic methods like ABR) for assessing hearing in newborns *via* a simple set-up. Otoacoustic emissions (OAEs) are sounds of cochlear origin recorded in the auditory meatus (ear canal), produced by the action of healthy outer hair cells. The emissions themselves serve no purpose and are simply a leakage of energy from the ear. Hearing is facilitated by hair cell activity in the cochlea and more specifically, the activity of outer hair cells. There are three rows of outer hair cells (OHCs) and one row of inner hair cells that sit on the basilar membrane, sandwiched by the tectorial membrane on top. This forms the organ of Corti. There are around 12000 motile OHCs working together to provide mechanical assistance to sound energy, amplifying the travelling wave to overcome the viscous nature of the cochlear fluid. As the 'W' shaped steriocilia are stimulated by fluid moving over them, it causes the cells to alternately contract and release, providing a pumping action. This mechanical system provides the frequency tuning within the cochlea. The inner hair cells are also stimulated and deflected by fluid flow; and at a specific threshold, the inner cells release a neurotransmitter which causes the auditory nerve to transmit a signal to the brain.

Cochlear damage is almost always apparent in the loss of outer hair cells. This is true regardless of the etiology–congential progressive hearing loss, ototoxic drugs, presbyacusis (Sensorineural hearing loss with aging), as well as noise-induced hearing loss. With damaged OHCs, there is no amplification or frequency tuning, thus the child will not only suffer a threshold shift but also have problems with frequency discrimination.

OAE test is performed *via* a small probe placed in the child's ear canal; click sounds are delivered and response is detected (Box 21.3). The child must be quiet.[10]

BOX 21.3: Details of screening tests

The two available techniques are Otoacoustic emissions (OAE) and Auditory Brain-stem response (ABR).

Otoacoustic emissions (OAE): Probe is kept in the ear and the machine is switched 'on' when click sounds are produced. Sound waves travel from the external ear to the inner ear and causes outer hair cells of the cochlea to move, producing sound detected by the machine probe at the external ear canal. This indicates that the baby has a normal cochlear (inner ear) function.

Cost of instrument: OAE Screener Otoportlite (Otodynamics, UK) cost ₹ 2.95 lakh + Tax; can be purchased locally.

Purchase and maintenance: Of the four basic parts of the OAE instrument (main body, probe, probe tips and couplers), it is the couplers which require replacement most often, when the debris in the ear canal or wax obstructs it. Couplers cost around ₹ 500. Probe tips may require frequent changes, cost ₹ 50. Main instrument and probe last long enough for two to three years. In addition, the batteries need to be replaced.

OAE may be affected by debris or fluid in the external and middle ear, decreased tympanic mobility, delayed cochlear maturation - resulting in referral rates of 5% to 20% when screening is performed in the first 24 hours after birth. Hence, OAE should be done on the day of discharge or 72 hours after birth. Referral rates <3% may be achieved when screening is performed during first 48 hours after birth. In a two step system using OAE as the first step, referral rates of 5% to 20% for repeat screening with ABR or OAE may be expected.

Due to automated OAEs, screening can be conducted by anyone after baseline training. However, the person should be educated till graduate level or preferably from medical field, so he/she can communicate results to caregivers.

Auditory Brainstem Response (ABR): ABR is an electro-physiologic measurement that is used to assess auditory function from the eighth nerve through the auditory brainstem; *via* placing disposable surface electrodes high on the forehead, mastoid and the nape of the neck.

Recommendations on Screening

- A two-stage screening protocol with OAE as the first screen, followed by ABR for those who fail the OAE screen.[11]
- It is advisable that all hospitals with level-3 neonatal care have OAE and ABR facilities. If not feasible, a centralized hearing screening with a portable OAE is suggested and all abnormal cases can be referred for ABR to the nearest centre.
- The program is to be coordinated by an audiologist and weekly assessment meeting is to be convened with the staff to discuss and sort out the issues, if any (held by the convenor). Usual issues could include non-compliance by parents to bring the child for repeat OAE or ABR. This usually can be tackled by phone calls made by screening personnel, coordinator, or in rare instances by the convenor himself. A medical social worker can be involved for problem-solving.
- Personnel with basic knowledge in computer and good communication skills are chosen. They should be provided basic training in hearing screening and also skills to gather information on high-risk criteria, if any, from parents/hospital staff/hospital records. This training is to be conducted over one day.
- The screening personnel should visit each hospital daily/on alternate days/twice a week/weekly depending upon the number of births in that particular hospital. Daily screening may be carried out in hospitals which have more than 200 births, alternate day screening in hospitals with 100–200 births and twice weekly or weekly screening in hospitals with births less than 100 per month.
- All screeners should maintain a register of all cases screened and those with abnormal results. Neonates with abnormal screening results should be evaluated. It is the duty of the screeners to call back all abnormal cases

for follow up, with the help of a coordinator. (Number of hospitals covered by a screener depends on the number of cases in a particular hospital and proximity of the hospitals)

- If abnormal OAE is detected, it is repeated at 6 weeks on the 1st immunization visit. If again abnormal, ABR is done for confirmation followed by full audiological evaluation and remediation with hearing aids (cochlear implant may be required in cases of profound hearing loss or poor response to hearing aids).
- All NICU babies undergo ABR testing to rule out auditory dyssynchrony/auditory neuropathy.
- In babies with abnormal ABR, detailed enquiry is made to identify and record any risk factors. Any baby missing screening before hospital discharge is called for OAE test on the first immunization visit.
- All babies with abnormal ABR should undergo detailed ENT evaluation hearing-aid fitting and auditory rehabilitation before 6 months of age. Systematic evaluation for ruling out syndromic associations such as ophthalmic, paediatric and cardiac assessments should be conducted.
- Children with neonatal meningitis should be treated as a special category and need investigations including imaging and intervention like cochlear implant (if needed) on a semi-emergency basis. Delay can result in cochlear ossification which may preclude subsequent intervention like a cochlear implant.

The goal is to screen newborn babies before 1 month of age, diagnose hearing loss before 3 months of age and start intervention before 6 months of age. Hurdles experienced in the screening process include: less motivated pediatricians; lack of awareness among parents/community; non-compliance by the family for evaluation, and stigma attached to hearing aids.

CONCLUSION

As normal hearing is critical for speech and language development, it is recommended that during first 6 months of life, clinicians identify infants with hearing loss, preferably before 3 months of age. Other important issues are:

- Evaluate infants before discharge from nursery, especially high risk babies
- Universal neonatal screening and not targeted 'high risk' screening is ideal since about 50% of infants with hearing loss have no known risk factors for hearing loss and are discharged from well-baby nursery
- Delayed onset hearing loss should be considered and followed up (if presence of language delays, infections, head trauma, stigmata of syndromes, ototoxic medications, recurrent otitis media, intrauterine infections, neurofibromatosis type II)
- Prevalence of hearing loss is more than twice that of the other newborn disorders combined, which can be screened
- Never delay hearing assessment in a suspected case; no child is too young to be tested or too young to be evaluated
- Never resort to rudimentary tests of hearing (like clapping hands) as confirmatory tests, and reassure parents that their child's hearing is normal.

Universal Newborn Hearing Screening (UNHS) has become a standard practice in most developed countries. The identification of all newborns with hearing loss before 6 months has now become an attainable and realistic goal. A concept of a centralized newborn hearing screening model existing in Ernakulam District Kerala to cater to all hospitals in the district is worth replicating.[12] It takes away the financial burden of each hospital investing for the screening equipment. Follow up of positive cases and drop-outs are made easier with the central reporting and monitoring system. With unified strength of pediatricians, IAP city/

Key Messages

- Hearing loss should be screened preferably before 1 month of age.
- Universal neonatal screening rather than targeted 'high risk' screening is ideal.
- If abnormal OAE detected, it is repeated at 6 weeks or on the first immunization visit. If again abnormal, ABR is done for confirmation followed by full audiological evaluation and remediation with hearing aids.
- All NICU babies should undergo ABR testing to rule out auditory dys-synchrony/ auditory neuropathy.

district branches could take initiative to replicate this model in their respective towns or districts and by collaborating with government agencies involved in implementation of Rashtriya Bal Swasthya Karyakram.

Newborn hearing screening will help to identify hearing loss at an earlier age and alleviate the double tragedy of inability to hear and speak. Forming a consensus and national level guidelines for hearing screening is very important to construct a healthy independent society. Early intervention is mandatory for best prognostic outcomes.

REFERENCES

1. Stevenson J, McCann D, Watkin P, Worsfold S, Kennedy C. The relationship between language development and behaviour problems in children with hearing loss. J Child Psychol Psychiatry. 2010;51:77–83

2. Yoshinaga-Itano C, Sedey AL, Coulter DK, Mehl AL. Language of early-and later-identified children with hearing loss. Pediatrics. 1998;102: 1161–71.

3. Dominguez M, Becker S, Bruce I, Read H. A spiking neuron model of cortical correlates of sensorineural hearing loss: Spontaneous firing, synchrony and tinnitus. Neural Comput. 2006; 18:2942:2958.

4. Wynbrandt J, Ludman MD. The Encyclopaedia of Genetic Disorders and Birth Defects. New York, USA: Infobase Publishing; 2009.

5. Berg AL, Spitzer JB, Towers HM, Bartosiewicz C, Diamond BE. Newborn hearing screening in the

NICU: profile of failed auditory brainstem response/passed otoacoustic emission. Pediatrics. 2005;116: 933–98.

6. Al-Kandar JM, Alshuaib WB. Newborn hearing screening in Kuwait. Electromyogr Clin Neurophysiol. 2007;47:305–13.

7. Joint Committee on Infant Hearing. Year 2007 Position Statement: Principles and Guidelines for Early Hearing Detection and Intervention Programs. Pediatrics. 2007;120:898–921.

8. Jones KL. Smith's Recognizable Patterns of Human Malformation 6th Edition, Philadelphia, USA: Elsevier; 2009.

9. Rashtriya Bal Swasthya Karyakram. Available from http://nrhm.gov.in/nrhm-components/rmnch-a/child-health-immunization/rashtriya-bal-swasthya-karyakram-rbsk/background.html. Accessed on February 6, 2015.

10. Kemp DT. Otoacoustic emissions, their origin in cochlear function, and use. Br Med Bull. 2002; 63:223–41.

11. Hunter MF, Kimm L, Cafarlli DD, Kennedy CR, Thornton AR. Feasibility of otoacoustic emission detection followed by ABR as a universal neonatal screening test for hearing impairment. Br J Audiol. 1994;28:47–51.

12. Paul AK. Early identification of hearing loss and centralized newborn hearing screening facility-the Cochin experience. Indian Pediatr. 2011;48: 355–9.

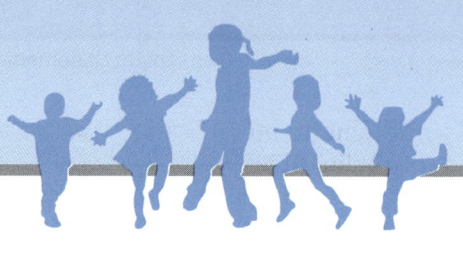

IAP Guidelines on Rickettsial Diseases in Children

Narendra Rathi, Atul Kulkarni, Vijay Yewale

There is a surge in the number of publications on rickettsial diseases from India in recent years. These infections have been reported from various states and union territories like Maharashtra, Delhi, Karnataka, West Bengal, Pondicherry, Kerala, Tamil Nadu, Himachal Pradesh, Jammu and Kashmir, Rajasthan, Meghalaya, Manipur, Goa and Uttarakhand.[1-4] Once thought to be diseases of rural population, these infections are increasingly reported from urban areas of India.

Rickettsial diseases pose multiple problems to clinicians.[5] Treatment of these infections is inexpensive and highly effective in early course of the disease but it is extremely difficult to make a diagnosis at this stage due to low index of suspicion, non-specificity of signs and symptoms and absence of low cost, rapid and widely available diagnostic test. Even if suspected by clinician, therapy is empirical as serological tests for diagnosis become positive around a week after onset of fever and early diagnostic test like polymerase chain reaction (PCR) is not freely available. Public health impact of these infections is enormous in India, and it differs in areas with low and high index of suspicion.[5] In areas with low index of suspicion, there is underdiagnosis,[6] and untreated cases have high morbidity (gangrene, Acute respiratory

distress syndrome, gastrointestinal bleed, neurological sequelae, disseminated intravascular coagulation etc.), high mortality (death rate up to 30%) and financial burden on families towards investigations and empiric treatment.[7] In endemic areas with high index of suspicion, there is rampant and irrational use of empiric doxycycline therapy for cases with undifferentiated fevers, with high propensity for adverse effects and drug resistance.

Rickettsia are obligate intracellular proteobacteria spread by eukaryotic vectors like ticks, mites, fleas and lice. Epidemiology of these infections is based on geographic and temporal distribution of their vectors. Rickettsia are divided into four biogroups namely spotted fever group (SFG) comprising Rocky Mountain spotted fever, Rickettsial pox, Indian tick typhus or Mediterranean spotted fever or Boutonneuse fever; Typhus group comprising Epidemic louse borne typhus, Brill–Zinsser disease and Endemic/Murine flea borne typhus; Scrub typhus group and miscellaneous group comprising Ehrlichiosis, Anaplasmosis, TIBOLA (tick borne lymphadenopathy) and DEBONEL (dermacentor borne necrosis eschar lymphadenopathy). Diffuse endothelial infection (infective vasculitis) leading to microvascular leakage and vascular lumen obstruction are basic pathogenetic mechanisms, which explain various clinical features of these infections. The most abundant surface protein of the rickettsia is OmpB and antibodies to OmpB could be a novel treatment tool in future.

Given the increasing reports of rickettsial infections in recent times, diagnostic dilemma in the minds of practicing pediatricians, lack of freely available, rapid and cheap diagnostic tests and enormous public health impact of these infections, Indian Academy of Pediatrics (IAP) felt the need to form practice guidelines on this topic to help pediatricians across India in the management of rickettsial diseases.

RECOMMENDATIONS

Case Definitions

Suspected case: A patient having compatible clinical scenario, suggestive epidemiological features and absence of definite alternative diagnosis should be termed as a suspected case of rickettsia. Definition of 'compatible clinical scenario' and 'suggestive epidemiological features' is provided in Boxes 22.1 and 22.2, respectively. Alternative diagnosis can be searched from (but not limited to) the list of differential diagnoses (Box 22.3).

Box 22.1: Compatible clinical scenario for rickettsial infection

One or more of the following:
- Undifferentiated fever of more than 5 days.
- Sepsis of unclear etiology.
- Fever with rash.
- Fever with edema.
- Dengue-like disease.
- Fever with headache and myalgia.
- Fever with hepatosplenomegaly and/or lymph-adenopathy.
- Aseptic meningitis/meningoencephalitis/acute encephalitic syndrome.
- Fever with cough and pulmonary infiltrates or community acquired pneumonia.
- Fever with acute kidney injury.
- Fever with acute gastrointestinal or hepatic involvement.

Box 22.2: Suggestive epidemiological features for rickettsial infections

One or more of the following within 14 days of illness onset:
- Tick bite.
- Ticks seen on clothes or in and around homes or in areas where children play
- Visit to areas which are common habitats of vectors like high uncut grass or weeds or bushes or rice fields or woodlands (where rodents share habitats with animals) or grassy lawns or river banks or poorly maintained kitchen gardens.
- Animal sheds in proximity of homes.
- Contact with pet or stray dog infested with ticks.
- Living in or travel to areas endemic for rickettsial diseases.
- Occurrence of similar clinical cases simultaneously or sequentially in family members, coworkers, neighbourhood or pets.
- Exposure to rodents.

Box 22.3: Differential diagnoses for rickettsial infections*

- Viral diseases: enteroviral diseases, measles, dengue fever, chikungunya, infectious mononucleosis.
- Bacterial diseases: meningococcemia, leptospirosis, typhoid fever, scarlet fever, secondary syphilis, infective endocarditis.
- Protozoal diseases: malaria.
- Vasculitis: Kawasaki disease, thrombotic thrombo-cytopenic purpura.
- Adverse drug reactions.
- Differential diagnoses pertaining to each systemic presentation.

* Not an exhaustive list

Probable case: Suspected case having either eschar, or having rapid (<48 hours) defervescence with anti-rickettsial therapy, or having suggestive laboratory features (*see later*), or having Weil-Felix test positive with titre of 1:80 or more in OX2, OX19 or OXK or positive IgM ELISA for rickettsia (optical density >0.5).

Confirmed case: Suspected case having rickettsial DNA detected in whole blood or tissue samples, or fourfold rise in antibody titres on acute and convalescent sera detected by immunofluorescence assay (IFA) or immuno-peroxidase assay (IPA).[8] In countries like India, where PCR and IFA are not commonly available, properly performed paired serological tests like ELISA have high positive predictive value.

ETIOLOGICAL AGENTS

Rickettsia conorii causing Indian tick typhus and *Orientia tsutsugamushi* causing Scrub typhus are common etiological agents in India. *Rickettsia kellyi candidiatus* like species are also reported.[10] Rarely murine flea borne typhus is reported.[8] Though there are differences in geographical distribution, vectors, host and clinical features, antibiotic treatment is same for both these groups.

EPIDEMIOLOGY AND PATHOGENESIS

- SFG is reported from Maharashtra, Karnataka and Tamil Nadu while scrub typhus is reported from almost all states and union territories of India.
- Rickettsial diseases can occur throughout the year, but more commonly seen from from May to February.[1]
- Due to low prevalence of rickettsial organisms in vectors, there is no role of doxycycline prophylaxis after tick bite.[11]
- Rickettsial diseases occur at all ages including neonates.[12,13]

CLINICAL FEATURES

Incubation period is 1 to 2 weeks. There is marked differences in disease severity and mortality due to remarkable genetic heterogeneity of rickettsial strains.

Fever: It is abrupt onset, high grade, may be associated with headache, myalgia and arthralgia.

Rash: Though rash is considered as a hallmark of these infections, it may be absent. Rash of SFG appears on day 2 to 5 of illness,[13] can be pruritic, is evolving (initially macular, becoming maculopapular, petechial, purpuric or gangrenous), has centripetal spread, and can involve palms and soles (considered typical of rickettsial diseases). Rash in these locations can also be seen in meningococcemia, infective endocarditis, adverse drug reactions, enteroviral diseases and syphilis. Rash in scrub typhus is maculopapular, uncommon than SFG, seen in 30 to 43% cases. The rash in typhus group is quite atypical, initially appearing on trunk, spreading centrifugally and usually sparing palms and soles.

Eschar: It is a crusty necrotic lesion with or without surrounding erythematous halo, which suggest the location of the vector bite. It is painless, nonpruritic and about 1 cm in diameter. Eschar is usually single but multiple eschars do occur. It resembles the skin burn of cigarette butt and is associated with regional lymphadenopathy. In fact, one should search for eschar in the draining area of regional lymphadenopathy, if the later is discovered, as regional lymphadenopathy is a marker of hidden or developing eschar.[14] It is recommended that eschars be carefully looked for, as those in intertriginous area may be missed. Eschar is considered as pathognomonic of rickettsial diseases, though it can be seen in anthrax, bacterial ecthyma, spider bite and rat bite fever. It is uncommon in SFG while more commonly seen in scrub typhus (7–97%).

Hepatosplenomegaly, lymphadenopathy and conjunctival injection

Edema: Periorbital or pedal edema or anasarca.

Systemic presentations: Apart from above mentioned clinical features, rickettsial infections have various systemic clinical features. Of particular importance is to realise that rickettsial infections can have initial presentations with these systemic features. It is recommended that clinicians should be aware of 4 systemic presentations of rickettsial diseases: central nervous system, respiratory, gastrointestinal and renal. Rickettsial diseases should be considered in the differential diagnosis of every patient with aseptic meningitis or meningoencephalitis or acute encephalitic syndrome with compatible epidemiological history.[15–18] Cough associated with pulmonary infiltrates or pneumonia is another common presentation of rickettsial diseases.[19] It is recommended to add empiric treatment for scrub typhus in addition to recommended regimen for the management of community acquired pneumonia, in regions where scrub typhus is likely to occur.[8] Gastrointestinal and hepatic presentation in the form of nausea, vomiting, diarrhea, abdominal pain, and hepatitis, severe enough to suggest diagnosis of acute gastroenteritis or surgical abdomen, is known in children with rickettsial infections, especially in the early part of the clinical course.[20,21] Acute renal failure (ARF) can be a presenting feature of rickettsial disease and is associated with a bad prognosis. The possibility of scrub typhus should be borne in mind, whenever a patient of fever presents with varying degrees of renal insufficiency, particularly if eschar exists along with the history of environmental exposure.[13,22,23]

Complications: Disseminated intravascular coagulation, Acute Respiratory Distress syndrome, Hemophagocytic Lymphohistiocytosis, purpura fulminans, gangrene[24] and myocarditis are various complications seen.

SCORING SYSTEM

The scoring system proposed by Rathi, *et al.*[13] for diagnosis of SFG rickettsioses using clinical, laboratory, and epidemiological features with a diagnostic cutoff score of 14 has high sensitivity (96.1%) and specificity (98.8%), similar to detection of specific IgM antibody by ELISA but needs revalidation in multicentric, prospective trials with larger sample size including both hospitalized and outpatient children.

LABORATORY DIAGNOSIS (Fig. 22.1)

Suggestive laboratory features: Presence of these features support the diagnosis and help to rule out some differential diagnoses. These

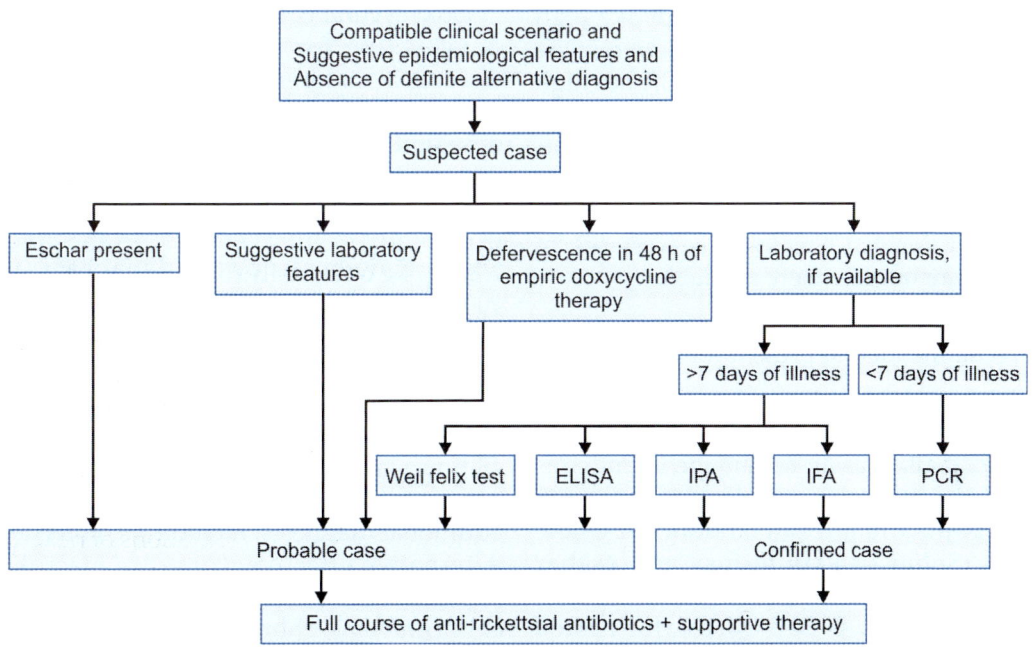

Fig. 22.1: Management Algorithm for Rickettsial Infections

Box 22.4: Suggestive laboratory features for rickettsial infections

- Normal to low total leukocyte count with a shift to left in early stages and leukocytosis later on
- Thrombocytopenia
- Raised ESR and CRP
- Hyponatremia
- Hypoalbuminemia and
- Elevated hepatic transaminases.

are enumerated in Box 22.4. In fact, clinicians must look for rash and eschar in all cases of fever and should collect serum sample for suggestive laboratory features before administration of empirical antibiotics.

Serology: These tests are usually positive after first week of illness. These are biogroup-specific and not species-specific. Four-fold rise in titers in two serum samples, 2–4 weeks apart, favours diagnosis. Weil Felix test is used if other tests are not available. It has advantages of being inexpensive, easily available, not requiring expertise and sophisticated instruments. It has lower sensitivity but better specificity. A single titre above 1:80 may indicate possibility of infection, but at a high cut-off titre (1:320) positive predictive value and specificity is better.[25] IgM ELISA has high sensitivity and specificity and hence preferred. IFA is gold standard test but has disadvantages of being expensive, not easily available and needing a lot of expertise and sophisticated instruments. Other tests like western blot and IPA are not routinely available.

RICT: Rapid immunochromatographic test is not recommended at present for diagnosis.

PCR: It is useful for diagnosis in the first week of illness and unlike serology, it is species specific. It also has an advantage in endemic areas with high background level of antibodies in the population. It can be done on whole blood, eschar or skin biopsy and eschar scrapings. Specificity of PCR is almost 100%, while sensitivity is 22.5–36.1% (for nested PCR) and 45–82% (for Real-time PCR).[26] Sensitivity is more in tissue specimen than blood and is decreased by doxycycline therapy.[27]

Isolation of organisms by cell culture and laboratory animals and immunostaining of skin rash or eschar biopsy are not useful for clinical purpose.

TREATMENT (Fig. 22.1)

Treatment must be initiated empirically in suspected cases without awaiting laboratory confirmation, as morbidity and mortality escalate rapidly with each day of treatment delay. Also treatment should not be discontinued solely on the basis of a negative test result.[27]

Patients with organ dysfunction, severe thrombocytopenia, mental status changes, need for supportive therapy, inability to take oral medications or unreliable caregiver and follow up should be hospitalized.

Concomitant empiric treatment for other conditions which are life threatening and cannot be reliably ruled out may need to be administered (e.g. meningococcemia) while awaiting laboratory results.

Doxycycline is the drug of choice. Use of doxycycline for treatment of rickettsial diseases in children of any age is no longer a matter of controversy. Doxycycline used at the dose and duration for these infections, even with multiple courses, do not result into teeth staining or enamel hypoplasia.[28,29] It should be used orally or intravenously in the dose of 2.2 mg/kg twice daily for children <40 kg and 100 mg twice daily for children above 40 kg, for 3 days after subsidence of fever or total 7 days. Severe or complicated cases may need 10 days therapy. The response to doxycycline is dramatic and fever persisting beyond 48 hours of initiation of doxycycline should prompt consideration of alternative or additional diagnosis, including coinfection.[27] Alternative effective drugs are macrolides (oral clarithromycin or oral/intravenous azithromycin), chloramphenicol and rifampicin. Azithromycin is used in the dose of 10 mg/kg/day for 5 days.

Rickettsial strains with reduced suscepti-bility to doxycycline are reported,[30,31] and alternative drugs can be used in such a situation.[32] It is recommended that rifampicin should not be routinely used for treatment of rickettsial diseases in India. Clinicians should monitor the progress of patients in the light of reports of drug resistance. Fluoroquinolones are not recommended for treatment.[33] Sulfonamides are contraindicated.

Supportive management: Severely ill patients may need other supportive measures as dictated by clinical situation.

POOR PROGNOSTIC FACTORS

G6PD deficiency, sulfonamide therapy, younger age, shorter incubation period, absence of rash, diabetes mellitus and delayed institution of anti-rickettsial drugs is asso-ciated with poorer outcome.

PREVENTION

Vaccine and post-exposure prophylaxis is not available for clinical use. Vector control, prevention of vector bite, prompt removal of attached ticks and pre-exposure chemopro-phylaxis are useful strategies to prevent rickettsial diseases.

Vector control: Short term vector control could be achieved by controlling rodents and cut-ting, burning and bulldozing vegetations with heavy spraying of insecticides such as lindane.

Preventing vector bite: This is the most effective strategy.
- Avoid exposure to vector infested habitats (described under suggestive epidemio-logical features in Box 22.2).
- Closed toe shoes and light coloured (for tick visibility) long pants and long sleeves cloths should be worn with shirt tucked into pants and pants tucked into socks or boots.
- Permethrin based (on cloths) and 20–50% DEET (N, N-diethyl-m-toluamide) based (on skin) insect repellants should be used.

- Hot water washing and hot drying effectively kills ticks on cloths.
- Pets should be protected with medications or tick collars and periodic de-ticking be done.
- Regular tick checks should be performed after spending time with tick infested animals or in tick infested habitats.

Prompt removal of attached ticks: This is a useful strategy as ticks need minimum 4–6 hours of attachment before they transmit infection.[11] Bathing soon after exposure is effective. It is recommended that proper technique of tick removal be used. Use tweezers, grasp ticks head as close to skin surface as possible and gently pull upwards with constant pressure. Attachment area should be immediately cleaned with soap and water or alcohol or an iodine scrub. Ticks should neither be removed nor be crushed with bare fingers. Gasoline, nail polish, kerosene, petroleum jelly or lit matchsticks should not be used for tick removal. Incine-ration of ticks after removal, rather than flushing down the sewer system is recommended.[27]

Pre-exposure chemoprophylaxis: It is recom-mended for short period, high- risk exposure. Weekly doxycycline started before and for 6 weeks after exposure is recommended.

REFERENCES

1. Dasari V, Kaur P, Murhekar MV. Rickettsial disease outbreaks in India: A Review. Ann Trop Med Public Health 2014;7:249–54.
2. Kamarasu K, Malathi M, Rajagopal V, Subramani K, Jagadeesh Ramasamy D, Mathai E. Serological evidence for wide distribution of spotted fevers and typhus fever in Tamil Nadu. Indian J Med Res 2007;126:128–30.
3. Bithu R, Kanodia V, Maheshwari RK. Possibility of scrub typhus in FUO cases: An experience from Rajasthan. Indian J Med Microbiol 2014;32: 387–90.
4. Narvencar KPS, Rodrigues S, Nevrekar RP, Dias L, Dias A, Vaz M, *et al.* Scrub typhus in patients

reporting with acute febrile illness at a tertiary health care institution in Goa. Indian J Med Res 2012;136:1020–4.

5. Rathi N. Rickettsial Diseases in India- A long way ahead. Pediatr Infect Dis 2015;7:61–3.

6. Kulkarni A. Childhood Rickettsiosis. Indian J Pediatr 2011;78:81—7.

7. Rathi N, Rathi A. Rickettsial infections: Indian perspective. Indian Pediatr 2010;47:157–64.

8. DHR-ICMR. Guidelines for Diagnosis and Management of Rickettsial Diseases in India. ICMR; 2015, February.

9. Mittal V, Gupta N, Bhattacharya D, Kumar K, Ichhpujani RL Singh S, et al. Serological evidence of rickettsial infections in Delhi. Indian J Med Res 2012;135:538–41.

10. Prakash JA, Sohan Lal T, Rosemol V, Verghese VP, Pulimood SA, Reller M, Molecular detection and analysis of spotted fever group Rickettsia in patients with fever and rash at a tertiary care centre in Tamil Nadu, India. Pathog Glob Health 2012;106:40–5.

11. Paul ML, Ross MJ. Rickettsial and Ehrlichial Diseases. In: Cherry J, Demmler-Harrison GJ, Kaplan SL. Steinbach W, Hotez P. Feigin and Cherry's Textbook of Pediatric Infectious Diseases, 7th ed. New York: Saunders Elsevier, 2013;2647–2666.e4.

12. Arthi P, Bagyalakshmi R, Krishna M, Krishna M, Nitin M, Madhavan HN, et al. First case series of emerging Rickettsial neonatal sepsis identified by PCR based DNA sequencing. Indian J Med Microbiol 2013;31:343–8.

13. Rathi N, Rathi A, Goodman MH, Aghai ZH. Rickettsial diseases in Central India: proposed clinical scoring system for early detection of spotted fever. Indian Pediatr 2011;48:867–72.

14. Narayanasamy DK, Arunagirinathan AK, Kumar RK, Raghavendran VD. Clinico-laboratory profile of scrub typhus-An emerging rickettsiosis in India. Indian J Pediatr 2016 Jun 29.

15. Sood AK, Chauhan L, Gupta H. CNS manifestations in Orientia tsutsugamushi Disease in North India. Indian J Pediatr 2016;83:634.

16. Rathi N, Maheshwari M, Khandelwal R. Neurological manifestations of rickettsial infections in children. Pediatric Infectious Disease 2016;7:64–6.

17. Tikare NV, Shahapur PR, Bidari LH, Mantur BG. Rickettsial meningoencephalitis in a child—a case report, J Trop Pediatr 2010;56:198–200.

18. Baldwin K, Rathi N. Rickettsial Disease. In: Editors: Robert L, Daniel T, William M. International Neurology, second edition. Wiley Blackwell: UK, 2016;291–5.

19. Watt G, Parola P. Scrub typhus and tropical rickettsiosis. Curr Opin Infect Dis 2003;16:429–36.

20. Mahajan SK. Rickettsial diseases. J Assoc Physicians India 2012;60:37–43.

21. Syed AZ, Carol S. Gastrointestinal and hepatic manifestations of tickborne diseases in US. Clin Infect Dis 2002;34:1206–12.

22. Yen TH, Chang CT, Lin JL, Jiang JR, Lee KF. Scrub typhus: a frequently overlooked cause of acute renal failure. Ren Fail 2003;25:397–410.

23. Kumar V, Kumar V, Yadav AK, Iyengar S, Bhalla A, Sharma N, et al. Scrub Typhus Is an Under-recognized Cause of Acute Febrile Illness with Acute Kidney Injury in India. PLoS Negl Trop Dis 2014;8:e2605.

24. Kulkarni A, Vaidya S, Kulkarni P, Bidri LH, Padwal S. Rickettsial disease-an experience. Pediatr Infect Dis 2009;1:118–24.

25. Batra HV. Spotted fevers & typhus fever in Tamil Nadu. Indian J Med Res 2007;126:101–3.

26. Kim DM, Park G, Kim HS, Lee JY, Neupane GP, Graves S, Stenos J. Comparison of conventional, nested, and real-time quantitative PCR for diagnosis of scrub typhus. J Clin Microbiol 2011; 49:607–12.

27. Biggs HM, Behravesh CB, Bradley KK, Dahlgren FS, Drexler NA, Dumler JS, et al. Diagnosis and Management of Tickborne Rickettsial Diseases, CDC. MMWR Recomm Rep 2016;65:1–44.

28. Volovitz B, Shkap R, Amir J, Calderon S, Varsano I, Nussinovitch M. Absence of tooth staining with doxycycline treatment in young children. Clin Pediatr (Phila) 2007;46:121–6.

29. Todd SR, Dahlgren FS, Traeger MS, Beltrán-Aguilar ED, Marianos DW, Hamilton C, et al. No visible dental staining in children treated with doxycycline for suspected Rocky Mountain spotted fever. J Pediatr 2015;166:1246–51.

30. Kim YS, Yun HJ, Shim SK, Koo SH, Kim SY, Kim S. A comparative trial of a single dose of azithromycin versus doxycycline for the treatment of mild scrub typhus. Clin Infect Dis 2004; 39:1329–35.

31. Watt G, Chouriyagune C, Ruangweerayud R, Watcharapichat P, Phulsuksombati D, Jongsakul K, et al. Scrub typhus infections poorly responsive to antibiotics in northern Thailand. Lancet 1996;348:86–9.

32. Liu Q, Panpanich R. Antibiotics for treating scrub typhus. Cochrane Database Syst Rev 2002; 3:CD002150.

33. Elisabeth BN, Cristina S, Didier R, Philippe P. treatment of Rickettsial spp. infections: a review. Expert Rev Anti Infect Ther 2012:10;1425–37.

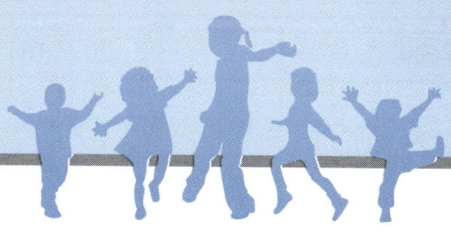

Consensus Statement of the IAP on Evaluation and Management of Autism Spectrum Disorder

Samir Dalwai, Shabina Ahmed, Vrajesh Udani, Nandini Mundkur, SS Kamath, MKC Nair

Framing guidelines for management of Autism Spectrum Disorder (ASD) in India is a pressing need due to the clinical complexity of the condition, high prevalence (1 in 65 children 2–9 years of age),[1] and the fact that ASD poses multiple limitations on schooling, adult capital and social inclusion.

The meeting on formulation of National consensus guidelines on neurodevelopmental disorders was organized by Indian Academy of Pediatrics in Mumbai, on 18th and 19th December, 2015. The invited experts included Pediatricians, Developmental Pediatricians, Psychiatrists, Pediatric Neurologists, Remedial Educators and Clinical Psychologists. The participants framed guidelines after extensive discussions and literature review. Thereafter, a committee was established to review the points discussed in the meeting.

Subsequent sections include the points of consensus on evaluation and management of ASD.

RECOMMENDATIONS

Clinical Evaluation

Empirically, it has been found that the earliest symptoms are absence of normal behavior (not presence of abnormal ones), i.e. absence of warm, joyful, reciprocating expressions or to-and fro babbling and jargoning; and, a 'very good' baby, i.e. quiet and undemanding. Other key signs include parental concerns about inconsistent hearing or unusual responsiveness, especially to name call; extremes of temperament and behavior ranging from marked irritability to alarming passivity; and regression of social skills and/ or speech.

Screening

All children should be screened by a standardized autism screening tool at 18 and 24 months of age.[2]

a. If the child is above 18 months, then administer the ASD—specific screening tool (discussed later).

b. If the child is below 18 months, then:
(i) evaluate social communication skills,
(ii) commence parental education and
(iii) reschedule next visit after 3 months (if child's age is less than 12 months) or after 1 month (if child's age is more than 12 months).

If concerns persist, then administer the ASD–specific screening tool.

c. *If screening results are positive or concerning then:* (i) continue parental education, (ii) refer the child for comprehensive ASD evaluation, (iii) initiate an early intervention program, (iv) evaluate hearing status, and

(v) schedule next follow-up visit after a month.

The Modified Checklist for Autism in Toddlers (M-CHAT) is a freely available and downloadable questionnaire (in multiple languages) to be completed by parents, which takes about 10 minutes to complete. It uses a simple scoring procedure based on passed/failed items. If the child screens positive, a follow up interview is conducted including only those items on which the child failed in initial screening, thus decreasing the likelihood of false-positive results.[3] The Social Communication Questionnaire is another tool that is also available in many Indian languages. Studies have looked at the sensitivity and specificity of these tools and found that they are more accurate for pervasive developmental disorders including ASD with lower intellectual and adaptive functioning.[4] The Trivandrum Autism Behavior Checklist was developed at the Child Development Centre at Trivandrum, Kerala and it was observed that the results of evaluation were comparable to those obtained by administering the Childhood Autism Rating Scale (CARS).[5]

Clinical Features

Symptoms of ASD must be present in the early developmental period, but they may not be apparent until later (i.e., when social demands exceed limited capacities). Hence, symptoms of ASD are most commonly recognized in the second year of life. However, symptoms in children with the least severe phenotypes of ASD may not be apparent to parents or teachers until four to six years of age or later. ICD-10 continues to require that symptoms be present before three years of age.[6-9]

Children may present with delays in core developmental areas in first year of life or may develop typically and then plateau. Approximately two-thirds of patients with ASD present with lack of acquisition of communication skills during the first two years of life; and one-fourth to one-third of children achieve early language milestones, but have regression of language, communication and/or social skills between 15 and 24 months of age.[8,10-13] Other reported features in literature are as varied as sensory and motor impairments, deficits in play and imitation skills, and gastrointestinal symptoms.[14-26]

Co-morbidities

Associated conditions with ASD could include intellectual or language impairment, known genetic conditions, catatonia, motor deficits (e.g. abnormal gait, clumsiness, toe-walking or hypotonia), macrocephaly, medical disorders (e.g. seizures, lead poisoning in children with pica); neurodevelopmental, behavioral and/or mental health co-morbidities (e.g. hyper-activity, anxiety, depression, behavioral dysregulation), sleep problems (e.g. late onset, frequent waking, restlessness) that may affect daytime function, gastrointestinal, feeding, and nutrition problems (e.g. constipation, restricted diet), and delays in acquisition of self-help skills (e.g. toileting, dressing, hygiene).

Diagnosis

Diagnosis of ASD is made as per the Diagnostic and Statistical Manual of Mental disorders-fifth edition,[27] and independent checklists (discussed below) serve the purpose of eliciting the diagnostic features. The INCLEN diagnostic tool for ASD (INDT-ASD) has high content validity, internal consistency, criterion validity, convergent validity and 4-factor construct validity.[28] The Indian Scale for Assessment of Autism (ISAA) has a sensitivity of 93.3, specificity of 97.4 and positive and negative predictive values of 35.5 and 0.08, respectively; with good reliability but sub-optimal validity. The role of ISAA is relevant to identification and certification of 3–9 year old children at high risk for Autism, with the cut-off being an ISAA score of above 70.[29] Another useful tool is the Childhood

Autism Rating Scale (CARS); CARS score of ≥33 (sensitivity, 81.4%, specificity, 78.6%; Area under the curve 81%) has been advised for diagnostic use in the Indian population. CARS has good inter-rater reliability (0.74) and test-retest reliability (0.81).[30] The Autism Diagnostic Observation Schedule (ADOS) has also been validated and translated into Hindi and Bengali.[31] In addition, the Autism Diagnostic Interview (ADI), with a sensitivity and specificity of 92% and 89% , respectively, is a tool that can be used for diagnosis, albeit having significant cost and usage-time implications.[32-35] Table 23.1 summarizes the various operational aspects of ISAA, INCLEN diagnostic tool, ADI and ADOS.

All children with ASD should undergo a physical examination, and screening for hearing and vision.[36] Assessment of cognitive ability and adaptive skills is recommended for planning intervention, with respect to observed social-communication difficulties relative to overall development. The child's strengths and weaknesses need to be charted.[37] Measurements of receptive and expressive vocabulary (using a tool like Receptive-Expressive Emergent Language Scale, REELS) and social-pragmatic skills (e.g. clinically or via a scale like ADOS) are essential to have a complete diagnostic impression and an informed intervention plan.[38] Occupational and physical therapy evaluations should be conducted to evaluate sensory and/or motor difficulties.[39] Based on family history, examination and any dysmorphic features, additional evaluations are recommended to probe for hypothyroidism, homo-cystinuria, head injury, fetal alcohol syndrome or chromosomal abnormalities. Landau-Kleffner syndrome should be ruled out (aphasia and distinctive EEG features). Neurologic consultation and EEG is required (including, MeCP2 gene for possible Rett's disorder if suspected). A Wood's lamp examination for signs of Tuberous sclerosis, as well as genetic testing including G-banded karyotype, Fragile X testing, or chromosomal microarray maybe done if clinically indicated.[36,40-42]

Intervention

Intervention should begin as early as possible, even while evaluation for a definitive diagnosis is ongoing. Intervention should target core features of autism and should be specific, evidence-based, structured and appropriate to the developmental needs of the child. Management should be provided through interdisciplinary teams, coordinated by a Developmental pediatrician/pediatrician and should include a child neurologist or psychiatrist, clinical psychologist, occupational therapist, speech and language therapist, special educator, nutritionist and social worker.[36]

Intervention Models

Many interventional models are established, such as Behavioral models (e.g., Applied Behavior Analysis or ABA), Structured teaching (e.g., The Treatment and Education of Autistic and related Communication-handicapped Children or TEACCH), Developmental/relationship-based models (e.g., Floor time) and Integrated programs that use a combination of strategies within the treatment program (e.g., Social Communication,

Name of the tool	Time taken (approx)	Age-group	Cost	Languages
INCLEN tool (INDT-ASD)	45-60 minutes	2–9 years (as per the validation study)	Free	Hindi, English, multiple regional languages
ISAA	20–30 minutes	3–9 years	Free	—do—
ADI	120 minutes	2 years and above	$ 261[*]	English
ADOS	40–60 minutes	12 months and above	$2095[*]	Hindi, Bengali, English

TABLE 23.1: Some diagnostic tools for autism

*Last accessed in January 2017

Emotional Regulation and Transactional Support or SCERTS).[36,38] In terms of co-morbidities, cognitive behavioral therapy has shown effectiveness for anxiety and anger management in high functioning young adults with ASD.[36] Pharmacotherapy may be offered to children with ASD when there is a specific target symptom or co-morbid condition.[36,38]

Effectiveness of an Intervention

A good educational program for autism depends on the child's chronological age and developmental level, specific strengths and weaknesses and family needs. A recommended program should preferably have[2]: 1:1 or 1:2 (child to therapist ratio), individualized for each child and with an interdisciplinary team that documents evaluation and intervention. Each professional should have specialized expertise in working with children with autism. A minimum of 25 hours per week of intervention is critical for effectiveness. Ongoing program evaluation and adjustment is necessary. A curriculum emphasizing attention, imitation, communication, play and social interaction is essential. Family involvement is a pre-requisite for the program's effectiveness.

The program goals should include: (a) enhancing eye contact, social orientation, nonverbal and verbal communication, (b) reducing the repetitive and restricted behaviors/activities/interests, sensory issues and hyperactivity (e.g., increasing sitting tolerance), (c) improving joint attention and (d) improving social, motor, and behavioral capabilities. Individuals with ASD should be offered interventions specifically targeting deficits in social communication/pragmatic language (group or individually focused) with a focus on social skills, based on empirically supported methods described in a protocol or manual.[43,44]

Parent-mediated Early Intervention

Parent-education and home-interventions are important but not necessarily a substitute to individual therapeutic intervention for each child; these are more likely to be effective if part of a multidisciplinary intervention program. There is not much scientific evidence for the efficacy of parent-mediated approaches (for outcomes like improved language and communication, improved child initiation and adaptive behavior, reduced parents' stress).[45,46] However, the evidence for positive change in patterns of parent-child interaction (e.g., shared attention or parent-child synchrony) is strong.[45,46] Active involvement of families and/or caregivers as a form of co-therapy is desirable but only with appropriate supervision, training and monitoring. Parents should help set goals and priorities for their child's treatment, and they should teach or reinforce new skills at home and in the community. Parent-mediated interventions are cost-effective and increase the sense of empowerment on the part of caregivers.[45,46]

Educational Management

Inclusion: Inclusion is the goal of educational management; though, it needs to be rationalized and practically implemented based on individual situation.

Special services: An appropriate Individualized Educational Plan (IEP) is central in providing effective service e.g., Early Start Denver Model, and the Treatment and Education of Autism and related Communication-handi-capped Children (TEACCH) program.[45-49]

Curriculum: Educational plan should reflect an accurate assessment of the child's strengths and vulnerabilities and their relation to academic skills. Modified or special curricula must be adapted and provided to meet optimum education needs of the child.

Provisions: Various boards provide for certification with special provisions for children with autism.[36]

Children with ASD need a structured educational approach with explicit teaching. Interventions should be planned, intensive and individualized with an experienced, interdisciplinary team of providers, and family involvement. An accurate assessment of the child's strengths and vulnerabilities is required, with an explicit description of intervention goals and procedures as well as monitoring of effectiveness. A parent-education and home component is important. Both ESDM and TEACCH programs have been found to be effective.[47-49]

Psychopharmacologic Interventions

Psychopharmacologic interventions can improve the child's functioning and the ability to participate in behavioral interventions. Medication should always be used in conjunction with appropriate behavioral and environmental interventions. Pharmacologic therapy may also be warranted for the treatment of co-morbid psychiatric or neurodevelopmental conditions, or for specific ('target') behavioral symptoms that interfere with overall functioning.[36] Specific pharmacological treatments have been summarized in Table 23.2 and an overview is provided below:

Stimulants for hyperactivity and inattention: Methylphenidate improves symptoms of hyperactivity and inattention in children with ASD, and may also have beneficial effects on social communication and self-regulation. It is recommended when impaired function persists (not due to other causes like anxiety); in spite of behavioral and/or environmental interventions. However, the response rate to methylphenidate is lower in children with ASD, than in children with Attention Deficit Hyperactivity Disorder without ASD. In the largest crossover trial, approximately 50% of children with ASD responded to methyl-phenidate (as measured on the hyperactivity subscale of the Aberrant Behavior Checklist); with greater improvement at higher doses (0.25 to 0.5 mg/kg versus 0.125 mg/kg per dose).[50-53] Adverse effects of methylphenidate include sleep disturbance, decreased appetite, irritability, tics, sadness, dullness and social withdrawal.[54,55]

Risperidone for maladaptive behaviors: In case of ineffectiveness of stimulants and/or presence of maladaptive behaviors, risperidone is recommended. Maladaptive behaviors in children with ASD include irritability, aggression, explosive outbursts (tantrums) and self-injury. These behaviors may occur in response to anxiety or frustration, which should be the first targets of management. Maladaptive behaviors can also occur due to anxiety/mood disorders or impulse control problems-if one of these conditions is identified as a cause for the behavior, then medications targeting that symptom should be used.

Risperidone is the most commonly used atypical antipsychotic drug for the treatment of maladaptive behaviors in children with ASD.[56] It is approved for treatment of irritability presenting with aggression, tantrums and/or deliberate self injury in children (≥5 years) with ASD. Randomized

TABLE 23.2: Drugs available for pharmacological management of autism spectrum disorders

Drug name	Indications	Dose	Side-effects
Methylphenidate	Impaired function in spite of behavioural and environmental interventions	10–40 mg each morning, extended release	Sleep disturbance, decreased appetite, irritability, tics, sadness, dullness and social withdrawal
Risperidone	Ineffectiveness of stimulants and/or maladaptive behaviors	0.5–3.5 mg/day	Weight gain, increased appetite, fatigue, drowsiness, drooling, dizziness
Atomoxetine	Methylphenidate not tolerated	1.2 mg/kg/day	Nausea, anorexia, fatigue, early awakening
Fluoxetine	Repetitive behaviors and rigidity	2.4–20 mg/day	None significant

controlled trials and systematic reviews indicate a positive response in individuals with ASD and disruptive behaviors. Risperidone does not significantly affect deficit in social interaction and communication.[57] Adverse effects are usually mild and resolve over a few weeks.[58] Risperidone is recommended to be given for children 5–16 years of age in the dose of maximum 3 mg per day.

Selective serotonin-reuptake inhibitors (SSRIs) for repetitive behaviors and rigidity: Repetitive behaviors, stereotypies, and rigidity in children often interfere with function. Potential treatments for repetitive behaviors in children with ASD include SSRI, clomipramine, atypical antipsychotics and valproate.[59] Fluoxetine (or another SSRI) can be used as the initial medication for repetitive behaviors that require pharmacologic intervention (maximum dose: 10 mg per day). SSRIs have fewer side effects than other agents and may be helpful in treatment of coexisting anxiety. Rigorous studies on use of SSRIs in children with ASD are lacking. The available evidence suggests that fluoxetine may be beneficial for repetitive behaviors and rigidity.[60]

Sleep disturbances: Many children with ASD have sleep disturbances, including late onset, frequent waking and restlessness.[62] Sleep disturbances may be related to abnormalities in melatonin, serotonin, or gamma-aminobutyric acid (GABA). The evaluation of sleep disturbances in children with ASD should include a thorough sleep history and screening for obstructive apnea and other sleep disorders. It is important to ensure appropriate sleep hygiene. Behavioral interventions to decrease sleep disturbances should be used, before considering pharmacologic interventions.[63] Medications are unlikely to be effective in the absence of an appropriate sleep schedule. There is little evidence for pharmacologic management of sleep disturbances in children. No medications are approved by the US Food and Drug Administration to address sleep in ASD.

However, several are used in clinical practice.

Melatonin is recommended for patients with ASD who have difficulty falling asleep and staying asleep, despite appropriate sleep hygiene and behavioral or environmental interventions. A low starting dose of 0.5 to 1 mg, 30 minutes before sleeping time, regardless of age and weight should be given (maximum dose: 10 mg).[63]

Gastrointestinal problems: The frequency and types of gastrointestinal (GI) disorders in children with ASD are similar to those in children without ASD. GI disorders in children with ASD generally should be managed in the same way as in children without an ASD.[64-66]

Anxiety: It is common in individuals with ASD and may contribute to aggressive, explosive, or self-injurious behaviors. Anxiety in children with ASD is treated with the same therapies that are used to treat anxiety in other children. Pharmacotherapy is one arm of a multimodal approach that may include individualized therapy, cognitive behavioral therapy, behavioral interventions/incentives, accommodations to address sensory sensitivities and special education services.[67] Components of the multimodal therapy may vary from patient to patient. Buspirone (an anxiolytic) is another agent that may be used to treat anxiety in children with ASD.[68]

Mood disorders: A number of agents have been used to treat symptoms related to dysregulated mood in children and adolescents with ASD. These include atypical antipsychotics (for maladaptive behaviors), SSRIs (for repetitive behaviors and anxiety) and mood-stabilizing agents (e.g., lithium). None of these agents have been studied specifically for mood regulation in children with ASD.

Depression: Antidepressant therapy, similar to its use in non-ASD children, may be indicated if depressive symptoms persist despite counseling and psychosocial interventions. Side effects include increased incidence of behavioral activation (e.g. impulsivity, silliness, agitation and dis-inhibition) and risk of suicidal ideation. Individuals with ASD may respond to very low doses of SSRI or serotonin norepinephrine reuptake inhibitors, but typical pediatric doses may be necessary. It is important to 'start low and go slow'.

Complementary and alternative therapies: There is no evidence for effectiveness of these therapies and pediatricians should be able to counsel caregivers to not opt for these therapies.[36]

Prognosis

In clinical experience, certain factors are known to be associated with positive outcomes; these include: presence of joint attention, functional play skills, higher cognitive abilities, mild severity of ASD symptoms, early identification, involvement in intervention, and a move towards inclusion with typical peers. However, in a recent systematic review, it was shown that less severe sub-types of ASD and early identification predicted favorable outcomes while other factors were inconclusive.[69] In another study, it was noted that development of communicative and language skills at an early age and high IQ could be key predictors of optimal outcomes.[70]

Disability Certification

According to the National Trust for the Welfare of Persons with Autism, Cerebral Palsy, Mental Retardation and Multiple

Disabilities Act, 1999; various schemes have been made available like Niramaya (Insurance), Aspiration (Early intervention) and Gyan Prabha (scholarship).[71] Moreover, the notification issued in April 2016 by the Department of Empowerment of Persons with Disabilities under the Ministry of Social Justice and Empowerment, detailed the guidelines for evaluation of Autism and procedure for its certification.[71-73] The IAP expert group recommends that ASD should be diagnosed using the DSM-5 and INCLEN tools and certified using the ISAA. Certification of disability for persons with Autism maybe executed by an Autism Certification Medical Board, duly constituted by the Central Government or the State Government, comprising of (a) a Clinical/Rehabilitation Psychologist; (b) a Psychiatrist and (c) a Pediatrician or General Physician, depending on the specific case. The Government guidelines have requested state governments to constitute these certification medical boards immediately and stated that the certificate should be valid for a period of five years for individuals below 18 years of age with temporary disability; and for those who have acquired permanent disability, should receive 'permanent' validity on their certificates.

CONCLUSION

Autism Spectrum Disorder is a complex condition with widely varying clinical manifestations, thus requiring evaluation and intervention by a range of professionals working in coordination. Behavioral and environmental interventions are the key to optimal outcomes, in conjunction with medications for specific symptoms. Parent involvement during intervention is incumbent to sustain therapeutic gains.

REFERENCES

1. Silberberg D, Arora N, Bhutani V, Durkin M, Gulati S, Nair M, et al. Neuro-Developmental disorders in India -from epidemiology to public policy. Neurology. 2014; 82:P7–P324.

2. Myers SM, Johnson CP. Management of children with autism spectrum disorders. Pediatrics. 2007; 120:1162–82.

3. Robins DL, Casagrande K, Barton M, Chen CMA, Dumont-Mathieu T, Fein D. Validation of the modified checklist for autism in toddlers, revised with follow-up (M-CHAT-R/F). Pediatrics.. 2014; 133;37–45.

4. Chandler S, Charman T, Baird G, Simonoff E, Loucas T, Meldrum D, et al. Validation of the social communication questionnaire in a population cohort of children with autism spectrum disorders. J Am Acad Child Adolesc Psychiatry. 2007;46:1324–32.

5. Nair MKC. Autism Spectrum Disorders. Indian Pediatr. 2004;41:541–3.

6. Chawarska K, Klin A, Paul R, Volkmar F. Autism spectrum disorder in the second year: Stability and change in syndrome expression. J Child Psychol Psychiatry. 2007;48:128–38.

7. Landa RJ, Holman KC, Garrett-Mayer E. Social and communication development in toddlers with early and later diagnosis of autism spectrum disorders. Arch Gen Psychiatry. 2007;64:853–64.

8. Landa RJ, Gross AL, Stuart EA, Faherty A. Developmental trajectories in children with and without autism spectrum disorders: the first 3 years. Child Dev. 2013;84:429–42.

9. McConachie H, Le Couteur A, Honey E. Can a diagnosis of Asperger syndrome be made in very young children with suspected autism spectrum disorder? J Autism Dev Disord. 2005;35:167–76.

10. Ozonoff S, Iosif AM, Young GS, Hepburn S, Thompson M, Colombi C, et al. Onset patterns in autism: correspondence between home video and parent report. J Am Acad Child Adolesc Psychiatry. 2011;50:796–806.

11. Thurm A, Manwaring SS, Luckenbaugh DA, Lord C, Swedo SE. Patterns of skill attainment and loss in young children with autism. Dev Psychopathol. 2014;26:203–14.

12. Johnson CP, Myers SM. Identification and evaluation of children with autism spectrum disorders. Pediatrics. 2007;120:1183–215.

13. Braun KV, Pettygrove S, Daniels J, Miller L, Nicholas J, Baio J, et al. Evaluation of a methodology for a collaborative multiple source surveillance network for autism spectrum disorders—Autism and Developmental Disabilities Monitoring Network, 14 sites, United States, 2002. MMWR. 2007;56:29–40.

14. Volkmar FR, Pauls D. Autism. Lancet. 2003;362: 1133–41.

15. De Giacomo A, Fombonne E. Parental recognition of developmental abnormalities in autism. Eur Child Adolesc Psychiatry. 1998;7:131–6.

16. Volkmar F, Wiesner L. Autism and related disorders. In: Carey WB, Crocker AC, Elias ER, Feldman HM, Coleman WL, editors. Developmental-Behavioral Pediatrics. 4th ed. Philadelphia: Saunders Elsevier; 2009. p.675.

17. Teplin SW. Autism and related disorders In: Levine MD, Carey WB, Crocker AC, editors. Developmental-Behavioral Pediatrics. 3rd ed. Philadelphia: WB Saunders, 1999. p.589.

18. Johnson CP. Recognition of autism before age 2 years. Pediatr Rev. 2008;29: 86.

19. Saint-Georges C, Mahdhaoui A, Chetouani M, Cassel RS, Laznik MC, Apicella F. et al. Do parents recognize autistic deviant behavior long before diagnosis? Taking into account interaction using computational methods. PLoS One. 2011;6: e22393.

20. Ming X, Brimacombe M, Wagner GC. Prevalence of motor impairment in autism spectrum disorders. Brain Dev. 2007;29:565–70.

21. Barrow WJ, Jaworski M, Accardo PJ. Persistent toe walking in autism. J Child Neurol. 2011; 26:619–21.

22. Stone WL, Lemanek KL, Fishel PT, Fernandez MC, Altemeier WA. Play and imitation skills in the diagnosis of autism in young children. Pediatrics. 1990;86:267–72.

23. Filipek PA, Accardo PJ, Ashwal S, Baranek GT, Cook EH, Dawson G, et al. Practice parameter: Screening and diagnosis of autism: Report of the Quality Standards Subcommittee of the American Academy of Neurology and the Child Neurology Society. Neurology. 2000;55:468–79.

24. Kientz MA, Dunn W. A comparison of the performance of children with and without autism on the Sensory Profile. Am J Occup Ther. 1997; 51:530–7.

25. McElhanon BO, McCracken C, Karpen S, Sharp WG. Gastrointestinal symptoms in autism spectrum disorder: a meta-analysis. Pediatrics. 2014;133: 872–83.

26. Bresnahan M, Hornig M, Schultz AF, Gunnes N, Hirtz D, Lie KK, et al. Association of maternal report of infant and toddler gastrointestinal symptoms with autism: evidence from a prospective birth cohort. JAMA Psychiatry. 2015; 72:466–74.

27. American Psychiatric Association. Diagnostic and statistical manual of mental disorders, fifth edition. Arlington, VA: American Psychiatric Association; 2013.

28. Juneja M, Mishra D, Russell PS, Gulati S, Deshmukh V, Tudu P, et al. INCLEN diagnostic tool for autism spectrum disorder (INDT-ASD): Development and validation. Indian Pediatr. 2014;51:359–65.

29. Mukherjee SB, Malhotra MK, Aneja S, Chakraborty S, Deshpande S. Diagnostic accuracy of Indian Scale for Assessment of Autism (ISAA) in chidren aged 2–9 years. Indian Pediatr. 2015;52:212–16.

30. Russell PS, Daniel A, Russell S, Mammen P, Abel JS, Raj LE, et al. Diagnostic accuracy, reliability and validity of Childhood Autism Rating Scale in India. World J Pediatr. 2010;6:141–147.

31. Rudra A, Banerjee S, Singhal N, Barua M, Mukerji S, Chakrabarti B. Translation and usability of autism screening and diagnostic tools for autism spectrum conditions in India. Autism Res. 2014;7:598–607.

32. Le Couteur A, Rutter M, Lord C, Rios P, Robertson S, Holdgrafer M, et al. Autism diagnostic interview: A standardized investigator-based instrument. J Autism Dev Disord. 1989;19:363–87.

33. Lord C, Rutter M, Le Couteur A. Autism Diagnostic Interview Revised: a revised version of a diagnostic interview for caregivers of individuals with possible pervasive developmental disorders. J Autism Dev Disord. 1994;24: 659–85.

34. Lecavalier L, Aman MG, Scahill L, McDougle CJ, McCracken JT, Vitiello B. et al. Validity of the autism diagnostic interview-revised. Am J Ment Retard. 2006;111:199–215.

35. Dalwai SH, Modak DK, Bondre AP, Gajria D. Analysis of tools for diagnosing autism spectrum disorder in the Indian context. Acad J Ped Neonatol. 2016; 1:555–62.

36. Volkmar F, Siegel M, Woodbury-Smith M, King B, McCracken J, State M. Practice parameter for the assessment and treatment of children and adolescents with autism spectrum disorder. J Am Acad Child Adolesc Psychiatry. 2014; 53:237-57. Available from: http://www.jaacap.com/article/S0890-8567(13)00819-8/pdf. Accessed January 14, 2017.

37. Volkmar FR, Wiesner LA. A Practical Guide to Autism: What Every Parent, Family Member, and Teacher Needs to Know. Hoboken, NJ: John Wiley; 2009.

38. Paul R, Sutherland D. Enhancing early language in children with autism spectrum disorders. In: Volkmar F, Klin A, Paul R, Cohen D, editors. Handbook of Autism and Pervasive Developmental Disorders. 3rd ed. New Jersey: John Wiley, Hoboken; 2005. p. 946–76.

39. Baranek GT, Parham LD, Bodfish JW. Sensory and motor features in autism: assessment and intervention. In: Volkmar FR, Klin A, Paul R, Cohen DJ, editors. Handbook of Autism and Pervasive Developmental Disorders. 3rd ed. New Jersey: John Wiley, Hoboken; 2005. p. 88–125.

40. American Psychiatric Association. Diagnostic and Statistical Manual of Mental Disorder, 4th ed, text rev. Washington, DC: American Psychiatric Press; 2000.

41. Camfield P, Camfield C. Epileptic syndromes in childhood: clinical features, outcomes, and treatment. Epilepsia. 2002;43:27–32.

42. Schaefer GB, Mendelsohn NJ. Genetics evaluation for the etiologic diagnosis of autism spectrum disorders. Genet Med. 2008;10:4–12.

43. Kendall T, Megnin-Viggars O, Gould N, Taylor C, Burt LR, Baird G. Management of autism in children and young people: summary of NICE and SCIE guidance. BMJ. 2013;347:f4865

44. Maglione MA, Gans D, Das L, Timbie J, Kasari C. Nonmedical interventions for children with ASD: Recommended guidelines and further research needs. Pediatrics. 2012;130:S169–S78.

45. Oono IP, Honey EJ, McConachie H. Parent mediated early intervention for young children with autism spectrum disorders (ASD). Evid Based Child Health. 2013;8: 2380–479.

46. Zwaigenbaum L, Bauman ML, Choueiri R, Kasari C, Carter A, Granpeesheh D, et al. Early interven-

tion for children with autism spectrum disorder under 3 years of age: recommendations for practice and research. Pediatrics. 2015; 136:S60–S81.

47. National Research Council. Educating Children with Autism. Washington, DC: National Academy of Sciences Press; 2001.

48. Dawson G, Rogers S, Munson J, Smith M, Winter J, Greenson J, *et al.* Randomized, controlled trial of an intervention for toddlers with autism: the Early Start Denver Model. Pediatr 2010;125:e17–e23.

49. Ozonoff S, Cathcart K. Effectiveness of a home program intervention for young children with autism. J Autism Dev Disord 1998;28:25–32.

50. Handen BL, Johnson CR, Lubetsky M. Efficacy of methylphenidate among children with autism and symptoms of attention-deficit hyperactivity disorder. J Autism Dev Disord. 2000;30:245–55.

51. Research Units on Pediatric Psychopharmacology (RUPP) Autism Network. Randomized, controlled, crossover trial of methylphenidate in pervasive developmental disorders with hyperactivity. Arch Gen Psychiatry. 2005;62: 1266–74.

52. Posey DJ, Aman MG, McCracken JT, Scahill L, Tierney E, Arnold LE, *et al.* Positive effects of methylphenidate on inattention and hyperactivity in pervasive developmental disorders: an analysis of secondary measures. Biol Psychiatry. 2007;61:538–44.

53. Jahromi LB, Kasari CL, McCracken JT, Lee LS, Aman MG, McDougle CJ, *et al.* Positive effects of methylphenidate on social communication and self-regulation in children with pervasive developmental disorders and hyperactivity. J Autism Dev Disord. 2009;39:395–404.

54. Towbin KE. Strategies for pharmacologic treatment of high functioning autism and Asperger syndrome. Child Adolesc Psychiatr Clin N Am. 2003;12:23–45.

55. Aman MG, Farmer CA, Hollway J, Arnold LE. Treatment of inattention, overactivity, and impulsiveness in autism spectrum disorders. Child Adolesc Psychiatr Clin N Am. 2008;17:713–38.

56. McVoy M, Findling R. Child and adolescent psychopharmacology update. Psychiatr Clin North Am. 2009;32:111.

57. McDougle CJ, Scahill L, Aman MG, McCracken JT, Tierney E, Davies M, *et al.* Risperidone for the core symptom domains of autism: results from the study by the autism network of the research units on pediatric psychopharmacology. Am J Psychiatry 2005;162:1142–8.

58. Barnard L, Young AH, Pearson J, Geddes J, O'brien G. A systematic review of the use of atypical antipsychotics in autism. J Psychopharmacol 2002;16: 93–101.

59. Huffman LC, Sutcliffe TL, Tanner IS, Feldman HM. Management of symptoms in children with autism spectrum disorders: A comprehensive review of pharmacologic and complementary-alternative medicine treatments. J Dev Behav Pediatr; 2011;32:56–68.

60. McPheeters ML, Warren Z, Sathe N, Bruzek JL, Krishnaswami S, Jerome RN, *et al.* A systematic review of medical treatments for children with autism spectrum disorders. Pediatrics. 2011;127: e1312–e21.

61. Frye RE, Rossignol D, Casanova MF, Martin V, Brown G, Edelson SM, *et al.* A review of traditional and novel treatments for seizures in autism spectrum disorder: findings from a systematic review and expert panel. Front Public Health. 2013;1:1–26.

62. Elrod MG, Hood BS. Sleep differences among children with autism spectrum disorders and typically developing peers: A meta-analysis. J Dev Behav Pediatr. 2015;36:166–77.

63. Melatonin and Sleep Problems in ASD: A Guide for Parents. Available from: https://www.autismspeaks.org/sites/default/files/docs/sciencedocs/atn/melatonin_guide_ for_parents.pdf. Accessed: January 23, 2016.

64. Buie T, Campbell DB, Fuchs GJ, Furuta GT, Levy J, VandeWater J, *et al.* Evaluation, diagnosis, and treatment of gastrointestinal disorders in individuals with ASDs: a consensus report. Pediatrics 2010; 125: S1–S18.

65. Scottish Intercollegiate Guidelines Network. Assessment, diagnosis and clinical interventions for children and young people with autism spectrum disorders. A national clinical guideline. Scottish Intercollegiate Guidelines Network, Edinburgh 2007. Available from: www.sign.ac.uk/guidelines/fulltext/98/index.html. Accessed May 7, 2016.

66. Buie T, Fuchs GJ, Furuta GT, Kooros K, Levy J, Lewis JD, *et al.* Recommendations for evaluation and treatment of common gastrointestinal problems in children with ASDs. Pediatrics. 2010;125:S19–S29.

67. White SW, Oswald D, Ollendick T, Scahill L. Anxiety in children and adolescents with autism spectrum disorders. Clin Psychol Rev 2010;29: 216–29.

68. Posey DJ, Guenin KD, Kohn AE, Swiezy NB, McDougle CJ. A naturalistic open-label study of mirtazapine in autistic and other pervasive developmental disorders. J Child Adolesc Psychopharmacol. 2001;11:267–77.

69. Steinhausen HC, Mohr Jensen C, Lauritsen MB. A systematic review and meta analysis of the long term overall outcome of autism spectrum disorders in adolescence and adulthood. Acta Psychiatr Scand. 2016;133:445–52.

70. Mukaddes NM, Tutkunkardas MD, Sari O, Aydin A, Kozanoglu P. Characteristics of children who lost the diagnosis of autism: A sample from istanbul, Turkey. Autism research and treatment. 2014; http://dx.doi.org/10.1155/2014/472120.

71. Bhargava A. School Education of Children with Special Needs in India with a Perspective on the Initiatives for Children with Autism. Available from: http://www.iccwtnispcanarc.org/upload/pdf/1494590016school%20edcation%20special%20needs%20india.pdf. Accessed: January 14, 2017.

72. Government of India. Guidelines for Evaluation and Assessment of Autism and Procedure for certification. Available from: http://disability affairs.gov.in/upload/uploadfiles/files/Autism%20Guidelines-%20Notification_compressed. pdf. Accessed: January 14, 2017.

73. Barua M, Kaushik JS, Gulati S. Legal provisions, educational services and health care across the lifespan for autism spectrum disorders in India. Indian J Pediatr. 2017; 84:1–7.

Consensus Statement of the IAP on Evaluation and Management of Attention Deficit Hyperactivity Disorder

Samir Dalwai, Jeeson Unni, Veena Kalra, Pratibha Singhi, Leena Shrivastava, MKC Nair

Attention-deficit/hyperactivity disorder (ADHD) is highly prevalent in children worldwide, and could be the most common neuro-behavioral disorder in children.[1,2] In India, the reported prevalence rates vary. A 2013 study from southern India reported prevalence of 11.3% in primary school children (sample size of 770 children, 6–11 years of age).[3] In terms of centre-based data, a retrospective study in Mumbai reviewed archival data (2009-2012) from case records of 1301 children presenting with developmental concerns (mean age: 6 years) and identified 422 children with ADHD (32.4%).[4] ADHD often co-exists with other developmental conditions such as Oppositional defiant disorder, Conduct disorder, learning disability and Anxiety. Given the public health burden and complexity of the condition, management of ADHD requires a systematic, multidisciplinary approach and therefore, evidence-based, standardized national guidelines are essential.

A meeting on formulation of national consultation guidelines on neurodevelopmental disorders was organized by Indian Academy of Pediatrics in Mumbai, on 18th and 19th December, 2015. The invited experts included pediatricians, developmental pediatricians, pediatric neurologists, psychiatrists, remedial educators and clinical psychologists. The participants framed guidelines after extensive discussions and review of literature. Thereafter, a committee was established to review the points discussed in the meeting, and the points of consensus on evaluation and management of ADHD are presented herein.

RECOMMENDATIONS

ADHD is a disorder that manifests in early childhood. The symptoms affect cognitive, academic, behavioral, emotional and social functioning. ADHD is a chronic condition and children and adolescents with ADHD are to be considered as children and youth with special health care needs.[5]

ADHD has a genetic and biochemical basis. Role of environmental factors is uncertain; they may influence symptoms of ADHD (sub-syndromic) rather than the syndrome of ADHD.[5]

Developmental Screening

Parent and teacher-rated scales are recommended for screening, which have been used globally as well as in studies conducted in India to screen ADHD, followed by a formal diagnosis using the Diagnostic and Statistical Manual of Mental Disorders (DSM). These scales include the Conners Index Questionnaire, and the vanderbilt ADHD diagnostic teacher rating scale.[6,7]

Core clinical features: Clinical sub-types include: predominantly hyperactive-impulsive, predominantly inattentive and combined ADHD.

Hyperactivity-impulsivity (HI): Although typically observed by 4 years of age, HI is increasingly being reported in children with younger age of presentation of symptoms. HI increases during the subsequent three to four years, peaks at 7–8 years of age and declines thereafter. By adolescence, it is difficult to identify HI, although the adolescent may feel restless or have difficulties in settling down.

In contrast, impulsivity usually persists throughout life and it is influenced by the child's environment. Adolescents with untreated ADHD and easy access to alcohol and substances of abuse are at greater risk of substance abuse, than adolescents without ADHD.[8]

Inattention: Children with predominantly inattentive ADHD have limited ability to focus and they are slow in cognitive processing and responding. Note that these symptoms are not due to defiance or lack of comprehension.[9] Inattention is usually identified late and not apparent until the child is 8–9 years of age.

Core symptoms must impair function in academic, social, or occupational activities for a child to be diagnosed with ADHD. Early diagnosis is essential to avoid further compromise of functional achievement.[5]

ADHD and Life-stage

Pre-school children: High activity level, poor inhibitory control and short attention span are common even in typically developing pre-school children. ADHD should be suspected in case of increased precarious behaviors and physical injuries or unmanageable behaviors across different settings. Combined type of ADHD is most common in this group and persists in 60–80% of children in school-age.

School children: School children have relatively stable attention levels and experience decrease in hyperactivity. However, 70% of these children have co-morbidities such as Oppositional defiant disorder and Specific learning disorder. ADHD has a major impact on peer and family interactions and academics, thereby influencing parent's reporting of presenting concerns.

Adults: At age 25 years; 15% individuals meet the full criteria for ADHD and ~65% are in partial remission. Symptoms of inattention persist more and show slower decline.[14]

Co-morbidities: Following co-morbidities have been identified with ADHD:[5] Oppositional defiant disorder (ODD); conduct disorders; learning disability; anxiety disorders; intermittent explosive disorder; substance abuse disorder; antisocial disorder; obsessive compulsive disorder; tic disorder; autism spectrum disorder and major depressive disorder.

Diagnosis

The fifth edition of the diagnostic and statistical manual of mental disorders[5] is used to diagnose ADHD. It is to be noted that diagnostic criteria (without subtyping) can be applied to children as young as 4 years of age.[11] On the other hand, adolescents may under-report core symptoms or functional impairment and may spend too little time at home for parents to be accurate informants. Hence, the pediatrician must obtain information from at least two teachers and/or other adults with whom the adolescent interacts (e.g., counselor, coaches, etc.).[11] The diagnostic tools mentioned (i.e. Child Behavior Check-List, Connors abbreviated rating scale and Vanderbilt ADHD diagnostic parent rating scale) have not been validated in the Indian population. The only freely available tool (based on fourth edition of DSM) that can be used for diagnosis of ADHD in the Indian context is the INCLEN Diagnostic Tool for ADHD (INDT-ADHD).[12] The sensitivity, specificity, positive and negative predictive values for the same are 87.7%, 97.2%, 98% and 83.3%, respectively. INDT-ADHD has an internal consistency of 0.91 and a moderate convergent validity with Conner's Parents Rating Scale (r =0.73).[12] The INCLEN tool is available in English, Hindi, Odia, Konkani, Urdu, Khasi, Gujrati, Telgu and Malayalam.[12] The time taken for its administration (excluding scoring time), as observed in clinic-settings, is 15–30 minutes (approx.).

Differential diagnosis: The symptoms of ADHD overlap with a number of other conditions, including developmental variations; neurologic or developmental conditions; emotional and behavioral disorders; psycho-social or environmental factors, and medical conditions.[11,13-14] Detailed history of the child and family, examination, psychometric testing, laboratory investigations, and genetic testing would help to establish the diagnosis. Few salient conditions to be differentiated include hyperactive/inattentive behaviors but within normal range for the child's developmental level and not impairing function, intellectual disability, learning disability, autism, language or communication disorder, anxiety disorder and motor incoordination disorder. Children with ADHD and with clinical features of autism should also receive genetic testing to rule out Fragile X syndrome. In areas that are known to be endemic for lead toxicity, a blood lead examination is indicated. Children in cities are at higher risk of lead toxicity due to vehicular traffic pollution and in case of use of leaded petrol. An audiological examination should also be conducted to rule out a hearing impairment.

Evaluation and Assessments

Any child 4 through 18 years of age, who presents with academic or behavioral problems and symptoms of inattention, hyperactivity, or impulsivity, should be evaluated.[11] Information should be obtained from parents or guardians, teachers, and other school and mental health clinicians involved in the child's care. Comprehensive evaluation for ADHD includes: (a) Confirmation of core symptoms for presence, persistence, per-vasiveness and functional complications; (b) Exclusion of differential diagnoses; and, (c) Identification of co-existing emotional, behavioral and/or medical disorders. Such a comprehensive evaluation requires review of medical, social, and family histories, clinical interviews with the parent and patient, and information on functioning in school or day-care.[11,15,16]

Medical evaluation: Important aspects of medical history include prenatal exposures (tobacco, drugs, alcohol), perinatal complica-tions or infections, head trauma, central nervous system infection, recurrent otitis media, history of sleep disturbances, medica-tions, family history of similar behaviors, and detailed child and family cardiac history before initiating medications.[11,16,17]

Physical examination: Physical examination is normal in most children with ADHD. Vision and hearing assessments are mandatory. It is essential to rule out differential diagnoses. Equally important is to document the following at each visit: height, weight, head circumference, and vital signs, assessment of dysmorphic features and neuro-cutaneous abnormalities, a complete neurologic examina-tion, and observation of the child's behavior in the clinic.[18]

Developmental and behavioral evaluation: This includes age of onset of core symptoms, their duration, settings in which the symptoms occur, and degree of functional impairment or functional impact of ADHD symptoms. Further information needed is developmental milestones, especially language milestones, school absences, psychosocial stressors, emotional, medical, and developmental events that may provide an alternative explanation for the symptoms (i.e., different diagnostic conditions). Observation of parent-child interactions in the office is an important component of assessment.

Information about core symptoms can be obtained through open-ended questions or from ADHD-specific rating scales. The pediatrician must document the presence of relevant behaviors from DSM-5.[16]

Educational evaluation: This includes completion of an ADHD-specific rating scale; a detailed summary of classroom behavior and interventions, learning patterns, and functional impairment at school; evaluation of copies of report cards and samples of schoolwork; and a review of school-based multidisciplinary evaluations (if performed).

The teachers who provide the information should have regular contact with the child for a minimum of four to six months, if they are to comment reliably on the persistence of symptoms. If there are discrepancies between parent and teacher reports, then information should be obtained from professionals working in after-school programs or other structured settings. Environmental factors (e.g. different expectations, levels of structure, or behavior management strategies) may be contributing to these symptoms.[11]

Management

Children with ADHD, 4 to 18 years of age, without co-morbid conditions can usually be managed by the primary pediatrician. Completion of ADHD rating scales by parents and teachers during the diagnostic evaluation helps to establish the presence of core symptoms in multiple settings.[19] Modalities of management of ADHD include behavioral interventions, medication and educational interventions (alone or in combination). Since children with ADHD or its symptoms are at an increased risk of intentional and unintentional injury, safety and injury prevention should be discussed during each visit.[5,11] Table 24.1 summarizes behavioral and educational interventions.

The teacher may submit a report card at regular intervals, which helps to monitor symptoms and the need for changes in the treatment plan.[24]

Age and Choice of Intervention

For children 4–6 years of age:

- Behavioral Intervention (BI), rather than medication, is the initial therapy.

TABLE 24.1: Behavioral and educational interventions

Type of intervention	Components	Age group
Behavioral intervention	a. Positive reinforcement; b. Time-out; c. Response cost (withdrawing rewards/ privileges when problem behavior occurs) and d. Token economy (combination of positive reinforcement and response cost)	For children 4–6 years of age as primary therapy and Children >6 years of age and adolescents, as therapy in addition to medication
Educational intervention	The classroom modifications and accommodations include 1. Having assignments written on the board 2. Sitting near the teacher 3. Having extended time to complete tasks 4. Being allowed to take tests in a less distracting environment 5. Receiving a private signal from the teacher when the child is 'off-task' 6. Being assigned a 'Study Buddy' 7. Being assigned a 'Shadow Teacher'	Children 5 years and above; depends on the child's capacity

- Addition of medication is indicated if target behaviors do not improve with BI and the child's functioning continues to be impaired.
- Methylphenidate is preferred rather than amphetamines or Atomoxetine.

For children >6 years of age and adolescents:[11,25]
- Treatment with medication rather than BI alone or no intervention.
- Stimulant drugs are the first line agents. Non-stimulants are second line agents.
- BI should be added to medication therapy.

Adding behavioral/ psychological therapy to stimulant therapy in school-aged children and adolescents does not provide additional benefit for core symptoms of ADHD, but has an impact on:
- Symptoms of coexisting conditions (e.g., oppositional/aggressive behavior)
- Educational performance
- Dose of stimulant therapy necessary to achieve the desired effects.

Behavioral Interventions

Parent-child behavioral therapy is aimed at improving parent-child relationships through enhanced parenting techniques. Behavioral interventions are most effective if parents understand the principles of behavior therapy (i.e. identification of antecedents and altering the consequences of behavior) and the techniques are consistently implemented.[11,20-22] Indications of behavioral intervention include: (a) Initial intervention for preschool children with ADHD (preferred to medication); (b) Adjunct to medication for school-aged children and adolescents with ADHD; (c) For children who have problems with inattention, hyperactivity, or impulsivity but do not meet criteria for ADHD (sub-syndromic). Specific interventions include: (a) Positive reinforcement; (b) Time-out; (c) Response cost (withdrawing rewards/privileges when problem behavior occurs) and (d) Token economy (combination of positive reinforcement and response cost).[22] Box 24.1 provides useful

> **Box 24.1:** Strategies for parents and teachers to regulate behaviors in children with ADHD
>
> 1. Maintaining a daily schedule (e.g., time table, post-its, reminders)
> 2. Using charts and checklists to help the child stay 'on task'
> 3. Keeping distractions to a minimum
> 4. Limiting choices
> 5. Providing specific and logical places for the child to keep his school books, toys, and clothes
> 6. Setting small, reachable goals
> 7. Rewarding positive behavior (e.g. with a 'token economy')
> 8. Identifying unintentional reinforcement of negative behaviors
> 9. Finding activities in which the child can be successful (e.g. hobbies, sports)
> 10. Using calm discipline (e.g. time out, distraction, removing the child from the situation)

strategies for parents and teachers to help children with ADHD regulate their own behavior.[11,23]

Educational Interventions

Children with ADHD may require changes in their educational program, including: (a) provision of tutoring or resource room support (either in a one-on-one setting or within the classroom), (b) classroom modifications, (c) accommodations, and (d) behavioral interventions.[11,23]

Pharmacologic Intervention

The drugs used for management of ADHD and their side-effects are detailed in Tables 24.2 to 24.4. The choice of medication depends on whether the child is in preschool in which case a stimulant (Methylphenidate) may be given, if indicated. For a school-aged child or adolescent, a stimulant is the first-line agent, followed by amphetamines or a monoamine reuptake inhibitor, i.e. Atomoxetine. Other medications (e.g. Alpha-2-adrenergic agonists) usually are used when children respond poorly to a trial of stimulants or Atomoxetine, or when children have unacceptable side

TABLE 24.2: Medications for ADHD

Type of drug	Name of the drug	Dosage forms	Duration of action	Dosage	Maximum dose
Stimulant	Methylphenidate	5 mg, 10 mg and 20 mg tablets	3–5 hours	Start with 5 mg/day for 1st day; then 5 mg twice a day	≤25 kg: 35 mg; >25 kg:60 mg.
Stimulant	Delayed onset methylphenidate	5 mg, 10 mg and 20 mg tablets	3–8 hours	5 mg/day twice daily dosing; increments of 20 mg per day, every 3–7 days	≤50 kg: 60 mg >50 kg: 100 mg.
Non-stimulant	Atomoxetine	10, 18 and 25 mg	10–12 hours	Start with 0.5 mg/kg per day for minimum 3 days and increase to 1.2 mg/kg per day after at least 3 days	100 mg per day or 1.4 mg/kg, whichever is lesser

TABLE 24.3: Side-effects of stimulant medications and management

Side-effects	Management
Decreased appetite	Counsel on high-protein, high-calorie diet and frequent snacks; advise on medication after meals
Tics	If distressing, taper or discontinue stimulant medication and consider guanfacine ER or clonidine ER monotherapy or augmentation
Poor growth	No action as ultimate adult height is not compromised
Dizziness	Self-resolving; symptomatic treatment
Insomnia/nightmares	Sleep hygiene; encourage natural sleep; melatonin as needed
Mood lability	Look for direct effect of medication (emotional symptoms correlate with expected time of medication effect) – if present, discontinue medication; if rebound effect (emotional symptoms occur later in day as medication expected to wearing off), then add short-acting stimulant in afternoon
Rebound symptoms	Add short-acting stimulant in afternoon; add slow-release tablets

TABLE 24.4: Side-effects of non-stimulant medications and management

Side-effects	Management
Gastrointestinal distress	Typically self-resolves; symptomatic care
Headache	Typically self-resolves; symptomatic care
Sedation (drowsiness)	Administer medication at bed-time
Transient growth effects	No action; adult height not affected
Elevated blood pressure or heart rate	No action if within age appropriate norms and asymptomatic
Suicidal ideation, hepatotoxicity, priapism (rare)	Counsel families on warning signs and symptoms of hepatotoxicity; discontinue medication; re-evaluation of the child

effects or significant coexisting conditions. The duration of action of the recommended drug and the child's ability to swallow pills also influence the choice of medication.

Stimulants are preferred to other medications because stimulants have rapid onset of action, and a long record of safety and efficacy. Individual differences in metabolism are more significant than weight-based dosing of stimulant medications. The optimal regimen is determined by changes in core symptoms and occurrence of side effects.[18,26]

Stimulant medications usually are started at the lowest dose that produces an effect and increased gradually (e.g., every 3–7 days) until core symptoms improve by 40–50% compared with baseline, or adverse effects become unacceptable. The frequency of stimulant medication (i.e., both, times per day and days per week) is based upon the type of ADHD and the functional domains in which improvement is desired. Onset of action is very important in a school-going child. At a therapeutic dose, the effects of stimulant medications on core symptoms usually are apparent in 30–40 minutes after administration and continue for the expected duration of action. Appetite suppression may indicate treatment response. Inadequate dose may be indicated by shorter than expected duration of action.[18]

A child with the predominantly inattentive type of ADHD may need medication only on school days. A child who has difficulty with peer relationships may need medication every day. A child who participates in after-school sports or activities on certain days of the week may require longer-acting preparations or more frequent dosing on those days. Optimal dose is the dose at which target outcomes are achieved with minimal side effects.

Parents should be advised that 2–6 weeks of medication maybe needed for any therapeutic effect to show and before dose-reduction is considered. If side-effects are severe, the clinician may decrease the dose of medication or change to another ADHD medication (stimulant or non-stimulant).[27]

After several years of medication, children and adolescents who have had stable improvement in ADHD symptoms and target behaviors are offered a trial off, of medication to determine whether medication is still necessary. If symptoms re-appear, after a period of remission, consider the risk factors/stressors that have led to the same and counsel parents on mitigating those; and resume medication. Children with ADHD may require changes in their educational programming. Combination therapy with medications and behavior/psychological therapy is superior to behavior/psychological therapy alone and necessary for restoration of function and inclusion.

Combination Therapy

Combination therapy uses both behavioral interventions and medications. Combination therapy may be warranted in preschool children who do not respond to behavioral interventions.

In a systematic review and a meta-analysis, combination therapy with medications and behavior/psychological therapy, was superior to behavior/psychological therapy alone. Children receiving combination therapy may require lower doses of medication and achieve greater improvement in non-ADHD symptoms (e.g., oppositional/aggressive, internalizing, teacher-rated social skills, parent-child relations and reading achievement) than children receiving medication alone. Cognitive behavioral therapy may be a helpful adjunct to medications for adolescents with ADHD. Dietary interventions are not recommended.

Referral to a developmental pediatrician, Child neurologist or child psychiatrist is needed in case of (a) Co-morbid conditions (e.g. oppositional defiant disorder, conduct disorder, substance abuse, emotional problems); (b) Coexisting neurologic or medical conditions (e.g. seizures, tics, autism spectrum disorder, sleep disorder); (c) Lack of response to a controlled trial of stimulant or Atomoxetine therapy.[25,28-30] Figure 24.1 provides a flowchart for the management approach to a child presenting with concerns regarding ADHD.

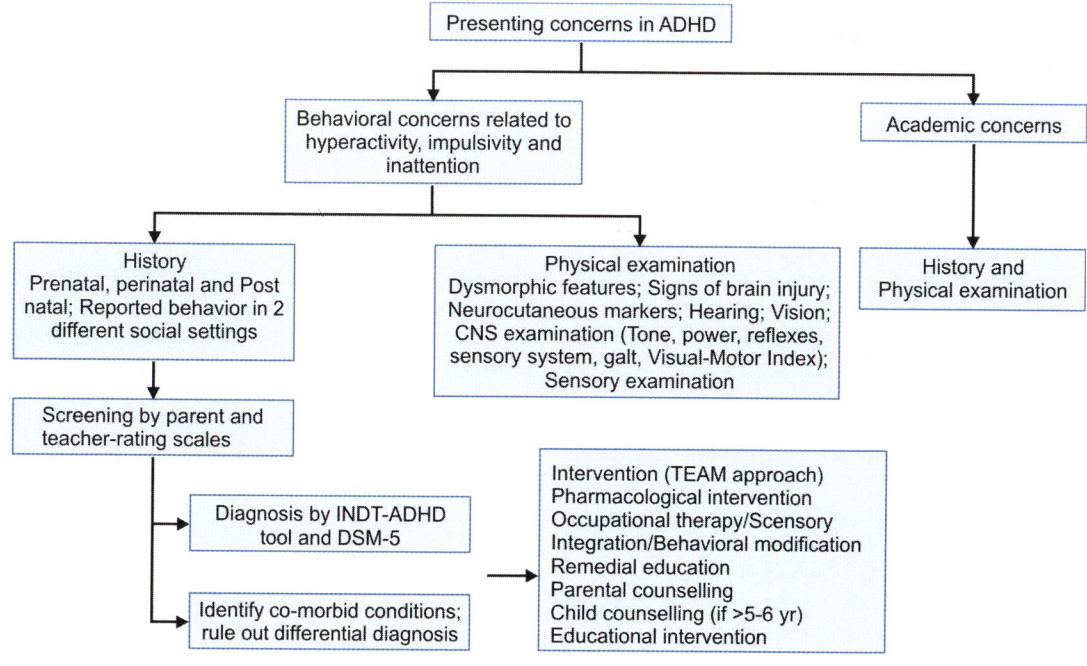

Fig. 24.1: Provides a flowchart for the management of ADHD

Disability Certification

Government organizations, the Persons with Disability Act (Equal Opportunities, Protection of Rights and Full Participation),1995, and the National Trust for the Welfare of Persons with Autism, Cerebral Palsy, Mental Retardation and Multiple Disabilities act, 1999, do not recognize ADHD as a neurodevelopmental disorder. Currently, there are no provisions for certifying children with ADHD. However, the Rashtriya Bal Swasthya Karyakram (RBSK) focuses on early detection and intervention of disease, disabilities, deficiencies and developmental problems including ADHD. Owing to the fact that it is the most common childhood neuro-behavioural disorder; high prevalence rates in India, and the dire need for affected children to receive sustained multidisciplinary interventions over a long period, the expert group strongly recommends disability certification for ADHD.

CONCLUSION

ADHD is characterized by behavioral, emotional and academic concerns, and requires a range of interventions such as medications, behavioural intervention, occupational therapy/sensory integration, remedial education, parent and child counselling and classroom modifications. A comprehensive inter-disciplinary approach leads to sustained alleviation of symptoms and greater capacity-building of caregivers and children to adjust with the disease over the long term.

REFERENCES

1. Faraone SV, Sergeant J, Gillberg C, Biederman J. The worldwide prevalence of ADHD: is it an American condition? World Psychiatry. 2003;2: 104–13.

2. American Psychiatric Association. Diagnostic and statistical manual of mental disorders. 4th ed. Washington, DC: American Psychiatric Association; 2000.

3. Venkata JA, Panicker AS. Prevalence of attention deficit hyperactivity disorder in primary school children. Indian J Psychiatry. 2013;55:338–42.

4. Duggal C, Dalwai S, Bopanna K, Datta V, Chatterjee S, Mehta N. Childhood Developmental and Psychological Disorders: Trends in Presentation and Interventions in a Multidisciplinary Child Development Centre. Indian J Soc Work. 2014; 75:495–522

5. American Psychiatric Association. Diagnostic and statistical manual of mental disorders, 5th edition. Arlington, VA: American Psychiatric Association; 2013.

6. Naik A, Patel S, Biswas DA. Prevalence of ADHD in a rural Indian population. Innovative J Med and Health Science. 2016;6:45–6.

7. Suvarna BS, Kamath A. Prevalence of attention deficit disorder among preschool age children. Nepal Med Coll J. 2009;11:1–4.

8. Levin FR, Kleber HD. Attention-deficit hyperactivity disorder and substance abuse: relationships and implications for treatment. Harv Rev Psychiatry. 1995;2: 246–58.

9. Weiler MD, Bernstein JH, Bellinger DC, Waber DP. Processing speed in children with attention deficit/hyperactivity disorder, inattentive type. Child Neuropsychol. 2000;6:218–34.

10. Faraone SV, Biederman J, Mick E. The age-dependent decline of attention deficit hyperactivity disorder: a meta-analysis of follow-up studies. Psychol Med. 2006; 36:159–65.

11. Subcommittee on Attention-Deficit/Hyperactivity Disorder, Steering Committee on Quality Improvement and Management. ADHD: clinical practice guideline for the diagnosis, evaluation, and treatment of attention-deficit/hyperactivity disorder in children and adolescents. Pediatrics. 2011.

12. Mukherjee S, Aneja S, Russell PS, Gulati S, Deshmukh V, Sagar R, et al. INCLEN diagnostic tool for attention deficit hyperactivity disorder (INDT-ADHD): Development and validation. Indian Paediatr. 2014;51:457–62.

13. Krull KR, Augustyn M, Torchia M. Attention deficit hyperactivity disorder in children and adolescents: Clinical features and evaluation. [cited 2012]. Available from: http://www.uptodate.com/contents/attention-deficit-hyperactivity-disorder-in-children-and-adolescents-clinical-features-and-evaluation? source=search_result&search=attention+deficit+hyperactivity+disorder+children&selected Title=2~150. Accessed January 23, 2016.

14. Gilger JW, Pennington BF, DeFries JC. A twin study of the etiology of comorbidity: attention-deficit hyperactivity disorder and dyslexia. J Am Acad Child Adolesc Psychiatry. 1992;31:343–8.

15. National Collaborating Centre for Mental Health, UK. Attention deficit hyperactivity disorder: diagnosis and management of ADHD in children, young people and adults. [cited 2009]. Available from: http://www.ncbi.nlm.nih.gov/pubmed-health/PMH0034228/toc/?report=reader. Accessed January 23, 2016.

16. Taylor E, Döpfner M, Sergeant J, Asherson P, Banaschewski T, Buitelaar J, et al. European Clinical Guidelines for Hyperkinetic Disorder–First Upgrade. Eur Child Adolesc Psychiatry. 2004;13:i7–i30.

17. Sedky K, Bennett DS, Carvalho KS. Attention deficit hyperactivity disorder and sleep disordered breathing in pediatric populations: a meta-analysis. Sleep Med Rev. 2014;18:349–56.

18. Wender EH. Managing stimulant medication for attention-deficit/hyperactivity disorder. Pediatr Rev 2001;23:234–6.

19. Collett BR, Ohan JL, Myers KM. Ten-year review of rating scales. V: scales assessing attention-deficit/hyperactivity disorder. J Am Acad Child Adolesc Psychiatry 2003;42:1015–37.

20. Charach A, Carson P, Fox S, Ali MU, Beckett J, Lim CG. Interventions for preschool children at high risk for ADHD: a comparative effectiveness review. Pediatrics 2013;131:1–21.

21. Kaplan A, Adesman A. Clinical diagnosis and management of attention deficit hyperactivity disorder in preschool children. Curr Opin Pediatr 2011;23:684–92.

22. Floet AL, Scheiner C, Grossman L. Attention-deficit/hyperactivity disorder. Paediatr Rev. 2010;31:56–69.

23. American Academy of Pediatrics. Understanding ADHD. Information for parents about attention-deficit/hyperactivity disorder. [cited 2001]. Available from: http://www.pediatricenter.org/docs/ADHD%20AAP%20hand out_HE0169.pdf. Accessed January 23, 2016.

24. Manansala MA, Dizon EI. Shadow teaching scheme for children with autism and attention deficit-hyperactivity disorder in regular schools. Educ Q. 2010;66:34–49.

25. Pliszka S. AACAP Work Group on Quality Issues. Practice parameter for the Assessment and Treatment of Children and Adolescents with Attention-deficit/hyperactivity Disorder. J Am Acad Child Adolesc Psychiatry. 2007;46: 894–921.

26. Kaplan G, Newcorn JH. Pharmacotherapy for child and adolescent attention-deficit hyperactivity disorder. Paediatr Clin N Am 2011;58:99–120.

27. Southammakosane C, Schmitz K. Pediatric psychopharmacology for treatment of ADHD, depression, and anxiety. Pediatrics 2015;136:351–9.

28. The MTA Cooperative Group. Multimodal Treatment Study of Children with ADHD. A 1 4-month randomized clinical trial of treatment strategies for attention-deficit/hyperactivity disorder. Arch Gen Psychiatry. 1999;56:1073–86.

29. Brown RT, Amler RW, Freeman WS, Perrin JM, Stein MT, Feldman HM, et al. American Academy of Paediatrics Committee on Quality Improvement; American Academy of Paediatrics Subcommittee on Attention-Deficit/Hyperactivity Disorder. Paediatrics. 2005;115:e749–e57.

30. Van der Oord S, Prins PJ, Oosterlaan J, Emmelkamp PM. Efficacy of methylphenidate, psychosocial treatments and their combination in school-aged children with ADHD: a meta-analysis. Clin Psychol Rev. 2008;28:783–800.

Consensus Statement of the IAP on Evaluation and Management of Learning Disability

MKC Nair, Chhaya Prasad, Jeeson Unni, Anjan Bhattacharya, SS Kamath, Samir Dalwai

Learning Disability (LD) in children is a well-recognized developmental disorder with profound academic and psychosocial consequences. Due to the complex nature of LD and the multiple disadvantages posed to the child due to LD, a multidisciplinary approach towards intervention is warranted. Given the paucity of published standardized treatment approaches for use in India, consensus guidelines for management of LD are needed.

The meeting on formulation of national consensus guidelines on neurodevelopmental disorders was organized by Indian Academy of Pediatrics in Mumbai, on 18th and 19th December, 2015. The invited experts included Pediatricians, Developmental pediatricians, Pediatric neurologists, Psychiatrists, Remedial educators and Clinical psychologists. The participants framed guidelines after extensive discussions. Thereafter, a committee was established to review and finalize the points discussed in the meeting. The following sections include the points of consensus on evaluation and management of LD.

Terminology: The term 'Learning Disability' (LD) is used synonymously with Specific Learning Disability and Specific Learning Disorder, the latter used by the fifth edition of Diagnostic and Statistical Manual of Mental Disorders (DSM-5).[1] However, in some countries, the term refers to intellectual disability (formerly called 'mental retardation').[2,3]

Definition: LDs are a heterogeneous group of disorders where the individual unexpectedly fails to competently acquire, retrieve and use information. The academic achievement is lower than expected, based on the child's overall intelligence.[2-4] LD has been defined as a neurodevelopmental disorder of biological origin manifesting in learning difficulties and problems in acquiring academic skills, which are markedly below age level. LD manifests during early school years and it is not attributed to intellectual disabilities, or neurological or motor disorders. The difficulties should last for at least six months, to warrant a diagnosis.[1]

The recommendations have been drafted for an age-range, based on current evidence. The diagnostic tool developed by the National Institute of Mental Health and Neurosciences (NIMHANS) for children with LD, is one of the recommended tools in India.[5] It includes two levels: Level-1 for children 5–7 years of age and Level-2 for children 8–12 years of age.[5] Hence, the recommendations pertain to children 5 years and above.

Prevalence: Approximately 5% of all students in public schools in the United States are identified as having LD;[4] while another study in US reported that 7% of children 3–17 years of age had LD.[6] The reported prevalence in India ranges from 1.6–15%, varying based on age-range, survey method, tool used, and region of the country.[7–10] A cross-sectional study conducted in Chandigarh (n=3600, grade 3 and 4 students) reported 3.08% of children with a diagnosis of LD.[8] Another study using informal assessment, conducted in five schools in Jaipur (n=1156, children 6–13 years of age) reported 12.8% with LD (21.6%, 15.5% and 22.3% of children with dyslexia, dyscalculia and dysgraphia, respectively).[9]

Types of Learning Disabilities

Dyslexia: Dyslexia or reading disability is a specific type of reading disorder caused by deficits in phonologic processing. These deficits are unexpected in relation to the student's overall intelligence and persist even after receiving appropriate (general educational) instruction. Dyslexia presents initially with problems in letter-sound relationships (i.e. decoding words and reading fluently in kindergarten or grade one). Problems in reading comprehension usually present in the latter part of the primary school years, when the focus is on reading to learn rather than learning to read-these can be identified by low overall reading achievement, or by low reading ability, relative to overall intelligence.

Dysgraphia: Dysgraphia or writing disabilities are caused by a range of neurodevelopmental weaknesses, including problems with handwriting (fine motor or grapho-motor) and visual-spatial perception. Children present with difficulties in copying efficiently from the board; may show excessive grammar and punctuation errors; may produce overtly simple written text and/or produce disorganized text that is difficult to follow. In contrast, problems exclusively in spelling (also called 'encoding', which is the ability to use letter-sound relationships effectively) in absence of problems in written expression is more indicative of a phonologic processing deficit (i.e., dyslexia), than a dysgraphia. Other problems include those in grammar and syntax as well as formulating, expressing and organizing ideas in writing.

Dyscalculia: Dyscalculia or mathematical disabilities may include problems with number sense, problems retrieving math facts (arithmetic combinations or calculations), difficulty with the language of math (correctly reading and understanding numbers and symbols), word problems in math (correctly reading and understanding the text of word problems) and the visual-spatial and organizational demands of math. Students may reverse numbers or make errors while reading them aloud. These problems are usually seen in conjunction with disabilities in reading or written expression. Math functions depend upon the ability of the student to understand words associated with arithmetic operations and word problems. Dyslexia can aggravate difficulties in acquiring math skills.

Co-morbid Conditions

These include Attention-deficit Hyperactivity Disorder (i.e. inattention, hyperactivity, impulsivity, having difficulty sustaining focus, being disorganized); Autism Spectrum Disorder (i.e. impairment in reciprocal social communication and social interaction; restricted repetitive patterns of behavior, interests or activities); Communication Disorders (i.e. deficits in language, speech and communication) and Developmental Coordination Disorders (i.e. impairment predominantly in gross and fine motor skills including handwriting skills, pedaling, buttoning shirts, completing puzzles, using zippers, playing ball games, etc.).

RECOMMENDATIONS

Diagnosis

The diagnosis of LD is made primarily by history. Diagnostic criteria and differential diagnoses (e.g. normal variations in academic achievement, ADHD, Intellectual disability, Learning disorders due to sensory or neurological impairments) have been provided in the DSM-5.[1] These conditions can be differentiated by history, examination, laboratory tests (e.g. blood lead level), hearing and vision assessment, specialized screening/referral.

Psychometric tests help to confirm the presence of LD and identify targets for intervention. An appropriate assessment for LD includes information from student's educational history, a description of classroom observations and standardized psychometric measures. LD can only be diagnosed after formal education starts, but can be diagnosed at any point afterward in children, adolescents, or adults, provided there is evidence of onset during the years of formal schooling. No single data source is sufficient for diagnosis. A mandatory vision and hearing assessment should be part of the protocol. Investigations for lead toxicity may be conducted, if suspected.

Assessments

Scales to diagnose LD take longer time to administer, which necessitates screening to identify 'at-risk' children. It is important to identify these children early, after school starts, for early intervention. Studies conducted in India to measure prevalence of LD have used screening questionnaires such as Specific Learning Disability-Screening Questionnaire (SLD-SQ)[8] or designed screening tools for class teachers to identify LD.[10] Pediatricians could use the SLD-SQ or focus on certain pointers in the latter to identify 'at-risk' children, in order to refer them for thorough evaluation by a developmental paediatrician. The pointers include: unexplainable absence from school, below average academic performance, poor writing ability, problems in reading ability, poor mathematical competence and problems in recall. Concerns in two or more of these areas, should warrant a referral.[10]

The language availability, cost, diagnostic performance and time taken to administer a range of tests more suitable for Indian children, especially those who are first-generation English learners, have been summarized in Table 25.1.[5,11–15]

NIMHANS index to assess children with LD.[5] The index comprises of the following tests: (a) attention test (number cancellation); (b) visual-motor skills (Bender-Gestalt test and developmental test of visual-motor integration); (c) auditory and visual processing (discrimination and memory); (d) reading, writing, spelling and comprehension tests; (e) speech and language assessments including auditory behaviour (receptive language) and verbal expression; and (f) arithmetic tests (addition, subtraction, multiplication and division).

The Rehabilitation Council of India (RCI) recommends informal assessment (i.e., parental interviewing after consent; gathering information from teacher/school; reviewing student's workbooks; and interviewing the child) and formal testing (i.e. criterion and norm-referenced tests). Tests for LD have two components: (a) testing for potential performance discrepancy–where a two-year discrepancy between potential and performance is an indicator of possible LD and, (b) testing of processing abilities.

One or more tests have to be administered based on the child's age and cognitive ability. The range of tests that can be administered are as follows:

Intellectual assessment: Woodcock Johnson Tests of Cognitive Ability (3rd edition; age two and above) or Malin's Intelligence Scale for Indian Children (for children 6 years and above), which is the Indian adaptation of

TABLE 25.1: Assessments for learning disability

Name of the test/battery	Age group/ grade	Cost	Note on diagnostic performance	Time taken	Available languages
NIMHANS	Level I: 5–7 yr Level II: 8–12 yr	Freely available	Test-re-test reliability: 0.53 ($p < 0.001$)	Variable (battery of tests)	English, Hindi, Kannada
GLAD	6 yrs or older	Freely available	Test-re-test reliability: 0.68 for Grade IV to 0.99 for grade III; Criterion validity: 0.74 to 0.89	Variable (curriculum-based)	English, Hindi
BKT	3–22 yrs	INR 2000[*]	IQs correlate highly with measures on Stanford-Binet Intelligence scales	2 hours	English; can be used with children not adequately exposed to English
WJ-III achievement	2 yrs and above	$2207[*]	Reliability: 0.81-0.94	60–70 minutes	English

*in January 2017; GLAD: Grade Level Assessment Device; BKT: Binet-Kamat test; NIMHANS: National Institute of Mental Health and Neurosciences

Wechsler intelligence scale for children (WISC).

Achievement: Woodcock Johnson III–tests of Achievement for children; Nelson Denny reading test for high school and college students.

Cognitive Processing Abilities: Woodcock Johnson Psycho-Educational Battery Revised (Part 1–tests of cognitive ability), Weschler Memory Scales Revised (age 16 years and above), Benton Visual Retention Test (age 8 years and above), Beery Visual-Motor Integration Test (age 2 years and above), Raven Colored Progressive Matrices (age 5 years and above) Rey Auditory-Verbal Learning Test (age ≥16 years), Bender Visual Motor Gestalt Test (age 4 years and above) and NIMHANS Index (Level I: 5–7 years and Level II: 8–12 years).

Assessment of intelligence is essential to exclude intellectual disability as a primary cause of difficulties in learning.

In a multi-linguistic country like India, it is important to develop scales to diagnose LD in non-English speaking students. As mentioned above, RCI has advised informal assessment for these students, in absence of standardized scales. Moreover, the Grade Level Assessment Device (GLAD) for children with learning problems in schools has been developed by the National Institute for the Mentally Handicapped (NIMH).[11]

It is essential to exclude other impairments as the primary cause of learning difficulties. Such impairments include low intellectual quotient; sensory deficits (visual and/or hearing impairment); physical impairments; history of multiple education settings; poor educational background or lack of prior learning; and cultural differences contributing to lack of experience with the English language (e.g. first-generation English learners). However, LD may co-exist with the above.

LD being a language-based disorder, it is imperative that tests for both receptive and expressive language be included in the comprehensive assessment. Other procedures include curriculum-based assessment; dynamic assessment; learning styles assessment and outcome-based assessment.

Intervention Approach

A basic intervention approach should focus on: (a) interpretation of evaluation reports; (b) description of specific skills that may be delayed (e.g. phoneme awareness and phonics, reading comprehension, spelling instruction, number sense, and organizational skills), and (c) identification of co-morbidities. The intervention should be inter-disciplinary and individualized to each child. Required services include: developmental pediatrics evaluation; neurological evaluation; ophthalmology and audiology evaluation; clinical psychology assessment; occupational therapy (e.g. handwriting, attention, hyperactivity, visual-motor coordination), remedial education (i.e. educational assessment and individualized education program), counseling for family, and career-counselling.

Remedial education includes educational assessment of the child for strengths and weaknesses in academic skills; development of an individualized education program (IEP) for each child having short-term and long-term goals, and monitoring the child's progress. Intervention sessions (i.e. twice- or thrice-weekly) could typically last for 45 minutes and continue for few years. Sessions could be offered in school or outside regular school hours. Parents need to be trained to adopt the strategies at home. Specific strategies include: (a) Review information about previous lesson on the topic before beginning the current lesson; (b) Clearly state what the student is expected to learn during the current lesson; (c) Describe how the student is expected to behave during the lesson e.g. tell the child not to talk with peers if the assigned task is found to be difficult, but to raise his/her hands to get the teacher's attention; (d) State all materials that the child will need during the lesson e.g. specify that the child needs crayons, scissors and coloured paper for an art project rather than leaving the child to figure out the use of materials; (d) Psycho-educational interventions (e.g. seating the child near the teacher to minimize classroom distractions), and

(e) Assigning a specific teacher to review daily assignments.

Intervention Strategies

Phoneme awareness-reading: During these sessions the child with dyslexia undergoes systematic and highly structured training exercises to learn that words can be segmented into smaller units of sound ('phoneme awareness'). During these sessions, the remedial teacher explicitly and directly teaches the following tasks: (i) Phoneme segmentation: e.g. what sounds do you hear in the word pot? What is the last sound in the word tap?; (ii) Phoneme deletion: e.g. What word would be left if the /m/sound was taken away from mat?; (iii) Phoneme matching: e.g. Do 'pen' and 'pipe' start with the same sound?; (iv) Phoneme counting: How many sounds do you hear in the word 'take'?; (v) Phoneme substitution: What word would you have if you changed the /p/ in pot to /h/?; (vi) Blending: What word would you have if you put these sounds together? /f/ /a/ /t/; (vii) Rhyming: Tell me as many words as you can that rhyme with the word eat.

Reading-phonics instruction: Phonics instruction begins only after phonemic awareness gets developed. The child is taught that these sounds ("phonemes") are linked with specific letters and letter patterns ("phonics"). The goal of teaching phonics is to link the individual sounds to letters, and to make that process fluent and automatic for both reading and spelling. In other words, phonics teaches students symbol-to-sound and sound-to-symbol linkages. Spellings are taught through 'phonics-based teaching' using colour-coded segmentation (e.g. bot/tle), word formation games and sight-word identification. However, the English language has words like 'any', 'because', 'island', 'enough', etc. which are impossible to spell from the sounds of their letters. These tricky words can be learned via 'mnemonics'. However, even after years of adequate remedial education, subtle deficiencies in reading, writing, and mathematical abilities do persist in many children. To develop reading fluency and automaticity should be a critical intervention goal for older children.

Basic principles–writing skills: All of the components of writing need to be considered to create an intervention plan for addressing the components that are most affected. Lower-order writing skills consist of printing/handwriting (transcription skills) and spelling skills (a phonics-based skill that requires sound-symbol relationships). Ultimately, the student should have memorized certain number of high-frequency words and spell them automatically (i.e. writing fluency), without which higher-order skills are more difficult to master. Higher-order writing skills require the ability to write sentences (e.g. understand language conventions related to punctuation, grammar, etc.) and produce a composition. Writing instruction involves drill and practice (explicit or direct instruction) of lower-order skills (transcription, spelling and writing fluency) in the service of higher-order skills (writing sentences and compositions). Direct instruction is required for the student to achieve accurate letter formation and fluency in writing, spelling, punctuation and grammar. Improvements in these lower-order skills can improve higher order performance. Specific types of instruction (e.g. strategy instruction) can be used to improve performance in higher order writing skills.

Basic principles–mathematics: Competence in mathematics depends upon mastery of lower-order skills which are then used in the service of higher order skills. In Mathematical disorder, primary deficits occur in number sense and math facts (arithmetic combinations or calculations). Performance in higher-order math skills also depends upon math fluency, i.e., the fluent application of number sense and math facts. Students with this disorder also have difficulty solving word problems. This can be due to problems in number sense and

calculation skills or a coexistent reading or language disability. Thus, effective remediation for reading and writing disability has to be primarily worked upon. Finally, visual-spatial and organizational problems can interfere with success in mathematics, which requires occupational therapy intervention.

Specific areas where intervention should focus have been described below:
Number sense: Number sense refers to having mental representation of quantity (i.e., ability to estimate and judge magnitude). It is an early-emerging skill that can fail to develop in students with Mathematical Disorder. Number sense is a prerequisite for math, and is a teachable skill. It can be compared to phonemic awareness, which is a prerequisite for reading (decoding), and is also a teachable skill. Number sense can be taught by (a) practicing identification or estimation of quantity (i.e. less and more); (b) 1:1 correspondence (e.g. correlating the number of coins being dropped into a box with the sound made by each of the coins, as it drops); (c) serial ordering (numbers are always counted in the same order); (d) "counting on" (i.e. identifying changes in quantity by adding up from a smaller quantity to create a larger quantity); (e) showing the link between addition and subtraction while using objects; (f) using more than one type of visual representation for numbers (e.g. both horizontal and vertical number lines); and (g) other visual representations that show differences in size, volume, etc.

Mathematical facts or calculation skills: Number sense is required to understand how to add, subtract, multiply, and divide numbers. However, these skills are also acquired by learning the rules for addition, subtraction, multiplication, and division. The strategies used include efficient and effective counting-strategy use, mathematic fluency, mathematic vocabulary and word problems, visual-spatial skills in mathematics and organization and planning in mathematics. They are detailed in Box 25.1.

Provisions and Advocacy

Advocacy of the rights of children with LD to achieve optimal potential via provisions is a necessity. Pediatricians as trustees and custodians of children are the strongest voices that children have.[16-18]

Presently, only few state governments (Maharashtra, Karnataka, Tamil Nadu, Kerala, Goa and Gujarat) and the National educational boards that conduct the Indian Certificate of Secondary Education and the Central Board of Secondary Education examinations have formally granted the benefit of availing the necessary provisions to children with LD.[19] Due to the central nervous system's higher plasticity in early years, remedial education should begin early when the child is in primary school.[16-18]

The cornerstone of treatment of LD is thorough comprehensive evaluation and outcome-based, documented multidisciplinary intervention. Screening of all children at the age of 7 years for LD in the pediatric clinic will be highly beneficial (2–3 years after school exposure). No Detention Policy (NDP) leads to delayed identification of learning problems, and needs to be seriously reviewed. Concept of multiple intelligence needs to be highlighted, i.e., students with LD can be poor

---

Box 25.1: Examples of interventions for mathematical disorders

Efficient and effective counting-strategy use: Counting strategies need to be taught explicitly alongside number facts. Students with Mathematical Disorder may not develop their own strategic learning. For example, they may not learn that "counting upward" from the larger addend (addend is a number that is added to another) can save time when doing addition problems (e.g. 5 + 4 = 9 is easier to understand than 4 + 5 = 9). Counting strategies can help develop both number sense and arithmetic combination skills. *Gradually,* students develop memory-based retrieval of answers, increasing their overall efficiency.

Mathematical fluency: Students have difficulties completing higher order Mathematical problems when they have not yet developed automaticity in basic arithmetic combinations and cannot retrieve memorized answers to basic arithmetic combinations quickly. Remediation is crucial at the beginning of third grade. Rote learning and memorization alone are not as effective as the combination of memorization with strategy instruction.

Mathematical vocabulary: Students have difficulties with the language of Mathematical. They may reverse numbers, or make errors when reading numbers aloud. Confusion about number symbols and signs is a distinguishing characteristic. In math, there are no context clues to help students decipher terms that they may not understand. The language of math must be taught directly and explicitly, not incidentally.

Word problems: Reading difficulties can aggravate difficulties in acquiring Mathematical skills. Students with reading and Mathematical difficulties, have greater difficulty with word problems than students with isolated Mathematical Disorder. They also have greater difficulty in understanding the meaning of the sentences describing the problem, understanding what the problem is asking and identifying extraneous or irrelevant information. General strategy instruction may be helpful in solving word problems.

Visual-spatial skills in Mathematical: Students may copy numbers incorrectly, write numbers illegibly, misalign numbers, have left-right disorientation of numbers, misplace digits in multi-digit numbers, skip rows or columns during calculations, fail to carry numbers (e.g., regrouping when appropriate), reverse number problems, start a calculation in the wrong place, or may not recognize operator signs. The use of lined or graph paper, or specific strategy instruction is effective. Visual-spatial weaknesses can also affect the student's understanding of volume and Mathematical problems in geometry.

Organization and planning in Mathematical: Due to planning and organizing difficulties, students may fail to verify answers and settle for the first answer they reach. Strategy instruction can help the student to follow a prescribed sequence when solving problems; check solutions using a computer; or prompt him/her to ask if the answer is a reasonable one.

Key Messages

- Intervention approach should focus on interpretation of evaluation reports, description of specific skills that may be delayed and identification of co-morbidities.
- It is essential to have an inter-disciplinary approach involving different specialities; regular and concise documentation facilitates the process.
- The intervention should be inter-disciplinary and individualized to each child.
- Remedial education includes assessment of the child's academic strengths and weaknesses and development of an individual education program (IEP) having short-term and long-term goals and monitoring of the child's progress.

in academic intelligence but may be better in other domains. Role of National Institute of Open Schooling is pertinent for children with LD in India.[20]

LD lowers the scores of a student's performance and provisions are intended to function as a corrective lens, which will deflect the distorted array of observed scores back to where they ought to be. These provisions aim to 'level the playing field' for these students as their academic performance would now be matching with their intellectual potential.[21-25]

Concessions for students with LD (all subtypes) include: (a) One hour or 25% extra time in public exams; (b) No mark reduction for grammar and spelling mistakes; (c) Use of calculator in Maths exam; (d) Exemption from writing one language exam; (e) Use of scribe or typing answers on a computer; and (f) 20% grace marks.[21-25]

In terms of inclusion, the following policy-level changes are conducive for children with LD: (a) Government of India launched the Sarva Shiksha Abhiyan in 2001 ('Education for All') that aims to provide useful and relevant education to all children, including children with disabilities in the mainstream ('inclusive education');[26] (b) Right of Children to Free and Compulsory Education 2009 (RTE Act) stresses on free and compulsory education for children 6 to 14 years of age, including children with special needs, and research has also looked at the challenges in its execution;[27] and (c) Rashtriya Bal Swasthya Karyakram (RBSK) focuses on early detection and intervention of disease, disabilities, deficiencies and developmental problems.[28]

Previously, learning disability was not included in the Persons with Disability Act (PWD, 1995). The recent bill (Rights of Persons with Disability Bill 2011 and passed as an Act in 2016) has included LD and recognized it as a disability.[25, 29]

REFERENCES

1. American Psychiatric Association. Diagnostic and statistical manual of mental disorders (DSM-5®). 5th ed. Washington, DC: American Psychiatric Pub. 2013

2. Adelman HS. Opinion papers toward solving the problems of misidentification and limited intervention efficacy. J Learn Disabil.1989;22:608–12.

3. Adelman HS. LD: the next 25 years. J Learn Disabil. 1992;25:17–22.

4. Lyon GR. Learning disabilities. Future Child. 1996; 6:54–76.

5. Kapur M, John A, Rozario J, Oommen A. NIMHANS Index of Specific Learning Disabilities. Psychological Assessment of Children in the Clinical Setting. Department of Clinical Psychology, National Institute of Mental Health and Neurosciences; Bangalore. 2002:88–126.

6. Boyle CA, Boulet S, Schieve LA, Cohen RA, Blumberg SJ, Yeargin-Allsopp M, et al. Trends in the prevalence of developmental disabilities in US children, 1997–2008. Pediatrics. 2011;127: 1034–42.

7. Mogasale VV, Patil VD, Patil NM, Mogasale V. Prevalence of specific learning disabilities among primary school children in a South Indian city. Indian J Pediatr. 2012;79:342–7.

8. Padhy SK, Goel S, Das SS, Sarkar S, Sharma V, Panigrahi M. Prevalence and patterns of learning disabilities in school children. Indian J Pediatr. 2016;83:300–6

9. Dhanda A, Jagawat T. Prevalence and pattern of learning disabilities in school children. Delhi Psychiatry Journal 2013;6:386–90.

10. Arun P, Chavan BS, Bhargava R, Sharma A, Kaur J. Prevalence of specific developmental disorder of scholastic skill in school students in Chandigarh, India. Indian J Med Res. 2013;138:89.

11. Narayan J. Grade Level Assessment Device for Children with Learning Problems in Schools (GLAD). Secunderabad: National Institute for the Mentally Handicapped (NIMH); 1997.

12. Kamat VV. A revision of the Binet scale for Indian children:(Kanarese and Marathi speaking). Br J Educ Psychol. 1934;4:296–309.

13. Woodcock RW, McGrew KS, Mather N, Schrank F. Woodcock-Johnson III NU tests of achievement. Rolling Meadows, IL: Riverside Publishing. 2001.

14. Panicker AS, Bhattacharya S, Hirisave U, Nalini NR. Reliability and validity of the NIMHANS Index of Specific Learning Disabilities. Indian J. Mental Health. 2015;2:175–81.

15. Malhotra S, Rajender G, Sharma V, Singh TB. Efficacy of cognitive retraining techniques in children with learning disability. Delhi Psychiatry J. 2009;12:100–6.

16. Lagae L. Learning disabilities: definition, epidemiology, diagnosis and intervention strategies. Pediatr Clin North Am. 2008;55:1259–68.

17. Shaywitx SE. Dyslexia. N Engl J Med. 1998;338: 307–12.

18. Karande S, Kulkarni M. Specific learning disability: the invisible handicap. Indian Pediatr. 2005; 42:315–9.

19. Karande S, Gogtay NJ. Specific learning disability and the right to education 2009 act: Call for action. J Postgrad Med. 2010;56:171–2.

20. Singal N. Inclusive education in India: International concept, national interpretation. Int J Disabil Dev Ed. 2006;53:351–69.

21. McDonnell L, LcLaughlin M, Morison P. Educating one and all: students with disabilities and standards-based reform. National Academy Press; Washington DC: 1997. p. 204.

22. Sandhu P. Legislation and the current provisions for specific learning disability in India-Some observations. Journal of Disability Studies. 2016; 1:85–8.

23. National Joint Committee on Learning Disabilities. Providing appropriate education for students with learning disabilities in regular education classrooms. J Learn Disabil. 1993;26: 330–2.

24. Hammill DD. On defining learning disabilities: an emerging consensus. J Learn Disabil. 1990; 23:74–84.

25. Unni JC. Specific learning disability and the amended "persons with disability act". Indian Pediatr. 2012;49: 445–7.

26. Kainth GS. A mission approach to Sarva Shiksha Abhiyan. Econ Polit Wkly. 2006;41:3288–91.

27. Mehrotra S. The cost and financing of the right to education in India: Can we fill the financing gap? Int J Educ Dev. 2012;32:65–71.

28. Operational Guidelines on Rashtriya Bal Swasthya Karyakram (RSBK). Ministry of Health and Family Welfare, Government of India. Available from: http://www.pbnrhm.org/docs/rbskguidelines. pdf. Accessed January 13, 2017.

29. Kamala R. Specific learning disabilities in India: Rights, issues and challenges. Indian J Appl Res. 2014; 4(5). Available from: https://www. worldwide journals.comindian-journal-of-applied-research-(IJAR)/file.php?val=May_2014_1398967503_e9548_190.pdf. Accessed January 13, 2017.

End-of-Life Care: Consensus Statement by Indian Academy of Pediatrics

Sudhir Mishra, Kanya Mukhopadhyay, Satish Tiwari, Rajendra Bangal, Balraj S Yadav, Anupam Sachdeva, Vishesh Kumar

Resuscitation is a common procedure performed in hospitals for all patients suffering from cardiac or respiratory arrest. Outcome of resuscitation is better in the pediatric age group than in adults. However, even in children, there are situations where hope for an intact survival is poor. Often, short term recovery and subsequent intensive care inflicts physical discomfort for patients and family alike. Family members also suffer mental and financial agony. This has been appreciated by healthcare providers across the world, and efforts have been made to provide meaningful care and graceful end to life, without painful life pending death for patients and feeling of guilt among the parents and family members.

DEFINITIONS

Euthanasia: This word is derived from Greek Eu and thanatos meaning good death. In medical parlance, it refers to acceleration of death by active intervention to alleviate suffering of a person who is in irretrievable situation. It has been amply clarified that euthanasia is essentially voluntary and any intervention against the will is equivalent to murder.[1] Euthanasia is 'active' when a deliberate intervention is undertaken with the express intention of ending life to relieve intractable suffering, and 'passive' when it involves withholding life support system for continuance of life.[2]

End-of-Life care: This refers to care of a person who has received a life-limiting diagnosis. It encompasses all aspects of care till the final outcome and care of mortal remains.[3]

Resuscitation: It is the process of restoring the cardiac or pulmonary function back to normal, fully or partially, after a cardiac or respiratory arrest.

Do-Not-Resuscitate (DNR) order: This is a treatment decision taken prior to event of cardiac or respiratory arrest, with the consent of patient, or where that is not possible, proxy consent of next of kin, where care providers will not provide requisite cardio-respiratory resuscitation. This does not preclude, or stop to any degree, normal care and treatment being given to the patient.[4]

THE LEGAL FRAMEWORK

The Constitution of India, Article 21, provides 'Protection of Life' and 'Personal Liberty'. It states that "no person shall be deprived of his life or personal liberty except according to procedure established by law." However, there have been several expansions of article 21 and in its expanded form it assures the right to live with human dignity. Death is universal but dying in a peaceful and dignified manner would be welcome by every individual.

Some persons interpreted the right to life as including right "not to live" or right to death (P. Rathinam *vs* Union of India, JT 1994(3) SC 392). However in this judgment, while accepting right-to-die, euthanasia was not considered viable and was not permitted. Several other judgments, (Gian Kaur vs State of Punjab, JT 1996 (3) SC 339; C.A. Thomas Master vs Union of India, Kerala HC, 2000 Cri LJ 3729) have held that right-to-life as enshrined in constitution article 21 does not confer right-to-death. In a recent judgment on a Public Interest Litigation (PIL), Rajasthan High court two judge bench upheld the PIL and held the Jain religious practice of "Santhara or Sallekhana — a practice of deliberate starvation to death" as unconstitutional, and to treat it as suicide punishable under section 309.[5]

WHY DO WE NEED END-OF-LIFE (EOL) DECISIONS?

There are many situations when patients with irreversible or end-stage diseases (where there is very little chance of recovery) remain, on assisted ventilation for days, weeks or months. This is associated with several conflicts:

1. This results in prolongation of 'vegetative life' that may be a source of misery for everyone, especially for the patient and the family.
2. There is a lowering of 'dignity of death' due to futile invasive procedures and unnecessary treatment.
3. There may not be any chance of improvement or survival leading to wastage of resources.
4. It may be a significant burden for the family or society–physically, financially and psychologically.

5. There may be situation where limited resources may be denied to a more 'deserving salvagable individual' because they are 'in use' for a vegetative individual.
6. In some specific situations, there may be need for withdrawing assisted respiratory support; e.g. in cases of brain-stem death that is certified by a board of medical experts.

In spite of the above situations—which happen quite frequently, especially in intensive care unit (ICU) set-up, cancer patients and in some irreversible chronic conditions – there are no legal guidelines in our country regarding withdrawal of care or EOL decisions. There is also no guideline regarding not to initiate resuscitation in conditions where life may not be meaningful after resuscitation.

PROCESS OF FORMING GUIDELINES

A National consultative meeting was organized at RML Hospital, New Delhi on 30th May 2014, where the participants included experts from various relevant fields like academicians from medical fraternity, practicing doctors, intensivists (adult, pediatric and neonatal), lawyers, persons with both legal and medical qualifications, administrators and members from regulatory bodies. Stakeholders like Government of India, Medical Council of India, social organizations, and legal and medical fraternity were represented. Representation from various medical disciplines included Pediatrics, Anesthesia, Oncology, Cardiology and Intensive care.

The consultative meet had four sessions: First session was on legal issues in relation to end-of-life care, protection of patient rights and rights of medical professional, laws related to right to life and deaths. Presentation included cases dealt by Hon'ble Supreme court including judgments. Second session focused on the issues related to care towards the end-of-life, especially in terminally ill patients.

Third session reviewed currently available guidelines and literature on the subject. In last session, issues on various aspects of the topic were discussed. Points agreed upon were reiterated and those lacking consensus were further discussed and a broad consensus was achieved. Summary guidelines were prepared and presented. A writing committee was designated. Draft of the write-up was prepared by two members of the writing committee, and was circulated among all members. Suggestions were incorporated in the final write-up.

END-OF-LIFE CARE

End-of-Life Care is defined by National Council for Palliative Care UK[6] as "Helps all those with advanced, progressive, incurable illness to live as well as possible, until they die. It enables the supportive and palliative care needs of both patient and family to be identified and met throughout the last phase of life and into bereavement. It includes management of pain and other symptoms and provision of psychological, social, spiritual and practical support."

This essentially means not taking up intensive care in the event of a cardiac or respiratory arrest but does not deny continued care, nutrition by oral or oro-gastric or naso-gastric route, pain relief, physiotherapy and other comfort care. It does not mean abandoning a patient after an EOL Care decision is taken.

Ethical Principles

While taking decisions for EOL in any critically sick patient, four ethical principles must be followed:[7]

Autonomy means an individual's rights of freedom and liberty to make changes that affect his or her life. In the right to self-determination, the informed patient has a right to choose the manner of his treatment. In pediatric and neonatal patients either the parents or a legal guardian can take such decisions.

Beneficence is acting in what is (or judged to be) in patient's best interest. The physician is expected to act in the best interests; his responsibility extends beyond medical treatment to ensure compassionate care during the dying process. The physician's expanded goals include facilitating (neither hastening nor delaying) the dying process, avoiding or reducing the sufferings of the patient and his family, providing emotional support and protecting from financial loss. "The best interest calculus generally involves an open ended consideration of factors relating to the treatment decision, including the patient's current condition, degree of pain, loss of dignity, prognosis and the risks, side effects and benefits of each treatment".[8]

Non-malfeasance means to do no harm, to impose no unnecessary or unacceptable burden upon the patient. This is subject to varied interpretation, as the same act may be considered as harmful or beneficial depending on the circumstances.

Distributive justice means treating patients truthfully and fairly. Physicians need to take a responsible decision and to make good use of the infrastructure, finances and human resources. The physician may thus provide treatment and resources to one with a potentially curable condition over another for whom treatment may be futile.

In cases of resuscitation of newborn, the autonomy of newborn and to take decision in life threatening emergency situations are both exceptions of general rules of ethics.

Dilemma in EOL Decisions

While dealing with a situation that may warrant EOL care decision or discussion, considering above mentioned principles, dilemma arise in the mind of treating doctor. These may be summarized as below:

Legal Dilemma

A reasonable amount of certainty is required to take decisions regarding EOL because the probability of dying is not always clear. In many countries, there are set guidelines about when to initiate EOL discussion; however, we do not have definite guidelines agreed upon by professional bodies. There can be questions in relation to which patients can be ascribed as 'approaching the end of life'. GMC guidelines[9] suggest that if a person is likely to die in a period of one year, he/she may be considered as 'approaching the end of life'.

Ethical Dilemma

Ethical dilemma arises when the opinions are at variance; e.g. one child or parent of the diseased may have difference of opinion from the other. It may so happen that the diseased person is a minor, but is old enough to understand and his/her opinion is different from parent(s). In another situation, opinion of the parent(s) may be detrimental to the baby.

Most of this dilemma can be solved with clear thought process, involvement of senior most physicians in the team, and good communication with the next of kin. However, in Indian social setup, where everyone wants to do 'the best' till the end for social reasons, it may still be difficult to achieve consensus among family members. In such situation, DNR or EOL should not be activated till consensus is achieved.

DO NOT RESUSCITATE

Do Not Resuscitate (DNR) is a clear concept in most developed countries.[10] It does not involve withdrawing life support system where a patient is already on ventilator or inotropes. It also does not involve discontinuing routine care like oxygen, nutrition, fluids (oral intravenous). DNR is like any other treatment decision, and must be adequately documented and communicated to all team members for effective implementation. In India, so far we do not have a clear legal guideline and accepted method of documentation of DNR.[11]

There are two more terms used in this relation; 'withhold LST (Life-sustaining Treatment Measures)', and 'withdraw LST'.

Witholding LST: LST, especially ventilation, central line placement and renal replacement therapy, require consent. Except in the event where none from family is available, and clinical condition of the patient is life-threatening, these should not be initiated without consent. While obtaining informed consent, it is required to inform the patients or attendants about the possible outcome, need or futility of the intervention, what can be expected as a result of such intervention and the cost likely to be incurred (where applicable – likely to be paid by the family) in the process. The same should be documented. Only after such informed consent, if the patient or relatives insist on continued intervention, these should be undertaken. Care should be exercised that refusal of such consent should not result in dilution of basic care to the patient and judgmental statements are not made by the staff working in the unit, which can result in feeling of guilt.

Withdrawing LST: Withdrawing life sustaining treatment is more difficult. It should always be done with clear and repeated discussion till parent(s) or next of kin understand the consequences and concur with the actions being taken and have given written consent for the same. Discussion should involve senior member of the medical team, preferably unit in-charge or the treating doctor. The withdrawal of support should never be done to facilitate use of equipment for another patient who may be potentially salvagable. This should never be used as an argument for counseling for withdrawal of support. The principles and components of 'good death' have been elaborated in Box 26.1. These have been modified from the guidelines of Indian Society of Critical Care Medicine and Indian Association of Palliative Care.[14,15]

Box 26.1: **Principles of good death**

- To understand the possible time of death
- To be in control of the situation at the time of death
- To die with dignity and privacy to the extent desired
- To be able to get pain relief, control over other symptoms and care including hospice care where available
- To be able to choose the place of death
- To have access to desired information and expertise
- To have access to support required including spiritual and emotional support
- To be able to decide about the presence of near and dear ones and who share the end
- To be able to issue advanced directive ensuring that one's wishes are respected*
- To avoid pointless prolongation of life
- Such provisions do not exist in India. At present, there is an appeal admitted to the Supreme Court on the issue of allowing advance directive.

*Modified from Reference number 14 and 15

Clinical Aspects of DNR

Who are the candidates for DNR?

It can be said that situations where resuscitation is not likely to lead to prolonged and useful survival, are the candidates for DNR (Box 26.2).

Box 26.2: Who are the candidates for DNR

- Where life sustaining treatment is likely to be ineffective or futile.
- Where patient has prolonged unconsciousness which is unlikely to recover.
- Where patient has a terminal condition for which there is no definitive therapy.
- Where patient has a chronic debilitating disorder where burden of resuscitation far outweighs the benefits.
- Where medical treatment appears futile. Futile medical treatment is generally defined as "where treatment is useless, ineffective or does not offer a reasonable chance of survival".[12]
- Such other factor that may be unique to the patient e.g., where patient has made an informed living will to refuse CPR.[13]

Who are not the candidates for DNR?

DNR should not be activated where:
- patient is unable to pay for advanced care
- the outcome is doubtful (may or may not improve situation)
- there is conflicting opinion among the family members
- responsible next of kin is not available for discussion
- written consent is not available

What is done and what is not done if DNR is activated[16] is listed in Box 26.3.

DNR Issues in Neonates

Neonates are in a special situation with respect to resuscitation and DNR orders. A clinician may face this situation right at the time of birth or subsequently during treatment. At the time of birth, condition of the baby may be anticipated or may not be anticipated and arise suddenly. Like in all other situations, social, emotional and cultural environment would affect DNR decisions.

Box 26.3: What is done and what is not done if DNR is activated[14]

Even with DNR orders, a health worker will provide basic support in the form of:
- Clear airway
- Provide Oxygen
- Position for comfort
- Splint
- Control bleeding
- Provide pain medication
- Provide emotional support
- Contact hospice or hospital (as hospice facility is hardly available in India)
- With DNR orders, a health care worker is not required to
- Perform chest compressions
- Insert advanced airway
- Administer Cardiac resuscitation drugs
- Provide ventilator assistance including noninvasive ventilation
- Defibrillate

Decisions at the Time of Birth

At the time of birth, two broad situations may demand a decision. First is a baby with congenital anomaly or anomalies that are incompatible or may be compatible with life, but the expected quality of life may be poor or a big drain on resources of family/society. Second situation is where the birth weight and gestational age is such that survival, especially intact survival, may be almost impossible. Where congenital anomalies are known before birth and the time permits, DNR decisions should be discussed with parent(s) and other family members, sometimes elders from society including religious leaders or family physician. If family desires that the baby should be resuscitated and subsequently reassessed for the status with respect to survival and treatment options, this must be honored. Where family agrees with DNR decision, it may be implemented if the baby is found to have expected situation/problem. The decision of DNR may be reversed if doctor finds baby's condition to be different from what was antenatally expected. This should also be explained to parent(s) during discussion on DNR.

Where there had been no opportunity for discussion with parents, baby should be resuscitated fully except in gross anomalies that are incompatible with life, e.g. anencephaly[17] or prematurity that is not compatible with life. Decision on prematurity depends on period of viability. With improving survival of babies with lower gestational age[18,19] definition of period of viability has become more difficult. This decision should be based on local survival data and possibility of intact survival in a given setup. However, as a general norm, it can be said that 24 weeks gestation babies are regularly surviving[18] in many centers in our country where tertiary care facilities are available and therefore any baby above this gestation age must be resuscitated in such centers. In centers where tertiary care facilities are not available, babies below 28 weeks gestation are not likely to survive. In such a situation, subsequent management options should be discussed with parents and a decision to resuscitate may be taken based on feasibility of transfer to a tertiary care neonatal unit. It would be prudent to attempt 'in utero' transfer in such situations.

Decision in Neonatal Units

DNR issues faced in neonatal units are qualitatively same as faced in other intensive care units. However, frequency of congenital anomalies in neonatal units is high and is a prominent reason for a DNR order. In a study from Oman,[20] lesions that will not allow meaningful survival (18 of 39) and lesions incompatible with life (15 of 39) were the reasons for a DNR order. Gestational age related reason (below 24 weeks gestation) was present in only 3 of 39 babies where DNR orders were given. This study also highlighted that parents were more comfortable accepting non-initiation of ventilator support (14 of 20 cases where it was proposed) than withdrawal of ventilator support (2 of 19 cases). In this study, 36% of deaths were preceded by a DNR order. This is far less than some of the western studies[21] where the frequency was as high as 68%.

In India, there are hardly any studies on this subject. However, wherever facilities for neonatal care are sparse, the requirement will be more and criteria for DNR order should be customized. While customizing and documenting these criteria, one should be cautious that lack of resources or inability to pay is not a criterion for DNR decisions in neonatal units, just as they are not in other intensive care units. Whereas tertiary neonatal intensive care units can use a gestational age criteria of 24 weeks, others like special care neonatal units being setup in district hospitals should use a gestational age cut-off of 28 weeks. Lesions incompatible with life or compatible with poor quality life are the criteria for all neonatal units to follow. It is strongly recommended that each unit should document its own criteria for DNR decisions.

Criteria for Brain Death in Children and Neonates

The diagnosis of brain death is often difficult but essential for counseling, more so while initiating discussion on withdrawal of support. The diagnosis of brain death is based on clinical examination and apnea test conducted twice at an interval of 24 hours for neonates and 12 hours for children beyond 1 month to 18 years of age. Wherever possible, $PaCO_2$ of 20 mm/Hg above the baseline should be documented. There is no role of ancillary tests like electroencephalography (EEG) or radionuclide scan for assessing cerebral blood flow for the diagnosis of brain death–either in neonates or children.[21–23]

Counseling

Preparation

Preparation for counseling involves unanimity in the health care team on appropriateness of DNR decision in the given circumstances.[24] Decision to invoke DNR order should first be discussed in the treating team including nurses.[24] Once agreed upon within health care team, further steps to initiate a discussion with the parents/patient or 'next of kin' should be undertaken.

Team needs to decide on competence of the patient to take a decision, in which case discussion should involve patient himself, unless he/she expresses his/her unwillingness to discuss matter related to death.[24,25] Where patient is not found competent, members of the family need to be taken into confidence and a next of kin should be identified. In Indian context, often the decision makers are not parents. They may be grandparents, local elders from community or other relatives. These persons must be included in the discussion process. In Indian social scenario, family may desire to include even a family physician or a doctor not working in health care facility where patient is currently being treated.[26] This should be permitted as it is more likely to be helpful

rather than a hindrance in taking appropriate decision. Pending such discussion, a DNR order should not be invoked and resuscitation carried out. However, finally only parents should be requested to sign on the papers.

Health care team leader (usually unit in charge or treating doctor) should be aware of all details about patient illness. The records related to patient's illness, including the progress notes, must be reviewed. It may be helpful to keep complete records of the patient, so that the progress (or lack of it) can be discussed based on clinical notes and investigation rather than being seen as the personal opinion of the treating physician.

It is a good social practice to formally introduce the members of health care team. This helps all concerned in understanding each other's perspective and help in breaking ice initially. Discussion should be initiated with the information on patient's illness (past and present), treatment being offered, future plan and benefits or futility of treatment and prognosis. Presence of a living will (though not really prevalent in Indian scenario) should be enquired about. The family members may be asked "what the patient would have done in such a scenario if he/she would have been competent. That may provide a clue to the attitude of the patient (and may be the person replying) towards life or death. This may help the 'next of kin' in decision-making.

Responsibility

It is difficult and stressful to undertake a conversation about death even for experienced clinicians.[25,27] Therefore, usually the senior most doctor (i.e. consultant in charge of the case) should take the responsibility for initiating and completing this discussion.[28,29] However, there may be situations where another member of the health care team has developed an excellent rapport with the patient. This may be junior doctor in the team or even a nurse. In such cases, responsibility may be given to that member and (s)he/she should be supported by other members.

Family and Social Issues Specific for Indian Situation

It is imperative for the counseling team to try and understand the social dynamics and identify the decision maker. In case of an old patient, an assessment of conflict of interest among family members should be explored. It is a common scenario to find that one person agrees with the decision of DNR and other(s) do not. In such situation, it is avoidable to press for the agreement, and it is prudent to call for another session. In Indian scenario and that of other developing countries, where hierarchy of community still exists, it may not be possible to give consent out of free will despite constitutional freedom to do so.[26] Financial issues may be involved, where the person responsible for the payment wants such a decision whereas others resist.[30] One such situation is where a newborn is delivered and is being taken care of at maternal grand-parents' cost. In these situations, it is not unusual to find a family member in agreement with the prognosis and futility of intensive treatment but out of social pressures and culture of 'doing best possible till the last' do not want to discontinue treatment.[27] Such situations should be handled with gradual re-enforcement of clinician's viewpoint and discussion on financial involvement in such situation may be of help, especially where the cost of hospitalization is to be borne out-of-pocket of an individual.

Another area of potential conflict can be where parents (or relatives where parents are not available) ask for abandoning treatment. Female gender of the child may confound this situation. In many parts of our country, first baby is delivered at maternal grandparents' place and at their cost. Here the father and relatives from his side may continue to press for continued treatment whereas maternal side that is bearing the cost of treatment may be more amenable to suggestions on DNR. Where doctors do not agree to DNR decisions, it should never be accepted based on suggestions of parents or relatives. In view of hierarchy of decision-making, which give first right to parents, no decision should be taken against the wishes of the father/mother of the baby.

Hierarchy for Decision Making[31–35]

There is no description of hierarchy for decision making; in Indian situation, only guidelines available on hierarchy are for inheritance of property. Though not meant for clinical decision-making, they do provide some guidance for similar situation[34] (Box 26.4). However, the hierarchy for consent in various situations (e.g. emergency treatment, clinical research) are clearly defined in some other countries and are logically acceptable for decision-making with respect to DNR decisions as well.

Process of Consent and Documentation

The process of taking consent involves preparation for discussion. All options in relation to possible alternative treatment strategies should have been discussed within the medical team and agreed upon.[24,25,28] It is useful to have privacy and uninterrupted time for discussion. Sensitivity and empathy are of paramount importance to achieve desired goal. Initiation of discussion should be by elaborating patient's current condition, which should be followed by a discussion on

---

Box 26.4: Hierarchy for decision-making*

1. Patient him(her)self so long he/she is competent.
2. Advanced health directive (will seldom be available in actual practice in India).
3. Enduring Guardian (In India, there is no law that recognizes this kind of arrangement. Therefore, this becomes invalid in Indian scenario)
4. Guardian
5. Spouse
6. Child
7. Parent
8. Sibling (who maintain close contact)
9. Unpaid provider of care
10. Anyone who maintains close contact

Same hierarchy could be valid for consent in situation of DNR

caregiver preference. Information provided should be free of jargon, in simple terms, and in language that relatives can understand. Uncertainties should be explained and also the fact that in the event of a cardio-respiratory arrest, there will not be enough time for discussion. Any distressing signal, verbal or in body language should be addressed. Realistic hope should be provided that is honest but not blunt. Realistic goals of care that is to be continued should be explained. Questions should be encouraged to clarify the situation. This also helps in assessing the mindset of the relatives.

Finally, after the discussion is over, a summary of the discussion should be documented (Box 26.5). If DNR is agreed upon, the order should be placed in the case records and the healthcare team should be informed of the same.

Review of DNR Orders

Every DNR order, even where it seems final, should be reviewed at predefined interval and continuation of DNR orders should be documented in the case records at least once in week.[25] However, patients' relatives may

---

Box 26.5: A checklist for the summary of discussion on DNR

- Name of the patient:
- Regd. No:
- Diagnosis:
- Prognosis:
- Names of persons involved in discussion:
- Likely outcome of CPR: Unsuccessful
- Preference of the patient: Against CPR/ Undecided / Not Known
- Views of the "person responsible": Against CPR/ Undecided / Not Known/ Wants CPR
- Reasons for decision of DNR / Not advising DNR:
- Goals of treatment: Palliation/ Symptom relief/ Recovery from present episode of illness
- Consultant Responsible for DNR order: Dr............
- Review Date: dd/mm/yyyy
- Remarks (if any)

*Same hierarchy could be valid for consent in situation of DNR

---

request review of the DNR orders. In such case, fresh documentation of discussion and decision taken should be documented. Another reason for revoking the DNR orders could be an unexpected improvement in patients' condition. Where a DNR order is revoked, the reasons for the same should be documented and informed to the relatives, preferably the same people who were present at initial discussion. It is of importance to note that if a patient is being transferred to another facility for care of the patient, DNR orders remains valid. However, it would be a good practice to re-communicate the same to the relatives.

EUTHANASIA

A detailed report was submitted to law ministry in 2012 regarding feasibility of making legislation on euthanasia, taking into the account of earlier 196th report of Law commission of India.[2] Supreme Court of India laid down the law on the subject of passive euthanasia in relation to incompetent patients who are in persistent vegetative state or in irreversible coma or of unsound mind. For safeguard purpose and to avoid misuse of law, permission from High court will be required before executing passive euthanasia. This law will continue till parliament makes a law on this subject that is now long pending. The commission supported passive euthanasia that is withdrawal of life support measures to dying patients which is different from euthanasia and assisted suicide. The bill entitled "The Medical Treatment of Terminally ill Patients (Protection of Patients and Medical Practitioners) Bill 2006" outlines safeguards to be maintained by attending doctors while taking such a decision.

Permission shall be sought from the jurisdictional District Court/High Court (wherever the latter has original jurisdiction) where treatment is being given to the patient, where the patient is in a persistently vegetative state and chances of revival seem remote.

However, according to report of Law commission of India, 2012, Supreme Court has laid the guidelines to seek high court's opinion as mandatory whenever any decision of withdrawal of life support is to be undertaken. The high court then should seek the opinion of three medical experts' committee and also put on notice the close relations and in their absence, the next friend of the patient and the state.

There is also a need to formulate policies on comfort care before death, palliative care and pain relief in terminally ill patients and nutrition policy of these patients.

Note: The guidelines may not be long lasting and will change with time. Significant legal issues may arise in the future and hence the guidelines may need revision. The guidelines are not mandatory or binding and the treating team may utilize the prevalent laws to make a decision.

REFERENCES

1. Viela LP, Caramelli P. Knowledge of definition of euthanasia. Study with doctors and caregivers of Alzheimer disease patients. Rev Assoc Med Bras 2009;55:263–7.

2. Passive Euthanasia-A relook: Law Commission of India 2012. Available from: http://lawcommissionofindia.nic.in/reports/report241.pdf. Accessed May 15, 2017.

3. Irish Hospice Foundation Definitions. Available from: http://hospicefoundation.ie/about-hospice-care/definitions. Accessed May 15, 2017.

4. Lofmark R. Do-not-resuscitate orders: Ethical aspects on decision making and communication among physicians, nurses, patients and relatives. Available from: http://lup. lub.lu.se/search/ws/files/5599819/1693395.pdf. Accessed May 15, 2017.

5. Nikhil Soni vs Union of India. Civil WP No. 7414/2006 Rajasthan High Court. Available from: https://indianka noon.org/doc/173301527/. Accessed May 15, 2017.

6. Commissioning End of Life Care- National Council for Palliative Care. Initial actions for new commissioners. Available from: http://www.ncpc.org.uk/sites/default/files/AandE.pdf. Accessed May 15, 2017.

7. Mohanty BK. Ethics in palliative care. Indian J Palliat Care 2009; 15:89–92.

8. Passive Euthanasia – A Relook- Report no 241. Available from: http://lawcommissionofindia.nic.in/reports/report 241.pdf. Accessed May 15, 2017.

9. Treatment and Care towards End of Life. Good Practice in decision making. GMC Guidelines 2010. Available from: http://www.gmc-uk.org/static/documents/content/Treatment_and_care_towards_the_end_of_life_-_English_1015.pdf . Accessed May 15, 2017.

10. Chen J, Flabouris A, Bellomo R. The medical emergency team system and not-for-resuscitation orders: results from the MERIT study. Resuscitation 2008;79:391–7

11. Salins NS, Pai SG, Vidyasagar M, Sobhana M. Ethics and medico-legal aspects of "Not for Resuscitation". Ind J Palliat Care 2010;16:66–9.

12. Mason JK, Laurie GT. Mason and McCall Smith's Law and Medical Ethics. 8th ed. Oxford: Oxford University Press, 2011;476.

13. Mcquoid-Mason DJ. Emergency Medical Treatment and 'Do Not Resuscitate' orders: When can they be used? South African Med J 2013; 103:1–7.

14. Myatra SN, Salins N, Iyer S. End of Life Care Policy: An integrated Care Plan for Dying. Indian J Crit Care Med 2014;18:615–635.

15. Macaden SC, Salins N, Muckaden M, Kulkarni P, Joad A, Nirabhawane V, et al. End of life care policy for the dying: Consensus position statement of Indian Association of Palliative Care. Ind J Palliat Care 2014;20:171–81.

16. Emergency Care Do Not Resuscitate order. State of Wisconsin. F-44763 (Rev 08/2015). Available from: https://www.dhs.wisconsin.gov/forms/f4/f44763.pdf. Accessed May 15, 2017.

17. Kattwinkel J, Perlman JM, Aziz K, Colby C, Fairchild K, Gallagher J, et al. Part 15: Neonatal Resuscitation: 2010 American Heart Association Guidelines for Cardio-pulmonary Resuscitation and Emergency Cardiovascular Care. Circulation 2010;122:S909–19.

18. Tyson JE, Parikh NA, Langer J, Green C, Higgins RD. Intensive care for extreme prematurity-moving beyond gestational age. N Engl J Med 2008;358:1672–81.

19. Kong XY, Xu FD, Wu R. Neonatal mortality and morbidity among infants between 24 to 31 complete weeks: A multicenter survey in China from 2013 to 2014. BMC Pediatr 2016;16:174–81.

20. da Costa DE, Ghazal H, Al Khusaiby S. Do not resuscitate orders and ethical decisions in a neonatal intensive care unit in a Muslim community. Arch Dis Child Fetal Neonatal Ed 2002;86:F115–9.

21. Mathur M, Ashwal S. Pediatric brain death determination. Semin Neurol 2015;35:116–24.

22. Sekar KC. Brain death in the newborns. J Perinatol 2007;27:59–62.

23. Tejedor Torres JC, Garcia AL. Making ethical decisions of limiting vital support to critical newborns. Ann Esp Pediatr 1997;46:53–9.

24. Clayton JM, Hancock KM, Butow PN, Tattersall MHN, Currow DC. Clinical practice guidelines for communicating prognosis and end-of-life issues with adults in the advanced stages of a life-limiting illness, and their caregivers. Med J Australia 2007;186(Suppl):S77-S108.

25. Treatment and Care Towards the End of Life: Good Practice in Decision Making. General Medical Council 2010. Available from: http://www.gmc-uk.org/End_of_life.pdf_32486688.pdf. Accessed May 15, 2017.

26. Kumar NK. Informed consent: Past and present. Perspect Clin Res 2013;4:21–25

27. Mani RK, Amin P, Chawla R. Guidelines for end-of-life and palliative care in Indian intensive care units: ISCCM consensus ethical position statement. Indian J Crit Care Med 2012;16:166–81.

28. Emanuel EJ, Fairclough DL,Wolfe P, Emanuel LL. Talking with terminally ill patients and their caregivers about death, dying, and bereavement: is it stressful? Is it helpful? Arch Intern Med 2004; 164:1999–2004.

29. Schachter L. Talking with terminally ill patients and their caregivers about death, dying, and bereavement: Is it stressful? Is it helpful? Arch Intern Med 2005;165:1437.

30. Jindal SK. End of life care: A curricular and practice need. J Postgrad Med Edu Res. 2012;46: 117–21.

31. Consent: Patients and Doctors Making Decisions Together. Available from: http://www.gmc-uk.org/static/documents/content/Consent_-_English_0414.pdf. Accessed May 15, 2017.

32. Guidelines for Withdrawal of Treatment of Irreversibly Critically ill Patients on Assisted Respiratory Support. Available from: http://pgimer.edu.in/PGIMER_PORTAL/AbstractFilePath?FileType=E&PathKey=MENUFILES_PATH&FileName=Guidelines04Mar2011152342.pdf. Accessed May 15, 2017.

33. Consent to Treatment Policy for the Western Australian Health System 2011. Available from: http://www.health. wa.gov.au/circularsnew/attachments/1135.pdf. Accessed May 15, 2017.

34. Jiloha RC. Mental Capacity/Testamentary Capacity. Indian Journal of Psychiatry Clinical Practice Guidelines 2009. Available from: http://www.indianjpsychiatry.org/cpg/cpg2009/article9.pdf. Accessed May 15, 2017.

35. Mental Capacity Act: Code of Practice. Available from: http://www3.imperial.ac.uk/pls/portallive/docs/1/51771696.PDF. Accessed May 15, 2017.

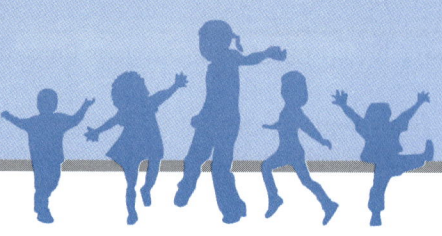

Consensus Guidelines on Management of Childhood Convulsive Status Epilepticus

Devendra Mishra, Suvasini Sharma, Naveen Sankhyan, Ramesh Konanki, Mahesh Kamate,
Sujata Kanhere, Satinder Aneja

Status epilepticus (SE) is a life-threatening emergency that requires prompt recognition and management.[1] Immediate treatment of status epilepticus is crucial to prevent adverse neurologic and systemic consequences.[2] Multiple protocols for management of SE in children are available both internationally[3–5] and from India.[6–8] It has previously been demonstrated that use of a pre-determined protocol for management of SE leads to favorable outcomes.[9] A single protocol for management of SE in children, suitable for use in the Indian setting, taking in consideration the common etiologies of SE and the drugs available, is thus the need of the hour.

PROCESS

A 'Multi-disciplinary Consensus Development Work-shop on Management of Status Epilepticus in Children in India' was organized by the Association of Child Neurology on 17th November, 2013 in New Delhi. The invited experts included General pediatricians, Pediatric neurologists, Neurologists, Epileptologists, and Pediatric intensive care specialists from all over India with experience in the relevant field. This group was designated as the 'Multi-disciplinary Group on Management of Status Epilepticus

in Children in India'. In addition, consultants and residents in Pediatrics were invited as observers. Experts had previously been divided into focus groups, and had interacted on telephone and e-mail regarding their group recommendations. During the meeting, each group presented its recommendations, which were deliberated upon by the house and a consensus reached on various issues. At the end of the meeting, it was decided to bring out guidelines on evaluation and management of Status epilepticus in children in India, and a Writing group designated for the purpose. Due to the lack of country-specific epidemiologic information and varying levels of care available at various centers, it was decided not to categorize the recommendations by either 'level of evidence' or 'strength of recommendation'.[10] The draft document was circulated by e-mail among all experts and suggestions received incorporated; the final document is presented here. It does not cover the management of neonatal SE and Super-refractory SE.

GUIDETLINES

A. Definition and Epidemiology

The most widely used definition for SE is "a seizure lasting more than 30 minutes or recurrent seizures for more than 30 minutes during which the patient does not regain consciousness".[11,12] More recently, an operational definition has also been suggested for adults and children older than 5 years[13] (Box 27.1). If we consider the duration for which most new-onset seizures in children last, once a seizure lasts for more than five to ten minutes, it is unlikely to stop spontaneously within the next few minutes, and intervention is indicated.[14] The use of the operational definition allows early treatment (starting at 5–10 min).[15] However, in view of most previous studies on SE having been done using the 30-minute definition, the group suggests that for research purposes, both the definitions be considered and data provided with respect to both time durations.

SE in children is commonly due to cryptogenic or remote symptomatic causes in older children, and febrile or acute symptomatic cause in younger children.[9,16] Majority of childhood convulsive SE in a UK study (56%) occurred in previously neurologically healthy children, a quarter of SE were prolonged febrile seizures, and 17% were acute symptomatic.[17] Epidemiological data on SE in India is limited to a few single-center studies,[18–20] with only one providing exclusive pediatric data.[18] The high proportion of acute symptomatic etiology, delayed presentation and poor outcome are the commonly reported findings. In an Indian pediatric intensive care unit (PICU) study over seven years, 53% had SE as their first seizure and only 60% had received any treatment prior to coming to the PICU.[18] A recent multi-centric study on SE in children across nine centers in India also reported similar findings: 82% acute symptomatic, <3% pre-hospital treatment, <20% deficit-free survival, and no uniform management protocol [unpublished data].

B. Pre-hospital Management

Treatment of SE needs to be initiated as early as possible since once seizures persist for 5 to 10 minutes, they are unlikely to stop on their own in the subsequent few minutes.[21] Moreover, the longer an episode of SE continues, the more refractory to treatment it becomes and the greater is the likelihood of complications.[22] Thus, the need for early treatment, preferably pre-hospital, is clear.

Pre-hospital management includes both first-aid during seizures, and pharmacotherapy. The initial care of a child with convulsions/coma is adequately described in Facility-based Integrated Management of Neonatal and Childhood Illnesses (F-IMNCI) guidelines of the Government of India[23] and will not be elucidated here further. Decision about pharmacotherapy must consider the drug and also the route of drug delivery (Box 27.2).

Benzodiazepines are the drugs that are currently in use for pre-hospital therapy for SE and include diazepam, lorazepam and midazolam. Pre-hospital treatment with benzodiazepines has been shown to reduce seizure activity significantly compared with seizures that remain untreated until the patient reaches the emergency department.[24] The various routes employed include per-rectal (diazepam, lorazepam, paraldehyde), intranasal (midazolam), buccal (midazolam,

---

Box 27.1: Important definitions

Status epilepticus (SE): A seizure lasting more than 30 minutes or recurrent seizures for more than 30 minutes during which the patient does not regain consciousness .

*Operational definition: Generalized, convulsive status epilepticus in adults and older children (>5 years old) refers to >5 min of (i) continuous seizures or (ii) two or more discrete seizures between which there is incomplete recovery of consciousness.[13]

Refractory SE: Seizures persist despite the administration of two appropriate anticonvulsants at acceptable doses, with a minimum duration of status of 60 minutes (by history or on observation).

Super-refractory SE: SE that continues 24 hours or more after the onset of anesthesia, including those cases in which the status epilepticus recurs on the reduction or withdrawal of anesthesia.

*For the purpose of initiating management.

Box 27.2: Recommendations for out-of-hospital management of seizures

Guiding Principles
- • Acute treatment with anticonvulsants should be commenced after continuous seizures or serial seizures >5 min in an out-of-hospital setting, and efforts made to transfer the patient to the nearest health care facility.
- Prolonged seizures should be treated with either nasal or buccal midazolam or rectal diazepam when intravenous line is not available or in the community setting.
- Rectal diazepam is safe and effective as first-line treatment of prolonged seizures in community setting or when intravenous access is not available.
- Buccal or intranasal midazolam is as effective as rectal diazepam and can be considered as a preferable alternative in community setting.

At Home: Parents
- First aid
- Rectal diazepam OR buccal midazolam OR intranasal midazolam
- Inform doctor/shift to hospital if >5 min (or if more than 2 min longer than previous seizure duration)

At Home/Out of Hospital by Paramedics
- First aid - Airway, breathing, circulation, oxygen
- Supportive care
- Intranasal midazolam OR buccal midazolam OR rectal diazepam
- Shift to hospital

First-level Health Facility (Clinic/PHC/Nursing home)
- ABC, Oxygen
- Intravenous access feasible:
  - Intravenous lorazepam (if refrigeration and electric supply), diazepam, or midazolam
- Intravenous access not feasible:
  - Intramuscular injection can be given: IM midazolam
  - Intramuscular injection not feasible: Intranasal/buccal midazolam, rectal diazepam
- Shift to higher center, if required.

---

lorazepam) and intramuscular (midazolam). Rectal diazepam is an approved out-of-hospital treatment for acute repetitive seizures in children. Response rates have been demonstrated to be similar to intravenous diazepam.[25] Multiple randomized, double-blind, placebo controlled studies have demonstrated that rectal diazepam given by caregivers at home is an effective and safe treatment for acute recurrent seizures.[26–28] Rectal administration may be difficult with wheel-chair users and larger patients. It can be socially unacceptable, and there is increasing concern about risk of sexual abuse allegations.[29,30] Therefore, non-rectal routes are gradually gaining favor for use by relatives/health workers in out-of-hospital settings. Rectal diazepam is the recommended drug for

control of seizures in the F-IMNCI guidelines, in situations where intravenous access is not available.[23]

In the past decade, research evidence has shown that buccal midazolam is more than or equally effective to rectal diazepam for children presenting to hospital with acute seizures, and is not associated with an increased incidence of respiratory depression.[29,31,32] Therefore, it may be considered as an acceptable alternative to rectal diazepam.[30] Intranasal midazolam has been shown to be as effective as intravenous diazepam in the treatment of prolonged febrile convulsions,[4,33–35] and may also be an alternative. More recent data from the RAMPART study[36] of prehospital management of SE in children and adults has shown intramuscular midazolam to be as safe and effective as intravenous lorazepam for pre-hospital seizure cessation. This may therefore emerge to be the agent of choice for out-of-hospital management of seizure by trained personnel.

Rectal and intranasal lorazepam have also shown efficacy for termination of acute convulsive seizures in children.[4,37] However, non-availability of a commercial preparation in India precludes any firm guidance on non-parenteral use of lorazepam in India.

Parents of all children at risk of seizure recurrence should be counseled for appropriate home management for seizure.[38]

C. Supportive Care and Stabilization

Although convulsive seizures are the most obvious manifestation, SE is in fact a multi-system phenomenon, i.e. prolonged and ongoing SE affects multiple organ systems. Hence, apart from attempts to rapidly control seizures, important goals of therapy are neuro-protection, and prevention and treatment of systemic complications associated with intravenous AEDs, anesthetic drugs and prolonged unconsciousness.[39] The supportive care should be tailored to the health care setting, the clinical presentations of SE, degree of encephalopathy, and degree of impairment of vital functions.

Airway, Breathing and Circulation

Assessment and care of vital functions is essential at all stages of managing any child with SE.[40] Adequate care of airway, breathing and circulaion takes precedence over any pharmacological therapy.

Airway: It is essential to maintain a patent airway during all stages of management of SE.
- In all children with brief seizures and altered sensorium, clearing the oral secretions (mouth, followed by nose) and keeping the child in recovery position is advisable to prevent aspiration. Cervical spine should be immobilized if trauma is suspected.

- In more severe degrees of altered sensorium, use an oral airway to prevent tongue from falling back.
- Endotracheal intubation in children whose airway is not maintainable with above measures.
- The airway compromise may occur at any stage; either as complication of prolonged or ongoing seizure, or due to respiratory depressant effect of medications.

Breathing: Hypoxemia may result from respiratory depression/apnea, aspiration, airway obstruction, and neurogenic pulmonary edema.[41]
- All children with SE should have their breathing and SpO$_2$ monitored continuously.
- All children with ongoing seizures should be given supplemental oxygen to ameliorate cerebral hypoxia, as it has been seen that the degree of hypoxia is often underestimated.
- Depending on the duration of SE and degree of altered sensorium, maintain oxygen saturation by: supplemental oxygen, AMBU bag, non-invasive continuous positive airway pressure (CPAP), and invasive ventilation by endotracheal intubation. Mechanical ventilation may also become necessary when children are started on continuous infusions of anesthetic agents.

Circulation: Continuous monitoring of pulse, blood pressure and perfusion should be done in all SE patients.
- Ensure good venous access (preferably have at least two venous lines); draw necessary blood samples, and start fluids and antiepileptic drugs as necessary.
- Maintain blood pressure in the normal range with necessary measures including: intravenous fluids, fluid boluses, and inotropes. Invasive blood pressure monitoring should be considered, if feasible, in children with hypotension and poor peripheral perfusion either spontaneously or following infusion of continuous anesthetic agents.

- The choice of IV fluids depends on the metabolic and glycemic status. If there is hyperglycemia (especially initial phase of catecholamine excess) it is preferable to give either dextrose normal saline (DNS) or normal saline. However, in general, hypotonic fluid should be avoided for initial resuscitation.

Precipitating Factors and Ongoing Complications

The treating team should anticipate one or more of the below mentioned problems depending on the duration of SE, age, underlying etiology, and the associated systemic co-morbidities. The cerebral and systemic metabolism undergoes changes described as initial phase of 'compensation', and if SE is sufficiently prolonged, later phase of 'decompensation'.[42,43] During the initial phase, prolonged seizures result in increased cerebral blood flow and metabolism, excessive catecholaminergic activity and cardiovascular changes. These in turn result in hyperglycemia, hyperpyrexia, tachycardia, sweating, hypertension, incontinence, cardiac arrhythmias, and lactic acidosis.[43–46] If the SE is prolonged, the cerebral autoregulation progressively fails and cerebral perfusion becomes dependent on systemic blood pressure resulting in hypoxia, cerebral ischemia, hypoglycemia, and lactic acidosis.[42,43] Management of these conditions is detailed in Table 27.1. Both hypernatremia

TABLE 27.1: Treatment of ongoing complications and precipitating factors

Condition	Management	Comments
Hypoglycemia	If present or if blood glucose cannot be measured, dextrose boluses with 2 ml/kg of 25% dextrose, maintain blood glucose >110 mg/dL[12]	Both hypoglycemia and hyperglycemia are deleterious to brain during SE. Hyperglycemia with resultant lactic acidosis may cause neuronal injury[13]
Hyperglycemia	During the initial compensatory phase (due to excess catecholamines) may normalize with control of seizures. If it is persisting, insulin infusion is required to maintain the blood glucose in the range of 140–180 mg/dL[12]	
Hypocalcemia	IV calcium gluconate: 1 mL/kg of 10% calcium gluconate diluted in 1 mL/kg of 5% dextrose; infuse over 20–30 min under close cardiac monitoring	Hypocalcemia in the context of SE should be treated with IV calcium
Hypomagnesemia	Magnesium: IM or slow IV at dose of 50–100 mg/kg per dose	If present, may make hypocalcemia refractory to treatment
Fever	Intravenous/intramuascular or rectal anti-pyretics. Other method of reducing temperature quickly is infusion of refrigerator-cold saline (4°C) boluses (20 mL/kg), although its effect is short-lived (30 minutes)[15]	May be due to continuing seizures or infections (either CNS infection or nosocomial infections); Uncontrolled, it may exacerbate neuronal injury.[14]
Hypernatremia	• Rapid fluid resuscitation is the first step, fluid of choice is normal saline; gradual correction is calculated based on standard formulas. • Hyperglycemia is often associated with hypernatremia, and requires treatment by change of IV fluids to dextrose-free solutions and/or insulin infusions	

Contd...

TABLE 27.1: Treatment of ongoing complications and precipitating factors *(Contd...)*

Condition	Management	Comments
Hyponatremia	• Rapid correction should be avoided except in cases with rapidly developing hyponatremia causing seizures and acute encephalopathy. • In symptomatic acute hyponatremia, boluses of hypertonic saline (3%) should be given at 1 ml/kg over one hour, and repeated till serum sodium reaches at least 125 meq/L. • In chronic hyponatremia, the correction has to be more gradual (over at least 48 h, and at rate of not more than 10–12 meq/L per day).	Causes include mannitol infusions, capillary leak associated with sepsis, SIADH, excessive diuretics usage, and external losses (diarrhea and vomiting)
Hypotension and cardiac dysfunction	• Early inotrope support with dobutamine or milrinone should be started in cases with cardiac-associated hypotension.[12] • In patients with cardiomyopathy or arrhythmias, invasive monitoring of blood pressure and central venous pressure for accurate fluid balance and titration of inotropes.	
Metabolic acidosis	• pH <7.2: Treat with fluid boluses and maintain systemic perfusion, along with aggressive control of seizures; it is infrequently associated with life-threatening arrythmia.[23] • More severe acidosis (pH <6.8), Sodium bicarbonate.[12]	Due to excessive muscle contraction, hypovolemia, distributive shock (with barbiturates), and propylene glycol toxicity[12,21,22]
Cerebral edema	• No benefit of empirical mannitol or cortico-steroids in children with SE in the absence of features of raised intracranial pressure (ICP). • Clinical features of raised ICP (decorticate posturing, hypertension associated with bradycardia, irregular breathing): Mannitol 5ml/kg bolus dose, followed by 2–3 mL/kg 6 hourly; in children with hypotension, 3% saline can be used at rate of 1 mL/kg/hour till serum sodium reaches to 165 meq/L.	Recent experimental studies have suggested the possibility of vasogenic edema mediated by tumor necrosis factor-alpha (TNF-α) and endothelin-1 with resultant breakage of blood-brain barrier (BBB) during SE.[26]
Infection	Appropriate culture specimens should be obtained, and empiric antibiotics should be started in those with high suspicion of nosocomial infection.	Risk of infections is increased in children with SE especially those with prolonged SE.

(serum sodium >145 meq/L) and hyponatremia (<135 meq/L) are deleterious for the brain. The major risks associated with hypernatremia are intracranial hemorrhage (subdural, subarachnoid and intraparenchymal) and osmotic demyelination (pontine or extrapontine) with rapid correction.

Risk of infections is greatly increased in those with SE, especially when the duration is prolonged. Ventilator-associated pneumonia, urinary tract infection, pseudomembranous colitis, oral candidiasis, and septicemia are the common infections.[47,48] Commonest organisms are *P. aeruginosa, A. spp, K. pneumoniae*, and Entero bacteriaceae.[48] Hyperpyrexia, rhabdomyolysis, and raised intracranial pressure are the other common accompaniments.[43,49,50] Rarely, SE is associated with ictal bradycardia, stress cardiomyopathy, neurogenic pulmonary edema, rhabdomyolysis and related renal failure, or bone fractures.[46] Hypotension is common due to prolonged seizures, IV benzo-diazepines, or anesthetic agent infusions, and stress cardiomyopathy (Takotsubo cardiomyopathy)[47,50-53] Cardiac arrhythmias are also common (up to 58%), with higher mortality in these patients.[54,55] Management depends on the cause of hypotension, hypovolemic shock, distributive shock, cardiomyopathy, or cardiac arrhythmias (Table 27.1).

Although in most cases it is mild, early identification and aggressive treatment of rhabdomyolysis prevents complications like renal failure and compartment syndrome. The initial fluids for resuscitation may include normal saline or 5% dextrose in water (approximately 2–3 times the daily maintenance). Sodium bicarbonate may be added to IV fluids, especially if there is associated metabolic acidosis and/or hyperkalemia.[56,57]

D. Investigations

The clinical scenario, including the history and physical examination, is the most important factor guiding the specific evaluation that each child will require.[58] The investigations usually considered include blood chemistries, complete blood count, antiepileptic drug (AED) levels, toxicological studies, lumbar puncture, electroencephalography, and neuroimaging (Computed tomography [CT] scan and Magnetic resonance imaging [MRI]). The major part of evaluation can be performed after the child has been stabilized in an intensive care setting, and the seizures have been completely or partially controlled.[58,59]

The investigations done are primarily to (i) determine the cause of status epilepticus, (ii) to look for complications of status epilepticus per se, and (iii) to identify the side-effects of drugs. Early identification of the etiology can result in aggressive specific management of cause. The investigations may vary depending on whether it is the first episode of SE in a normal child, or SE in a child with pre-existing epilepsy and already receiving AEDs.[16,58] The tests are detailed below (in no specific order), and listed in Table 27.2 in the order of importance.

TABLE 27.2: Investigations in a child with status epilepticus	
First Line	*Second Line**
SE in a child without history seizures	
Ionic/total calcium (especially <2 years)	MRI
Random blood sugar	EEG
Sodium (especially <6 months)	If clinical suspicion: Urine toxicology
Add, if febrile: Complete blood count; Lumbar puncture#	
SE in known epilepsy patient	
• Known non-compliance/Missed dose/Recent drug or dose changes	
Anti-epileptic drug level	Random blood sugar
Consider, if febrile	Ionic/total calcium (especially <2 y)
– Complete blood count	Sodium (especially <6 m)
– Lumbar puncture#	If clinical suspicion: Urine toxicology
• No known precipitating event	
Ionic/total calcium (especially <2 years)	If clinical suspicion: Urine toxicology
Random blood sugar	Anti-epileptic drug level (if feasible)
Sodium (especially <6 months)	
Add, if febrile: Complete blood count; Lumbar puncture#	
If refractory SE or Persistent encephalopathy: Video-EEG monitoring	

SE: Status epilepticus; *EEG and Neuroimaging should be done later, after stabilization of the patient; #A central nervous system infection may be considered even in afebrile infants (<6 mo) and lumbar puncture done, based on clinical setting.

Blood Chemistries

Electrolyte and glucose abnormalities have been reported to be present in 1–16% of children with SE, although it is unclear whether they were the etiology in all and did treatment lead to cessation of the SE.[16]

Serum calcium: Hypocalcemia as a cause of seizures is common in our country,[60,61] usually due to vitamin D deficiency, and presents as a cluster of seizures in infancy. Early recognition avoids unnecessary treatment with AEDs and other interventions. Ionic calcium is more reliable as a guide for treatment and levels are usually <0.8 µmol/L in symptomatic children. However, all children with SE and subnormal ionized calcium levels (<1.2 µmol/L) should be treated. Total serum calcium, if done, should always be combined with estimation of phosphorous, serum alkaline phosphatase and serum albumin, for proper interpretation. Serum calcium estimation is an essential investigation for all children younger than 2 years with status epilepticus, irrespective of presence or absence of suggestive features.

Random blood sugar: Should be done in all children at presentation (especially in children less than 5 years),[58] as hypoglycemia may be responsible for seizures, and both hypo- or hyper-glycemia cause brain damage. When hypoglycemia is documented, urine ketones and reducing sugar should also be evaluated. Serum sodium: Hyponatremia has been reported to be a cause in 1% of new-onset childhood convulsive SE.[62] However, most children with this abnormality were found to have suggestive features on history and clinical examination.[63] As this finding has important therapeutic implications,[58] serum sodium estimation should be done in all, if feasible.

Metabolic disorders: Metabolic disorders are reportedly present in around 4.2% of children with SE.[16] though their etiological significance is unclear. Routine metabolic workup therefore, appears unwarranted. However, arterial blood gas estimation should be done in all

children with established SE, if facilities are available; or when transferring to the Intensive Care Unit (ICU).

Workup for Infections

Blood counts: May be done routinely in children presenting with SE,[16] especially those with associated fever. Infants with infection may not have fever and blood counts should be considered in them, even if afebrile.

Similarly, send blood cultures if the child is febrile (and above 6 months), or in a younger child, even if afebrile, if an infection is suspected.

Cerebrospinal fluid (CSF) examination: A central nervous system (CNS) infection is reported in 12.5% of pediatric convulsive SE.[16] CNS infections are also an important cause of SE in Indian children.[18] A CSF examination should be done by lumbar puncture in a febrile child, after stabilizing the child and excluding raised intracranial tension.[16] In infants younger than 6 months, signs of meningitis may not be clearly demonstrated and fever also may not be present. In such a situation, whenever there is a clinical suspicion of a CNS infection or sepsis, lumbar puncture should be done.

If done, CSF should be subjected at least to cell count (total and differential), biochemistry (protein, sugar, CSF: blood sugar ratio), bacterial culture, and gram stain. CSF pleocytosis, if present, should not be ascribed to a febrile SE.[64] Additional investigations on the CSF should be individualized. Systemic illness is a common trigger for convulsive SE in a patient who is already at risk, and, therefore, fever itself is not an indication to perform a lumbar puncture in a patient with epilepsy presenting with SE.[58]

Antiepileptic Drug Levels

Inadequate AED drug levels (whether due to non-compliance, missed dose, or recent drug-dose alterations) are associated with a significant proportion of SE in children,[9] although some studies found contradictory results.[65] Low AED levels were found in more than 30% childhood SE, although this was not necessarily the cause of SE.[16]

AED levels should be done, if feasible, in all patients receiving AED and presenting with SE, as it has both etiologic (non-compliance/low drug-level as a cause) and therapeutic (loading dose of the previously effective drug for management) implications. However, availability of required facilities is likely to act as a bottleneck.

Electroencephalography (EEG)

While considering EEG in SE, two situations need to be considered, viz. an isolated, short-duration single EEG recording, or continuous EEG monitoring. No Indian studies on usefulness of EEG in pediatric SE are available. EEG abnormalities have been reported in ~90% children presenting with SE, though these were done hours to days later.[16] The information whether the seizure is focal or generalized is an important one when deciding chronic AED therapy for the patient. EEG monitoring has been shown to be extremely useful, but under-utilized in SE management. After convulsive SE, one-third of children who undergo EEG monitoring are reported to have electrographic seizures, and among these, one-third experience entirely electrographic-only seizures.[66,67]

An EEG should be considered in every child presenting with new-onset SE, although it can be delayed till the control of SE. An EEG should also be done if there is suspicion of non-convulsive SE (child not returning to the pre-SE state or remaining persistently encephalo-pathic even after the control of convulsive SE) or pseudostatus is suspected. Continuous EEG monitoring optimizes the management of SE and should be used, if feasible.

Neuroimaging

Neuroimaging can identify structural causes for SE, especially to exclude the need for neurosurgical intervention in children with new-onset SE without a prior history of epilepsy, or in those with persistent SE despite appropriate treatment. MRI is more sensitive and specific than CT scanning, but CT is more widely available and quicker in an emergency setting.

A meta-analysis reported structural lesions in 7.8% of childhood SE, commonly CNS malformations, trauma, and stroke/hemor-rhage.[66] In a more recent study,[68] the yield of MRI to detect structural lesions in convulsive SE was 31%. In the Indian setting, where inflammatory granulomas are a common cause of seizures,[69] neuroimaging is likely to provide a higher yield.

Neuroimaging should be done, if feasible, in all children with SE, in whom no definitive etiology has been found. It should only be done after the child is appropriately stabilized and the seizure activity controlled. Emergent neuroimaging may be considered if there are clinical indications (new-onset focal deficits, persistent altered awareness, fever, recent trauma, history of cancer, history of antico-agulation, or a suspicion of AIDS).

Special Tests

Metabolic and genetic testing: Inborn errors of metabolism account for about 4% of SE in children.[59] The common metabolic causes are listed at Table 27.3. SE usually occurs during an inter-current illness or metabolic stress.[16,70,71] Pyridoxine dependency can present even after the neonatal period,[72] and is reported in around 0.3% of pediatric SE.[16] This needs to be excluded by either getting the specific test done (elevated urinary a-aminoadipic semial-dehyde or the mutations in the ALDH7A1 gene), or giving a trial of intravenous pyridoxine.[72]

Metabolic and genetic testing should be considered when no etiology is revealed in initial evaluation and/or the preceding history is suggestive of a metabolic disorder. The specific studies to be obtained should be guided by the history and the clinical examination.

TABLE 27.3: Metabolic conditions associated with status epilepticus

Group/Disorders

Mitochondrial diseases
Myoclonic epilepsy with red ragged fibers (MERRF), Alpers syndrome, pyruvate dehydrogenase complex deficiency

Lipid storage disorders
Tay Sachs-Sandhoff disease, Krabbe disease, neonatal adrenoleukodystrophy, Zellweger syndrome, infantile Refsum disease, punctuate rhyzomelic chon-drodysplasia, Niemann-Pick disease type A and C, Neuronal ceroid lipofuscinosis

Amino-acidopathies
Serine metabolism disorders, hyperpolinemia type II, untreated phenylketonuria, Maple urine syrup diseases, congenital glutamine deficiency, Non-ketotic hyper-glycinemia

Organic acidopathies
Propionic, methylmalonic, D-2- hydroxyglutaric and isovaleric acidurias; 2-methyl-3-hydroxybutyril-CoA dehydrogenase deficiency

Other diseases
Vitamin-dependent epilepsies, creatine metabolism dysfunctions, Menkes disease, disorders of purine and pyrimidine metabolism

Toxicology: Toxin or drug-ingestion is a cause of SE that requires urgent specific treatment. Specific serum toxicology testing should be considered if initial assessment does not yield the etiology and/or a suggestive history is elicited.

Work-up for autoimmune encephalitis: Patients of any age who develop rapidly progressing symptoms presenting or accompanied by seizures or status epilepticus, usually including behavioral change and memory deficits, with CSF lymphocytic pleocytosis and/or oligoclonal bands of unclear etiology, and EEG findings of encephalopathy and/or epileptic activity, should have serum and CSF studies for antibodies. In some of these disorders, the MRI is often normal. The diagnosis is established by demonstrating antibodies in serum and CSF, though occasionally antibodies are detectable only in the latter.[73]

Investigations to detect SE complications and drug side-effects: The major complications are altered glucose metabolism, dyselectrolytemias, and metabolic acidosis.[62] Propylene glycol toxicity (vehicle in diazepam/lorazepam and barbiturates), Propofol infusion syndrome, immunosuppression due to barbiturate use, and liver toxicity due to AEDs[62,63] are the major drug side-effects seen. These are detailed in Table 27.4.

E. Pharmacotherapy

The goal of treatment is the immediate termination of seizures. For this, drugs should be used in quick succession, and if possible, rapid institution of pharmacological coma should be done in refractory cases. In the acute setting, anticonvulsants are best administered by the intravenous route. Alternative routes can be employed, to avoid delay in institution of therapy, especially in the pre-hospital settings. Pharmacotherapy of SE includes drug-management in the hospital, and management of refractory and super-refractory SE. Before starting pharmacotherapy for SE in the hospital, the pre-hospital drugs and doses should be taken in consideration, e.g. a child who has received one dose of midazolam during transfer should receive only one more dose of midazolam before moving on to the next drug. Table 27.5 provides the guidelines for using various AEDs for SE management, and Table 27.6 shows the recommended protocol, with Box 27.3 providing supplementary management options.

Status Epilepticus

A number of anticonvulsants are available and one can choose the drugs based on availability and cost, and the monitoring facilities available.

Benzodiazepines: Benzodiazepines are first line drugs for treatment of SE in children.[4,74,75] The choice within the benzodiazepines is based on side-effects and pharmacokinetic properties. Several RCTs and systematic

TABLE 27.4: Investigations to identify side-effects of drugs and to pick-up complications of status epilepticus

Condition	Drugs	Test
Propylene glycol toxicity	Lorazepam and barbiturates	Lactic acidosis, and osmolar gap calculation
Propofol infusion syndrome	Propofol	ABG, lactate, CPK, ECG monitoring, Serum electrolytes, creatinine clearance
Immunosuppression	Barbiturates	Screening for infections: Culture of body fluids, C-reactive protein level, procalcitonin level, white blood cell count, and differential count
Valproate toxicity	Valproate	Liver function tests, Platelet count
Hyperglycemia	RBS-6th hourly; Maintaining blood glucose 140–180 mg/dL	Massive increase in catecholamine can lead to hyperglycemia and damages the brain through worsening lactate acidosis. Glucose is controlled, preferably with insulin infusion, starting at a thresh-old not higher than 180 mg/dL; levels <110 mg/dL not safe
Metabolic acidosis	ABG every 6–8 hourly	
Dyselectrolytemia	Serum electrolytes at least daily	To identify SIADH and hyperkalemia
Renal failure	Urea, creatinine daily and calculation of creatinine clearance	Acute nonoliguric renal failure can result due to rhabdomyolysis, may become apparent with acutely rising serum creatinine, hyperkalemia, and hyperphosphatemia
Respiratory complications	Chest radiograph/ USG	To look for pneumonia and pleural effusions
Cardiac arrhythmia	ECG	Continuous or twice a day
Hypotension	Echocardiography	For apical ballooning cardiomyopathy (Takutsubo cardiomyopathy) due to massive release of catecholamines
Rhabdomyolysis	ABG	Metabolic acidosis not entirely explained by lactate accumulation, hyperkalemia, increased serum aldolase, hypocalcemia, and myoglobinuria
Infections	As per suscpicion	Common are pneumonia, sepsis, pseudomembranous colitis, and urinary tract infections. Gastrointestinal problems may be seen and often lead to adynamic ileus.

reviews have concluded that lorazepam is the agent of choice among the benzodiazepines.[4,74,75] More recent data; however, suggests that the efficacy and side-effect profile of lorazepam and diazepam is similar in children, when efficacy is defined as cessation of status epilepticus by 10 minutes without recurrence within 30 minutes.[76] Children receiving lorazepam are less likely to:

require additional doses of anticonvulsants to stop seizures, develop respiratory depression, and require admission to intensive care unit.[77] If lorazepam is not available, midazolam or diazepam can be used for aborting the seizure (Table 27.6). These two drugs are shorter acting and thus need to be followed up with longer-acting non-benzodiazepine anticonvulsants. When using benzodia-zepines, there is a risk

TABLE 27.5: Anticonvulsant usage in status epilepticus

Drug	Dosage and route	Comments
Lorazepam	0.1 mg/kg/IV (max 4 mg) @ 2 mg/min	Long acting benzodiazepine, Side effects: sedation, respiratory depression and hypotension.
Midazolam	0.15–0.2 mg/kg;/IV or IM (max 5 mg) Buccal/Nasal: 0.2–0.3 mg/kg (max 5 mg)	Can be used by IM route.
Diazepam	0.2–0.3 mg/kg (max 10 mg) IV 0.5 mg/kg per rectal (max 10 mg)	IV dose should be given slowly over 2–5 min under careful monitoring.
Phenytoin	20 mg/kg (max: 1000 mg) in NS @ 1 mg/kg/min (max 50 mg per min)	Must be diluted in saline. Side effects include; hypotension, cardiac arrythmias, 'purple glove syndrome', skin rashes. Contraindicated in severe hypotension and grade II AV block.
Fosphenytoin	20 PE/kg, Rate: 3 PE/kg/min	Fewer side effects compared with phenytoin. Can be given IM.
Valproate	20 mg/kg-IV infusion over 15 min, max rate-6 mg/kg/min. Followed by an infusion of 1–2 mg/kg/h	Avoid in presence of liver disease, coagulopathy, thrombocytopenia, suspected metabolic disease, and in infants.
Phenobarbitone	20 mg/kg in NS @ 1.5 mg/kg/min	Side effects: sedation, respiratory depression, and hypotension
Levetiracetam	20–30 mg/kg, over 15 min	Considered safe in children with metabolic diseases, oncology patients, and in those with liver disease or coagulopathy.
Thiopentone	Induction: 3 mg/kg bolus, repeated after 2 min, followed by maintenance 1–5 mg/kg/hr (increasing 1 mg/kg/hr every 2 min) to control seizures and/or to achieve "suppression-burst" EEG activity	Causes respiratory depression. Can also induce hypotension and heart failure, associated with an increased rate of nosocomial infections. Contraindicated in the presence of hypotension, cardiogenic shock and sepsis.
Topiramate	Initial dose: 5–10 mg/kg/day orally, maintenance dose of 5 mg/kg/day, if effective	Side effects: metabolic acidosis, decreased sweating and glaucoma.

NS- normal saline, PE: phenytoin equivalents, max-maximum, IV –intravenous, IM- intramuscular, @- at the rate

of respiratory depression or arrest, which increases with repeated doses of the drug.[78]

Pheytoin/Fosphenytoin: After using short-acting benzodiazepines, phenytoin is one of the preferred second-line anticonvulsant.[74] The loading dose of the drug offers long-duration seizure-suppression. Major precautions in its use are monitoring for hypotension and arrhythmias. In addition, local irritation and phlebitis are common with intravenous administration of phenytoin. Respiratory depression is exceedingly rare with its use and

it does not cause sedation. In children, care has to be taken to adequately dilute it in normal saline and as far as possible use a large caliber vessel. As a second-line AED in SE after benzodiazepines, phenytoin has been evaluated against phenobarbitone, valproate and levetiracetam.[74,79,80] However, recent evidence[80] does not support the first line use of phenytoin.

Fosphenytoin is a water-soluble pro-drug of phenytoin which has a more favorable side-effect profile and can be given intramuscularly. It is preferred over phenytoin, when

TABLE 27.6: Drug management of status epilepticus in a health facility[*]

Timeline	Drug treatment
0 min	*IV Access available:* Inj Lorazepam—0.1 mg/kg/IV (max 4 mg) @ 2 mg/min OR Inj Diazepam—0.2–0.3 mg/kg/IV (max 10 mg) Slow IV OR Inj Midazolam—0.15–0.2 mg/kg/IV (max 5 mg)
	IV access not available: Buccal/Nasal Midazolam 0.2–0.3 mg/kg (max 5 mg) OR PR Diazepam 0.5 mg/kg (max 10 mg) OR IM Midazolam 0.2 mg/kg (max 5 mg)
5 min	Repeat Benzodiazepine once
10 min	IV Phenytoin 20 mg/kg (max: 1000mg) in NS @ 1 mg/kg/min (max 50 mg per min), OR Inj Fosphenytoin 20 mg PE/ kg, Rate: 3 mg PE/kg/min

PICU bed Available
IV Midazolam infusion

PICU bed/PICU not-Available (following management may be done sequentially)	
Drug treatment	Additional action
IV Valproate 20 mg/kg–IV @ max 6 mg/kg/minute	Shift to PICU, if feasible
IV Phenobarbitone 20 mg/kg in NS @ 1.5 mg/kg/min	Shift to PICU, if feasible
Alternate drug: IV Levetiracetam (If Liver disease/Metabolic disease/ coagulopathy/on chemotherapy)—20–30 mg/kg @ 5 mg/kg/min infusion	Shift to PICU, if feasible
IV Midazolam infusion	Shift to PICU, if feasible

Details available in the text; #from the time child came to medical attention; AED- Anti epileptic drugs, PE- Phenytoin equivalent, NS- normal saline; Valproate and Levetiracetam can be interchangeably used in the sequence of drugs; Max-maximun dose; @- at the rate of.

Special situations
- If the child is already on anti epileptic drugs (AED) : Give half the loading dose of the respective AED.
- IV Pyridoxine: To be used in children with Isoniazid overdose AND in children <2 years of age without a clear etiology for seizures (IV Pyridoxine 100 mg infusion); B6 trial may also be given to any child with super-refractory status and neonatal onset of seizures, who has not received pyridoxine before.
- Liver failure or Chronic liver disease: prefer levetiracetam, avoid valproate; Liver failure- Avoid long acting benzodiazepines, Phenobarbitone; preferred drugs- Phenytoin, Levetiracetam.
- Renal Failure: Levetiracetam accumulates in patients with renal failure; Valproate and benzodiazepines are better options.
- Suspected or proven neurometabolic disorder or Inborn error of metabolism: prefer- Levetiracetam.
- Porphyria: Check drug list for safe agents in prophyria, avoid Phenobarbitone.
- Child less than 2 years : Avoid Valproate.
- Child with severe PEM: consider deficiency states aggravating or causing seizures - Magnesium, Calcium, Vitamin- B6, Vitamin B1.
- Child with neuromuscular disease and respiratory or bulbar weakness: Caution in using respiratory depressants like Benzodiazepines, Phenobarbitone; Prefer Phenytoin, Valproate, Levetiracetam.

available, but its higher cost and limited availability precludes its widespread use.

Phenobarbitone

Intravenous phenobarbitone is an effective alternative to phenytoin in benzodiazepine unresponsive seizures. The perceived risk of higher rate of respiratory depression after its use has not been seen in randomized trials.[74,80] Still, one needs caution in using it after two or more doses of benzodiazepines. It is particularly effective in infants younger than one year. When using this drug, personnel trained in intubation and resuscitation should be available. Hypotension, respiratory depression and sedation are the major side-effects. High dose phenobarbitone has also been used for refractory status epilepticus in intensive care setting.[81]

Valproic Acid (Sodium valproate)

The efficacy of valproic acid is similar to phenytoin after failure of benzodiazepines,[82] though a recent meta-analysis found it to have superior efficacy.[80] In a recent trial in children, intravenous valproic acid was shown to be equally effective as phenobarbitone with significant fewer adverse effects.[83] A recent systematic review of studies with mainly adult patients concluded that intravenous valproate was as effective as intravenous phenytoin for SE control.[84] It has also been shown to be effective in children with status epilepticus refractory to phenytoin.[85] The major advantage of valproic acid is the relative lack of sedation, respiratory depression or adverse hemodynamic events. On the other hand, caution needs to be exercised in its use in infants, and in those with liver disease, bleeding diathesis and suspected metabolic disorders.

Levetiracetam

This is another emerging drug in the management of status epilepticus. Presently there are no randomized trials reporting its use in children. Data in adults suggest that it is as effective as valproic acid.[80,84] This drug too has the advantage of relative lack of sedation, respiratory depression or adverse hemodynamic events. Additionally, it can be used in liver failure and in presence of bleeding

diathesis. It also has the advantage of relatively few drug-interactions.

An ongoing multi-centric trial is expected to clarify regarding the best drug (amongst valproate, fosphenytoin and levetiracetam) to be used after benzodiazepines.[86]

Refractory Status Epilepticus

SE is considered refractory if seizures persist despite the administration of two appropriate anticonvulsants at acceptable doses.[87] Earlier definitions also mentioned duration of the status (60 min or 120 min).[88,89] For the multi-centric Pediatric Status Epilepticus Research Group (pSERG) study, the definition described is prolonged seizures that fail to terminate after administration of two anti-epileptic drugs with different mechanisms of action or that require continuously administered medication to abort seizures, regardless of seizure duration.[90] These definitions highlight the concepts that the potential for neuronal injury is positively correlated with time, and pharmaco-resistance increases with time and is reflected in the number of drugs administered.[87] Refractory status epilepticus comprises around 10–40% of patients with status epilepticus.[87–91] Predictive factors for development of intractability in patients with SE include encephalitic etiology, severe impairment of conscious-ness at presentation, absence of a history of epilepsy, and low anticonvulsant levels (in patients with known epilepsy).[92,93]

EEG monitoring, if available, is important both to monitor for electroclinical seizures or non-convulsive electrographic seizures, and to titrate therapy and the depth of anesthesia, if necessary.[87] Additional investigations, other than those previously described, include a high resolution (3 Tesla) MRI to look for cortical dysplasias, metabolic work-up (blood Tandem mass spectrophotometry and/or blood/urine Gas chromatography mass spectrophotometry) in young children, and work-up for autoimmune encephalitis in patients with de novo status epilepticus associated with fever.

Refractory status epilepticus must be managed in the intensive care unit. These children require careful cardiorespiratory monitoring and may also require mechanical ventilation.

Agents available for treatment are anti-epileptic drugs (non-anesthetic agents) and intravenous anesthetic agents.[87] Non-anesthetic agents include pheno-barbitone, valproic acid, levetiracetam, topiramate, and lacosamide. Intravenous preparations for all the above-mentioned drugs, except topiramate are available. Intravenous anesthetic agents include midazolam, pentobarbital, thiopental sodium, and propofol. Pentobarbital is not available in India. Propofol has been used extensively in adult status epilepticus. However, the risk of propofol infusion syndrome is high in children and hence propofol is not approved for the treatment of pediatric status epilepticus in many countries.[94] Given the absence of clear evidence, the decision to use one or other anesthetic medications must take into account the patient's general condition, weighing the benefits against the potential adverse effects of the medication, and the medical staff's experience in the use of these drugs and their ability to manage the side effects.[95]

Second-line Anticonvulsants: After the failure of phenytoin/fosphenytoin, trial of any of the following: phenobarbitone, sodium valproate or levetiracetam may be given. In children below 2 years of age, pyridoxine (100 mg intravenously) may be tried. If the seizure continues despite this third agent, the patient must be shifted to the intensive care unit where facilities for mechanical ventilation and cardiorespiratory monitoring are available. If however, there is a delay in transfer or intensive care unit is not available, a fourth drug (phenobarbitone, sodium valproate or levetiracetam; whichever has not been tried

earlier) may be tried before proceeding to midazolam infusion.

There are reports of use of topiramate in children with refractory SE leading to rapid resolution of status with no hemodynamic or sedative side effects. As intravenous preparation is not available, it should be administered through nasogastric tube.[96] Anecdotal reports of efficacy of Lacosamide in children with SE exist;[97] however, more data is needed before its use can be recommended.

Intravenous Anesthetic Agents: Midazolam infusion is the most preferred initial treatment in children with refractory status epilepticus, effective in seizure control in 76% of these patients.[5] Midazolam is a short-acting benzodiazepine that rapidly equilibrates across the blood-brain barrier and has a short elimination half-life. It has a favorable pharmacokinetic profile which allows for repeat bolus dosing, aggressive titration of the infusion, and relatively fast recovery time [98]. It causes little hypotension, and vasopressors are usually only needed when high doses of midazolam are used.

Initial effectiveness in terminating pediatric RSE has been shown in several studies with efficacy rates of approximately 80–90%.[99,100] Midazolam should be given as a 0.2 mg/kg bolus then infusion at the rate of 1 µg/kg/min, increasing 1 µg/kg/min, every 5–10 min, till seizures stop, up to a maximum of 12 µg/kg/min.[101] Larger initial bolus doses (0.5 mg/kg) and more aggressive upward dose titration (up to 2 mg/kg/hour) may result in faster termination of status epilepticus.[87,98,100] Doses up to 36µg/kg/min have been used in previous studies, and may be tried provided it is being used in an ICU setting and appropriate monitoring and management facilities are available. Tapering should be started 24–48 hours after seizure stops at the rate of 1 µg/kg/min, every 3–4 hours. Although generally effective and well tolerated, a drawback of midazolam is the apparent increased propensity for seizure recurrence on tapering, compared with other intravenous anesthetic agents.

Thiopental sodium penetrates the central nervous system rapidly, allowing for rapid titration to EEG burst-suppression. It has multiple actions: activation of the GABA receptor; inhibition of N-methyl-D-aspartate (NMDA) receptors; and, alteration in the conductance of chloride, potassium, and calcium ion channels.[5] Its prolonged infusion results in a transition from the usual first-order elimination kinetics seen with bolus doses to the unpredictable zero-order kinetics and a prolonged elimination half-life because of distribution in lipid. This phenomenon makes recovery time prolonged and the drug effect can last days, even with short infusion periods of 12 to 24 hours.

Induction of barbiturate coma is done with bolus of 3 mg/kg, repeated after 2 min, followed by maintenance (1–5 mg/kg/hr) to control seizures and/or to achieve "suppression-burst" EEG activity (increasing 1 mg/kg/hr every 2 minutes).[95] The subsequent maintenance infusion should continue for 12–48 hours. Thiopental usually causes respiratory depression. It can also induce hypotension and heart failure, and inotropic support is frequently needed. Thiopental is associated with an increased rate of nosocomial infection, especially pneumonia, and ileus.[102] It is contra-indicated in the presence of hypotension, cardiogenic shock and sepsis.[95] It is reported to control seizures in 65% of the refractory SE patients not responding to midazolam.[97]

Super-Refractory Status Epilepticus

Around 15% of all those presenting to hospital in SE develop super-refractory status epilepticus and the mortality is 30–50%.[102,103]

Therapies for this entity have not been well studied. Treatment modalities depend on the availability of resources, and experience and familiarity of the treating physicians with the various modalities. Other than the previously mentioned drugs; the agents and modalities that have been tried in super-refractory status epilepticus include ketamine,[104] inhalational halogenated anesthetics,[105] magnesium infusion,[106] steroids and immunotherapy,[103] ketogenic diet,[107] hypothermia,[108] electrical and magnetic stimulation therapies,[103] electroconvulsive therapy,[109] and CSF drainage.[110] Emergency neurosurgery may be considered in children in whom a lesion has been detected as the cause of status epilepticus, e.g. cortical dysplasia.[111]

F. Febrile Status Epilepticus

It is defined as status epilepticus in a child aged 1 month to 5 years that also meets the definition of a febrile seizure.[112] Thus it is clear that febrile central nervous system infections associated with status epilepticus will not be included in febrile SE. Febrile SE occur in 5% of febrile seizures.[113] Western studies report febrile SE as the most common cause of status epilepticus in children (up to 50%),[114] although Indian studies have reported it to be less common (10%),[18] or have not characterized it separately.[8] Many of the issues related to investigations in febrile SE and its outcome are being explord by the FEBSTAT study.[112]

CSF changes in Febrile SE: Pleocytosis due to SE or febrile SE has long been a controversial issue, and probably the definitive answer is now available with the results of the FEBSTAT study.[112] The CSF results from this large group of patients with prolonged febrile seizure were usually normal: 96% had ≤5 WBCs/mm³; CSF glucose and protein levels were also unremarkable.[64] Human herpesvirus-6B has been reported to be the most common cause of febrile SE.[115]

Management of febrile SE is similar to that recommended for SE in these guidelines; however, there is evidence to show that phenytoin is less efficacious in this situation.[116]

G. Management Following Status Epilepticus

It is well-established that the duration of the first seizure does not affect the risk of

Box 27.4: Guidelines for follow-up management of children with status epilepticus

New-onset SE: Further treatment decisions should be similar to that for a First seizure.

Acute symptomatic seizures: Further treatment depends on the control of the precipitating event.

SE in known epilepsy:

• After control of SE for 24 hours, tapering of drugs should be started with 'last in, first out' as the guiding principle.

• All the AEDs should preferably be stopped during hospital stay and the child discharged on:
  – Augmented dose of the previous AED/s (if levels were sub-therapeutic or prescribed dose was less than maximum dose); and
  – Introduction of another appropriate AED (either replacement or addition), if previously receiving maximum doses of AED/s.

recurrence, whether it is a single seizure or a status epilepticus. Moreover, remission rates are also not different in those who present with an episode of SE.[117] Brief recommendations for follow-up management after control of SE are provided in Box 27.4.

H. Research Needs

During the deliberations, the group also tried to identify the areas requiring research in the Indian context. These are listed in Box 27.5, and are expected to provide guidance to the researchers about issues needing evidence-support.

Box 27.5: Research needs for status epilepticus in children

• Epidemiology of SE in India
• Role of hypocalcemia in SE, especially in infants
• Role of phenobarbitone and phenytoin as the initial AED after benzodiazepine
• Management of SE-associated with neuroinfections
• Outcome of SE in Indian children

REFERENCES

1. Pellock JM. Status epilepticus in children: update and review. J Child Neurol. 1994;9:27-35.

2. De Lorenzo RJ. Status epilepticus: concepts in diagnosis and treatment. Semin Neurol 1990;10: 396–405.

3. Abend NS, Gutierrez-Colina AM, Dlugos DJ. Medical treatment of pediatric status epilepticus. Semin Pediatr Neurol 2010;17:169–75.

4. Appleton R, Macleod S, Martland T. Drug management for acute tonic-clonic convulsions including convulsive status epilepticus in children. Cochrane Database Syst Rev 2008;3: CD001905.

5. Wilkes R, Tasker RC. Pediatric intensive care treatment of uncontrolled status epilepticus. Crit Care Clin 2013;29:239–57.

6. Expert Committee on Pediatric Epilepsy, Indian Academy of Pediatrics. Guidelines for diagnosis and management of childhood epilepsy. Indian Pediatr 2009;46:681–98.

7. GEMIND. Guidelines for management of epilepsy in India. Available from: www.epilepsy india.com/gemind-book/. Accessed on 23 July, 2013.

8. Sasidaran K, Singhi S, Singhi P. Management of acute seizure and status epilepticus in pediatric emergency. Indian J Pediatr 2012;79:510–7.

9. Morton LD, Pellock JM. Status Epilepticus. In: Swaiman KF, Ashwal S, Ferriero DM, Nina F Schor NF. Swaiman's Pediatric Neurology: Principles and Practice, 5e; Elsevier 2012; 798–810.

10. Sharma S, Mishra D, Aneja S, Kumar R, Jain A, Vashishtha VM, et al. for the Expert Group on Encephalitis, Indian Academy of Pediatrics. Consensus guidelines on evaluation and manage-ment of suspected acute viral encephalitis in children in India. Indian Pediatr 2012;49:897–910.

11. Epilepsy Foundation of America's Working Group on Status Epilepticus. Treatment of con-vulsive status epilepticus. Recommendations of the Epilepsy Foundation of America's Working Group on Status Epilepticus. J Am Med Assoc 1993;270:854–59.

12. Commission on Epidemiology and Prognosis, International League Against Epilepsy. Guide-lines for epidemiologic studies on epilepsy. Epilepsia 1993;34:592–96.

13. Lowenstein DH, Bleck T, Macdonald RL. It's time to revise the definition of status epilepticus. Epilepsia 1999; 40:120–2.

14. Shinnar S, Berg AT, Moshe SL, Shinnar R. How long do new-onset seizures in children last? Ann Neurol 2001;49:659–64.

15. Capovilla G, Beccaria F, Beghi E, Minicucci F, Sartori S, Vecchi M. Treatment of convulsive status epilepticus in childhood: Recommendations of the Italian League Against Epilepsy. Epilepsia 2013;54:23–34.

16. Riviello JJ, Ashwal S, Hirtz D, Glauser T, Ballaban-Gil K, Kelley K, et al. Practice Parameter: Diagnostic Assessment of the Child With Status Epilepticus (an evidence-based review). Report of the Quality Standards Subcommittee of the American Academy of Neurology and the Practice Committee of the Child Neurology Society. Neurology 2006;67: 1542–50.

17. Chin RF, Neville BG, Peckham C, Bedford H, Wade A, Scott RC. Incidence, cause, and short-term outcome of convulsive status epilepticus in childhood: prospective population-based study. Lancet 2006;368:222–29.

18. Gulati S, Kalra V, Sridhar MR. Status epilepticus in Indian children in a tertiary care center. Indian J Pediatr 2005;72:105–8.

19. Tripathi M, Vibha D, Choudhary N, Prasad K, Srivastava MV, Bhatia R, et al. Management of refractory status epilepticus at a tertiary care centre in a developing country. Seizure 2010;19: 109–11.

20. Sinha S, Satishchandra P, Mahadevan A, Bhimani BC, Kovur JM, Shankar SK. Fatal status epilepticus: A clinico-pathological analysis among 100 patients: from a developing country perspective. Epilepsy Res 2010;91:193–204.

21. Pellock JM. Overview: definitions and classifications of seizure emergencies. J Child Neurol 2007;22:9S–13S.

22. Chin RF, Verhulst L, Neville BG, Peters MJ, Scott RC. Inappropriate emergency management of status epilepticus in children contributes to need for intensive care. J Neurol Neurosurg Psychiatry 2004;75:1584–8.

23. Facility Based IMNCI (F-IMNCI) Participants Manual. Government of India. Available from: www.unicef.org/india/FBC_Participants_ Manual. Accessed August 31, 2014.

24. Alldredge BK, Gelb AM, Isaacs SM, Corry MD, Allen F, Ulrich S, et al. A comparison of lora-zepam, diazepam, and placebo for the treatment of out-of-hospital status epilepticus. N Engl J Med 2001;345:631–7.

25. Ahmad S, Ellis JC, Kamwendo H, Molyneux E. Efficacy and safety of intranasal lorazepam versus intramuscular paraldehyde for protracted convulsions in children: an open randomized trial. Lancet 2006;367:1591–7.

26. Dreifuss FE, Rosman NP, Cloyd JC, Pellock JM, Kuzniecky RI, Lo WD, et al. A comparison of rectal diazepam gel and placebo for acute repetitive seizures. N Engl J Med 1998;338:1869–75.

27. Cereghino JJ, Mitchell WG, Murphy J, Kriel RL, Rosenfeld WE, Trevathan E. Treating repetitive seizures with a rectal diazepam formulation: a randomized study. The North American Diastat Study Group. Neurology 1998;51:1274–82.

28. Pellock JM. Safety of Diastat, a rectal gel formulation of diazepam for acute seizure treatment. Drug Saf 2004;27:383–92.

29. Holsti M, Sill BL, Firth SD, Filloux FM, Joyce SM, Furnival RA. Prehospital intranasal midazolam for the treatment of pediatric seizures. Pediatr Emerg Care 2007;23:148–53.

30. Kutlu NO, Dogrul M, Yakinci C, Soylu H. Buccal midazolam for treatment of prolonged seizures in children. Brain Dev 2003;25:275–8.

31. Scott RC, Besag FM, Boyd SG, Berry D, Neville BG. Buccal absorption of midazolam: pharmacokinetics and EEG pharmacodynamics. Epilepsia 1998;39:290–4.

32. Ashrafi MR, Khosroshahi N, Karimi P, Malamiri RA, Bavarian B, Zarch AV, et al. Efficacy and usability of buccal midazolam in controlling acute prolonged convulsive seizures in children. Eur J Paediatr Neurol 2010;14:434–8.

33. Wiznitzer M. Buccal midazolam for seizures. Lancet 2005;366:182–3.

34. Kendall JL, Reynolds M, Goldberg R. Intranasal midazolam in patients with status epilepticus. Ann Emerg Med 1997;29:415–7.

35. Jeannet PY, RouletE, Maeder-Ingvar M, Gehri M, Jutzi A, Deonna T. Home and hospital treatment of acute seizures in children with nasal midazolam. Eur J Paediatr Neurol 1999;3:73–7.

36. Silbergleit R, Durkalski V, Lowenstein D, Conwit R, Pancioli A, Palesch Y, Barsan W; NETT Investigators. Intramuscular versus intravenous therapy for prehospital status epilepticus. N Engl J Med 2012;366:591–600.

37. Arya R, Gulati S, Kabra M, Sahu JK, Kalra V. Intranasal versus intravenous lorazepam for

control of acute seizures in children: a rando-mized open-label study. Epilepsia 2011;52:788–93.

38. Ma L, Yung A, Yau Ee, Kwong K. Clinical Guidelines on Management of Prolonged Seizures, Serial Seizures and Convulsive Status Epilepticus in Children. HK J Paediatr (New Series) 2010;15:52–63.

39. Shorvon S, Ferlisi M. The treatment of super-refractory status epilepticus: a critical review of available therapies and a clinical treatment protocol. Brain J Neurol 2011;134:2802–18.

40. Capovilla G, Beccaria F, Beghi E, Minicucci F, Sartori S, Vecchi M. Treatment of convulsive status epilepticus in childhood: Recommen-dations of the Italian League Against Epilepsy. Epilepsia 2013;54:23–34.

41. Wijdicks E. Neurologic catastrophies in the emergency department. Boston: Butterworth-Heinemann; 2000.

42. Lothman E. The biochemical basis and patho-physiology of status epilepticus. Neurology 1990;40:13–23.

43. Shorvon SD. Emergency treatment of acute seizures, serial seizures, seizure cluster and status epilepticus. In: Shorvon SD. Handbook of Epilepsy Treatment. Oxford: Blackwell Science; 2000.

44. Fountain NB. Status epilepticus: risk factors and complications. Epilepsia 2000;41:S23–30.

45. Fountain NB, Lothman EW. Pathophysiology of status epilepticus. J Clin Neurophysiol. 1995;12:326–42.

46. Simon RP. Physiologic consequences of status epilepticus. Epilepsia 1985;26:S58–66.

47. Wijdicks EFM. The multifaceted care of status epilepticus. Epilepsia 2013;54:61–3.

48. Sutter R, Tschudin-Sutter S, Grize L, Fuhr P, Bonten MJ, Widmer AF, et al. Associations between infections and clinical outcome para-meters in status epilepticus: a retrospective 5-year cohort study. Epilepsia 2012;53:1489–97.

49. Bleck TP. Intensive care unit management of patients with status epilepticus. Epilepsia. 2007;48:59–60.

50. Vespa PM, Miller C, McArthur D, Eliseo M, Etchepare M, Hirt D, et al. Nonconvulsive electrographic seizures after traumatic brain injury result in a delayed, prolonged increase in intracranial pressure and metabolic crisis. Crit Care Med 2007;35:2830–6.

51. Weeks SG, Alvarez N, Pillay N, Bell RB. Takotsubo cardiomyopathy secondary to seizures. Can J Neurol Sci 2007;34:105–7.

52. Stöllberger C, Wegner C, Finsterer J. Seizure-associated Takotsubo cardiomyopathy. Epilepsia 2011;52:e160–7.

53. Lemke DM, Hussain SI, Wolfe TJ, Torbey MA, Lynch JR, Carlin A, et al. Takotsubo cardiomyo-pathy associated with seizures. Neurocrit Care 2008;9:112–7.

54. Boggs JG, Painter JA, DeLorenzo RJ. Analysis of electrocardiographic changes in status epilep-ticus. Epilepsy Res 1993;14:87–94.

55. Manno EM, Pfeifer EA, Cascino GD, Noe KH, Wijdicks EFM. Cardiac pathology in status epilepticus. Ann Neurol 2005;58:954–7.

56. Luck RP, Verbin S. Rhabdomyolysis: a review of clinical presentation, etiology, diagnosis, and management. Pediatr Emerg Care 2008;24:262–8.

57. Gunn V, Nechyba C. The Harriet Lane Hand-book. 16th Ed. St Louis, MO: Mosby Elseiver, Inc; 2002.

58. Freilich ER, Zelleke T, Gaillard WD. Identification and evaluation of the child in status epilepticus. Semin Pediatr Neurol 2010;17:144–9.

59. Mastrangelo M, Celato A. Diagnostic work-up and therapeutic options in management of pedia-tric status epilepticus. World J Pediatr 2012;8:109–15.

60. Mehrotra P, Marwaha RK, Aneja S, Seth A, Singla BM, Ashraf G, et al. Hypovitaminosis D and hypocalcemic seizures in infancy. Indian Pediatr 2010;47:581–6.

61. Balasubramanian S, Shivbalan S, Kumar PS. Hypocalcemia due to vitamin D deficiency in exclusively breastfed infants. Indian Pediatr 2006;43:247–51.

62. Shorvon S, Ferlisi M. The treatment of super-refractory status epilepticus: a critical review of available therapies and a clinical treatment protocol. Brain 2011;134:2802–18.

63. Wijdicks EFM. The multifaceted care of status epilepticus. Epilepsia 2013;54:61–3.

64. Frank LM, Shinnar S, Hesdorffer DC, Shinnar RC, Pellock JM, Gallentine W, et al. FEBSTAT Study Team. Cerebrospinal fluid findings in children with fever-associated status epilepticus: results of the consequences of prolonged febrile seizures (FEBSTAT) study. J Pediatr 2012;161: 1169–71.

65. Maytal J, Novak G, Ascher C, Bienkowski R. Status epilepticus in children with epilepsy: the

role of antiepileptic drug levels in prevention. Pediatrics 1996;98:1119–21.

66. Greiner HM, Holland K, Leach JL, Horn PS, Hershey AD, Rose DF. Nonconvulsive status epilepticus: the encephalopathic pediatric patient. Pediatrics. 2012; 129:e748-55.

67. Sánchez Fernández I, Abend NS, Arndt DH, Carpenter JL, Chapman KE, Cornett KM, et al. Electrographic seizures after convulsive status epilepticus in children and young adults: a retrospective multicenter study. J Pediatr 2014; 164:339–46.

68. Yoong M, Madari R, Martinoss R, Clark C, Chong K, Neville B, et al. The role of magnetic resonance imaging in the follow-up of children with convulsive status epilepticus. Dev Med Child Neurol 2012;54:328–33.

69. Singhi P. Neurocysticercosis. Ther Adv Neurol Disord 2011;4:67–81.

70. Eriksson KJ, Koivikko MJ. Status epilepticus in children: Aetiology, treatment, and outcome. Dev Med Child Neurol 1997;39:652–8.

71. Hussain N, Appleton R, Thorburn K. Aetiology, course and outcome of children admitted to paediatric intensive care with convulsive status epilepticus: a retrospective 5-year review. Seizure 2007;16:305–12.

72. Yeghiazaryan NS1, Zara F, Capovilla G, Brigati G, Falsaperla R, Striano P. Pyridoxine-dependent epilepsy: An under-recognised cause of intractable seizures. J Paediatr Child Health 2012;48: E113–5.

73. Davis R, Dalmau J. Autoimmunity, seizures, and status epilepticus. Epilepsia 2013;54:46–9.

74. Treiman DM, Meyers PD, Walton NY, Collins JF, Colling C, Rowan AJ, et al. A comparison of four treatments for generalized convulsive status epilepticus. Veterans Affairs Status Epilepticus Cooperative Study Group. N Engl J Med 1998; 339:792–8.

75. Sreenath TG, Gupta P, Sharma KK, Krishnamurthy S. Lorazepam versus diazepam-phenytoin combination in the treatment of convulsive status epilepticus in children: A randomized controlled trial. Eur J Paediatr Neurol 2010;14:162–8.

76. Chamberlain JM, Okada P, Holsti M, Mahajan P, Brown KM, Vance C, et al. Pediatric Emergency Care Applied Research Network (PECARN). Lorazepam vs diazepam for pediatric status epilepticus: A randomized clinical trial. JAMA 2014;311:1652–60.

77. Appleton R, Sweeney A, Choonara I, Robson J, Molyneux E. Lorazepam versus diazepam in the acute treatment of epileptic seizures and status epilepticus. Dev Med Child Neurol 1995;37: 682–8.

78. Stewart WA, Harrison R, Dooley JM. Respiratory depression in the acute management of seizures. Arch Dis Child 2002;87:225–6.

79. Agarwal P, Kumar N, Chandra R, Gupta G, Antony AR, Garg N. Randomized study of intravenous valproate and phenytoin in status epilepticus. Seizure 2007;16:527–32.

80. Yasiry Z, Shorvon SD. The relative effectiveness of five antiepileptic drugs in treatment of benzodiazepine-resistant convulsive status epilepticus: A meta-analysis of published studies. Seizure 2014;23:167–74.

81. Crawford TO, Mitchell WG, Fishman LS, Snodgrass SR. Very-high-dose phenobarbital for refractory status epilepticus in children. Neurology 1988;38:1035–40.

82. Misra UK, Kalita J, Patel R. Sodium valproate vs phenytoin in status epilepticus: a pilot study. Neurology 2006;67:340–2.

83. Malamiri RA, Ghaempanah M, Khosroshahi N, Nikkhah A, Bavarian B, Ashrafi MR. Efficacy and safety of intravenous sodium valproate versus phenobarbital in controlling convulsive status epilepticus and acute prolonged convulsive seizures in children: A randomised trial. Eur J Paediatr Neurol 2012;16:536–41.

84. Liu X, Wu Y, Chen Z, Ma M, Su L. A systematic review of randomized controlled trials on the theraputic effect of intravenous sodium valproate in status epilepticus. Int J Neurosci. 2012; 122:277–83.

85. Mehta V, Singhi P, Singhi S. Intravenous sodium valproate versus diazepam infusion for the control of refractory status epilepticus in children: A randomized controlled trial. J Child Neurol 2007;22:1191–7.

86. Cock HR; ESETT Group. Established status epilepticus treatment trial (ESETT). Epilepsia. 2011;52:50–2.

87. Owens J. Medical management of refractory status epilepticus. Semin Pediatr Neurol. 2010; 17:176–81.

88. Mayer SA, Claassen J, Lokin J, Mendelsohn F, Dennis LJ, Fitzsimmons BF. Refractory status epilepticus: Frequency, risk factors, and impact on outcome. Arch Neurol 2002;59:205–10.

89. Stecker MM, Kramer TH, Raps EC, O'Meeghan R, Dulaney E, Skaar DJ. Treatment of refractory status epilepticus with propofol: Clinical and pharmacokinetic findings. Epilepsia 1998;39: 18–26.

90. Sánchez Fernández I, Abend NS, Agadi S, An S, Arya R, Carpenter JL, et al. Gaps and opportunities in refractory status epilepticus research in children: A multi-center approach by the Pediatric Status Epilepticus Research Group [pSERG]. Seizure 2014;23:87–97.

91. Abend NS, Dlugos DJ. Treatment of refractory status epilepticus: Literature review and a proposed protocol. Pediatr Neurol 2008;38: 377–90.

92. Drislane FW, Blum AS, Lopez MR, Gautam S, Schomer DL. Duration of refractory status epilepticus and outcome: Loss of prognostic utility after several hours. Epilepsia. 2009;50: 1566–71.

93. Holtkamp M, Othman J, Buchheim K, Meierkord H. Predictors and prognosis of refractory status epilepticus treated in a neurological intensive care unit. J Neurol Neurosurg Psychiatry 2005; 76:534–9.

94. Wilkes R, Tasker RC. Pediatric intensive care treatment of uncontrolled status epilepticus. Crit Care Clin 2013;29:239–57.

95. Capovilla G, Beccaria F, Beghi E, Minicucci F, Sartori S, Vecchi M. Treatment of convulsive status epilepticus in childhood: recommendations of the Italian League Against Epilepsy. Epilepsia 2013;54:23–34.

96. Shiloh-Malawsky Y, Fan Z, Greenwood R, Tennison M. Successful treatment of childhood prolonged refractory status epilepticus with lacosamide. Seizure 2011;20:586–8.

97. Wilkes R, Tasker RC. Intensive care treatment of uncontrolled status epilepticus in children: Systematic literature search of midazolam and anesthetic therapies. Pediatr Crit Care Med. 2014 Jun 3. [Epub ahead of print]

98. Koul R, Chacko A, Javed H, Al Riyami K. Eight-year study of childhood status epilepticus: Midazolam infusion in management and outcome. J Child Neurol 2000;17:908–10.

99. Morrison G, Gibbons E, Whitehouse WP. High-dose midazolam therapy for refractory status epilepticus in children. Intensive Care Med 2006;32:2070–6.

100. Raj D, Gulati S, Lodha R. Status epilepticus. Indian J Pediatr 2011;78:219–26.

101. Holmes GL, Riviello JJ Jr. Midazolam and pento-barbital for refractory status epilepticus. Pediatr Neurol 1999;20:259–64.

102. Shorvon S, Ferlisi M. The treatment of super-refractory status epilepticus: a critical review of available therapies and a clinical treatment protocol. Brain 2011;134:2802–18.

103. Ferlisi M, Shorvon S. The outcome of therapies in refractory and super-refractory convulsive status epilepticus and recommendations for therapy. Brain. 2012;135:2314-28.

104. Rosati A, L'Erario M, Ilvento L, Cecchi C, Pisano T, Mirabile L, Guerrini R. Efficacy and safety of ketamine in refractory status epilepticus in children. Neurology 2012;79:2355–8.

105. Mirsattari SM, Sharpe MD, Young GB. Treatment of refractory status epilepticus with inhalational anesthetic agents isoflurane and desflurane. Arch Neurol 2004;61:1254–9.

106. Visser NA, Braun KP, Leijten FS, van Nieuwenhuizen O, Wokke JH, van den Bergh WM. Magnesium treatment for patients with refractory status epilepticus due to POLG1-mutations. J Neurol 2011;258:218–22.

107. Cobo NH, Sankar R, Murata KK, Sewak SL, Kezele MA, Matsumoto JH. The ketogenic diet as broad-spectrum treatment for super-refractory pediatric status epilepticus: challenges in implementation in the Pediatric and Neonatal Intensive Care Units. J Child Neurol. 2014 Jan 23. [Epub ahead of print]

108. Guilliams K, Rosen M, Buttram S, Zempel J, Pineda J, Miller B, Shoykhet M. Hypothermia for pediatric refractory status epilepticus. Epilepsia. 2013;54:1586–94.

109. Lambrecq V, Villéga F, Marchal C, Michel V, Guehl D, Rotge JY, Burbaud P. Refractory status epilepticus: electroconvulsive therapy as a possible therapeutic strategy. Seizure 2012;21:661–4.

110. Köhrmann M, Huttner HB, Gotthardt D, Nagel S, Berger C, Schwab S. CSF-air-exchange for pharmacorefractory status epilepticus. J Neurol 2006;253:1100–1.

111. Vendrame M, Loddenkemper T. Surgical treatment of refractory status epilepticus in children: candidate selection and outcome. Semin Pediatr Neurol 2010;17:182–9.

112. Hesdorffer DC, Shinnar S, Lewis DV, Nordli DR, Pellock JM, Moshe SL, Shinnar RC, et al. for the FEBSTAT Study Team. Risk factors for febrile status epilepticus: A case-control study. J Pediatr 2013;163:1147–51.

113. Berg AT, Shinnar S. Complex febrile seizures. Epilepsia 1996;37:126–33.

114. Nishiyama I, Ohtsuka Y, Tsuda T, Kobayashi K, Inoue H, Narahara K, et al. An epidemiological study of children with status epilepticus in Okayama, Japan: incidence, etiologies, and outcomes. Epilepsy Res 2011;96:89–95.

115. Theodore WH, Epstein L, Gaillard WD, Shinnar S, Wainwright MS, Jacobson S. Human herpes virus 6B: a possible role in epilepsy? Epilepsia 2008;49:1828–37.

116. Ismail S, Lévy A, Tikkanen H, Sévère M, Wolters FJ, Carmant L. Lack of efficacy of phenytoin in children presenting with febrile status epilepticus. Am J Emerg Med 2012;30:2000–4.

117. Shinnar S, Berg AT, Moshe SL, O'Dell C, Alemany M, Newstein D, et al. The risk of seizure recurrence after a first unprovoked afebrile seizure in childhood: an extended follow-up. Pediatrics. 1996;98:216–25.

Chapter

28

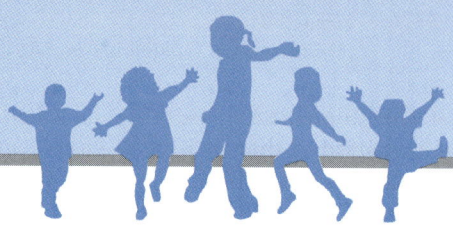

Infant and Young Child Feeding Guidelines, 2016

Satish Tiwari, Ketan Bharadva, Balraj Yadav, Sushma Malik, Prashant Gangal, CR Banapurmath, Zeeba Zaka-Ur-Rab, Urmila Deshmukh, Visheshkumar, RK Agrawal

The under-five population of India stands at a staggering 112.8 million.[1] However, despite all the advances in health, education and agriculture sectors as well as vast improvements in the country's economy, India figures in the list of countries that have made insufficient progress towards meeting the Millennium Development Goals.[2] It has the largest numbers of under-five children who are moderately or severely stunted, accounting for 38% of the global burden. India also has the highest numbers of children with moderate and severe wasting.

According to National Family Health Survey-3 data, about 20 million children are not able to receive exclusive breastfeeding (EBF) for the first 6 months, and about 13 million do not get good, timely and appropriate complementary feeding along with continued breastfeeding. Over the past several years, India has failed to witness any remarkable progress in infant feeding practices, with only a small increment being recorded in EBF rates amongst infants 0–6 months of age–from 41.2% in 1998–99 (NFHS-2) to 46.3%% in 2005–2006 (NFHS-3).[3] The rate of early initiation of breastfeeding stands abysmally low at 24.5%, while the median duration of EBF among last-born children is as brief as two months. Further, the rate of EBF drops

progressively from 51% at 2–3 months of age to 28% at 4–5 months of age. In a recent Annual Health Survey conducted in India from 2010 to 2013 covering all the 284 districts (as per 2011 census) of 8 Empowered Action Group (EAG) States (Bihar, Uttar Pradesh, Uttarakhand, Jharkhand, Madhya Pradesh, Chhattisgarh, Odisha and Rajasthan) and Assam,[4] the percentage of children breastfed within one hour of birth was observed to vary from 30% in Bihar and Uttar Pradesh to around 70% in Assam and Odisha. Children exclusively breastfed for at least 6 months ranged from 17.7% in UP to 47.5% in Chhattisgarh. Complementary feeding is introduced in only 53% infants between 6–8 months, with only about 44% of breastfed children being fed at least the minimum number of times recommended.[3] Overall, only 21% of breastfeeding and non-breastfeeding children are fed in accordance with the infant and young child feeding (IYCF) recommendations.

TECHNICAL GUIDELINES

Breastfeeding

WHO/UNICEF have emphasized the first 1000 days of life, i.e. the 270 days *in utero* and the first two years after birth as the critical window period for nutritional interventions.

As the maximal brain growth occurs, malnutrition in this critical period can lead to stunting and suboptimal developmental outcome. The optimal and appropriate infant and young child nutrition practices and strategies are enumerated in Box 28.1; the others are:

a. Breastfeeding should be promoted as the gold standard feeding options.

b. Antenatal counseling individually or in groups organized by maternity facility or mother support group (MSG) should prepare expectant mothers for successful breastfeeding.

c. For all normal newborns (including those by caesarean section) skin-to-skin contact should be initiated in about 5 minutes of birth in order that baby initiates breast-feeding in an hour of birth. The method of 'Breast crawl' can be adopted for early initiation.[5] In case of operative birth, the mother may need extra motivation and support. Skin-to-skin contact between the mother and new born should be encouraged by 'bedding in the mother and baby pair'. Mother should communicate, look into the eyes, touch and caress the baby while feeding. The new born should be kept warm by promoting Kangaroo Mother Care and promoting local practices to keep the room warm.[6]

d. Baby should be fed "on cues". The early feeding cues include sucking movements and sucking sounds, hand to mouth movements, rapid eye movements, soft cooing or sighing sounds, lip smacking, restlessness, etc. Crying is a late cue and may interfere with successful feeding. Babies should be breastfed at least 8 to 10 times in 24 hours till lactation is established (1 to 2 weeks) indicated by frequent urination, stooling and adequate weight gain. A sleepy baby can be easily woken up by removing blankets, removing clothes, changing loin cloth if wet, skin-to-skin contact in kangaroo position and gently massaging the back and the limbs. Periodic feeding is practiced in certain situations like in the case of a very small infant who is likely to become hypo-glycemic unless fed regularly, or an infant who 'does not demand' milk in initial few days. Adequacy of breastfeeding in this critical period should be monitored by clinical parameters complemented by weighing on digital weighing scale (minimum sensitivity of 5 g) on Day 1, 4, 7, 14 and 28. Maternity service should have a protocol to manage post-discharge follow ups along with protocols for management of excessive weight loss (>10%) and weight-faltering.

e. Every mother, especially the primipara, should receive support from doctors, nursing staff or community health workers (in case of non-institutional birth) with regards to correct positioning, latching and treatment of problems, such as engorge-ment, nipple fissures and delayed 'coming-in' of milk. If available, dedicated skilled supports like Lactation Consultants/Mother Support Counselors/Peer Coun-selors should be facilitated to support the mother in the antenatal, immediate postnatal period, post discharge follow-ups and in neonatal care units.

f. Mothers need skilled help and confidence-building during all health contacts and at home through home visits by trained community worker, especially after the baby is 3 to 4 months when a mother may begin to doubt her ability to fulfill the growing needs and demands of baby.

Box 28.1: The optimal and appropriate infant and young child nutrition practices and strategies

- EBF should be practiced till end of 6 months (180 days).
- After completion of 6 months, introduction of optimal complementary feeding should be practiced preferably with energy dense, home-made food.
- Breastfeeding should be continued minimum for 2 years and beyond.
- Mother should communicate, look into the eyes, touch and caress the baby while feeding. Practice responsive feeding.
- WHO Growth Charts recommended for monitoring growth.

g. The main reason given by majority of working mothers for stopping breast-feeding is their return to work following the maternity leave. Mothers who work outside should be assisted with obtaining adequate Maternity/Baby Care/Breastfeeding leave, should be encouraged to continue EBF for 6 months by expressing milk while they are out at work. They may be encouraged to carry the baby to a work place/crèche wherever such facility exists. The concept of "Hirkani's rooms" may be considered at work places (Hirkani's rooms are specially allocated room at the workplace where working mothers can express milk and store in a refrigerator during their work schedule). Every such mother leaving the maternity facility should be taught manual expression of her breast milk; however, for a working mother, this skill would prove invaluable.

h. If the breastfeeding was temporarily dis-continued due to an inadvertent situation, re-lactation should be tried as soon as possible.[7] Supplemental Suckling Tech-nique (SST) is a technique which can be used as a strategy to initiate re-lactation in mothers who have developed lactation failure or Mother's Milk Insufficiency (MMI). WHO recommends re-lactation through Supplemental Suckling technique. The drip and drop method helps to sustain the infant's interest of suckling at the breast.[8]

i. The possibility of induced lactation shall be explored according to the situation, e.g. adoption, surrogacy. It helps to create mother-infant bonding apart from security and comfort for the baby. The technique involves motivating the surrogate mother, having a willing and vigorously sucking infant, and an adequate support group. Prolactin and oxytocin, the hormones which govern lactation, are pituitary and not ovarian. Hence, stimulation of nipple and areola and repeated suckling by the baby are important. Lact-aid as nursing trainer is

also useful.[9] A course of prolactin enhancing drugs such as Metoclopromide or Dom-peridone is initiated.[10] Non-puerperal lactation in surrogate mothers has been successfully demonstrated among Indian mothers.[11]

j. Nursing in Public (NIP): Mothers should feel comfortable to nurse in public. All efforts should be taken to remove hurdles impeding breastfeeding in public places, special areas/rooms shall be identified/constructed or established in places like Bus stands, Railway stations, Air ports etc.

k. Adoption of latest WHO Growth Charts is recommended for monitoring growth.[12]

Complementary Feeding[13]

a. Appropriately thick homogenous comple-mentary foods home-made from locally available foods should be introduced at six completed months while continuing breast-feeding ad libitum.[14,15] During this period, breastfeeding should be actively supported and the term 'weaning' should be avoided.[16] Complementary feeding should be projected as the bridge that the mother has to make between liquid to solid transition and to empower the baby to 'family pot feeding'.

b. To address the issue of a small stomach size, each meal must be made energy dense by adding sugar/jaggery and ghee/butter/oil. To provide more calories from smaller volumes, food must be thick in consistency– thick enough to stay on the spoon without running off, when the spoon is tilted[17]

c. Foods can be enriched by making a fermented porridge, use of germinated or sprouted flour and toasting of grains before grinding.[16,18]

d. Adequate total energy intake can also be ensured by addition of one to two nutritious snacks between the three main meals. Snacks are in addition and should not replace meals. They should not to be con-fused with foods such as sweets, chips or other processed foods.[18]

e. Parents must identify the staple homemade food (as these are fresh, clean and cheap), comprising of cereal-pulse mixture in the ratio 2:1, and make them caloric and nutrient rich with locally available products.

f. Research has time and again proved the disadvantages of bottle feeding. Hence bottle feeding shall be discouraged at all levels.

g. The food should be a balanced diet consisting of various (as diverse as possible) food groups/components in different combinations. Easily available, cost-effective seasonal uncooked fruits, green and other dark colored vegetables, milk and milk products, pulses/legumes, animal foods, oil/butter, sugar/jaggery may be added in the staples gradually.[16,17]

h. Hygienic practices are essential for food safety during all the involved steps viz. preparation, storage and feeding. Hand washing with soap and water at critical times- including before eating or preparing food and after using the toilet.[17,18]

i. Practice responsive feeding. Self-feeding should be encouraged despite spillage. Each child should be fed under supervision in a separate plate to develop an individual identity. Forced feeding, threatening and punishment interfere with development of good/proper feeding habits.[17] Along with feeding, mother and care givers should provide psycho-social stimulation to the child through ordinary age-appropriate play and communication activities to ensure early childhood development.

j. Consistency of foods should be appropriate to the developmental readiness of the child in munching, chewing and swallowing. 'Neophobia' is the rule in them and any item may have to be offered several times for acceptance. Avoid foods which can pose choking hazard. Introduce lumpy or granular foods and most tastes by about 9 to 10 months. The details of food including; texture, frequency and average amount are summarized in Table 28.1.

HIV AND INFANT FEEDING

The following guidelines of HIV and infant feeding are based on recommendations given by WHO and NACO in 2013:

a. The best time to counsel HIV-positive mothers is during antenatal period. They should be informed about infant feeding options, *viz.* exclusive breastfeeding or exclusive replacement feeding that is recommended by the national authority so to improve HIV free survival of exposed infants. Exclusive breastfeeding is superior to exclusive replacement feeding in developing countries because it maximizes the chances of survival of the infant.[20]

b. Prevention of parent-to-child transmission (PPTCT) interventions should begin early in the pregnancy for all HIV infected pregnant women.[21]

c. In resource-limited settings, HIV-infected mothers of HIV-uninfected infants often have difficulty in deciding about feeding options, breastfeeding risks transmission of HIV to their infants and formula feeding is not always a feasible option due to high cost, lack of clean water or stigma associated with not breastfeeding. Recent clinical studies have proven that the risk of transmission through breastfeeding is minimal provided mother and the infant receive appropriate antiretroviral prophylaxis.

d. WHO 2013 guidelines recommend two options:
   - Providing lifelong antiretroviral treatment (ART) (one simplified triple regimen) to all pregnant and breastfeeding women regardless of CD4 count or clinical stage.
   - To provide ART to pregnant and breastfeeding women with HIV during the period of risk of mother-to-child HIV transmission and then continuing lifelong ART only for those women who are eligible according to their own health.[20,22]

TABLE 28.1: Options or treatment plans if mother is known to be HIV exposed

	Mother Exposed to HIV					
	Infant uninfected/status unknown	Mother diagnosed during labor/post-partum		Infant diagnosed after birth		Mother's ART regimen getting interrupted
			Not breastfeeding		Not breastfeeding	
EBF	Six months	Six months	Not breastfeeding	Six months	Not breastfeeding	EBF Six months
Complementary feeding	Start at six months	Start at six months	Start at six months	Start at six months	Start at six months	Start at six months
Maternal ART	Yes	Yes	Yes	Yes	Yes	Counseling for regular ART. Consider alternative ART.
Infant	NVP	NVP	NVP	NVP	No NVP	NVP six weeks after restarting.
Prophylaxis	Six weeks	Twelve weeks	Six weeks	Twelve weeks		Maternal ART.
Continue breast-feeding	Yes, For 1 year in EID negative infants	Yes, For 1 year in EID negative infants and 2 years for EID positive infants	No BF	Yes, For 2 years for EID positive infants	No BF	Yes, For 1 year in EID negative infants and 2 years for EID positive infants
Infant evaluation and treatment	EID: Do DBS (Dried Blood Spot) for DNA/PCR at 6 weeks for all HIV exposed babies; if positive do WBS (Whole blood specimen). If WBS positive, start Paediatric ART irrespective of CD4% for babies less than 2 years. Final confirmation of the HIV status in the baby should be done at 18 months by doing all 3 Rapid Tests irrespective of earlier EID status					

EBF: exclusive breastfeeding; NVP: Nevirapine; ART: Antiretroviral treatment; EID: early infant diagnosis

e. The global target is "elimination of new HIV infections among children" by 2015 and government of India is actively working towards it. Following the new guidelines from WHO (June 2013), National AIDS control organization (NACO) has decided to provide life-long ART (triple drug regimen) to all pregnant and breastfeeding women living with HIV. With this step, all pregnant women living with HIV should receive a triple drug ART regimen regardless of CD4 count or WHO clinical stage. This would also help in increasing the coverage for those needing treatment to keep them alive and for their own health, avoiding stopping and starting drugs with repeat pregnancies, provide early protection against mother-to-child transmission in future pregnancies and avoiding drug resistance. These recommendations can potentially reduce the risk of mother-to-child-transmission to less than 5% in breast-feeding populations. These guidelines have been implemented across India from January, 2014.[21]

f. Providing an optimized, fixed-dose combination once daily first-line ARV regimen of Tenofovir (TDF), Lamivudine (3TC) (or Emtricitabine [FTC]) and Efavirenz (EFZ) to all pregnant and breastfeeding women HIV has important programmatic and clinical benefits. Where access to CD4 testing is limited, WHO prefers that all pregnant and breastfeeding HIV-infected women, regardless of CD4 cell count, should continue antiretroviral treatment for life (sometimes called "Option B+").[22-24]

g. Exclusive breastfeeding is the recommended infant feeding choice in the first 6 months, irrespective of the fact that mother is on ART early or infant is provided with anti-retroviral prophylaxis for 6 weeks.

h. No Mixed Feeding is to be done during the first 6 months.

i. Mothers known to be infected with HIV and whose infants are HIV uninfected or of unknown HIV status should exclusively breastfeed their infants. Complementary foods should be appropriately introduced thereafter, and breastfeeding should be continued for the first 12 months of life. Initiate maternal ART and give Nevirapine (NVP) for 6 weeks. The treatment options, if mother is known to be infected with HIV, are presented in Table 28.2.

j. Mothers known to be infected with HIV and whose infants are HIV infected should exclusively breastfeed for the first 6 months of life, complementary foods

TABLE 28.2: Amounts of foods to offer [18,19]

Age	Texture	Frequency	Average amount each meal
6–8 months	Start with thick porridge, well mashed foods	2–3 meals per day plus frequent BF	Start with 2–3 table spoonfuls
9–11 months	Finely chopped or mashed foods, and foods that baby can pick up	3–4 meals plus BF. Depending on appetite offer 1–2 snacks	1/2 of a 250 mL cup/ bowl
12–23 months	Family foods, chopped or mashed if necessary	3–4 meals plus BF. Depending on appetite offer 1–2 snacks	3/4 to one 250 mL cup/bowl

If baby is not breastfed, give in addition: 1-2 cups of milk per day, and 1–2 extra meals per day.

The amounts of food included in the table are recommended when the energy density of the meals is about 0.8 to 1.0 kcal/g. If the energy density of the meals is about 0.6 Kcal/g, recommend to increase the energy density of the meal (adding special foods) or increase the amount of food per meal. Find out what the energy content of complementary foods is in your setting and adapt the table accordingly.

should be appropriately introduced thereafter, and breastfeeding should be continued for 24 months of life. Initiate maternal ART and give NVP for 6 weeks.

k. Mothers who are diagnosed with HIV during labor or in the immediate post-partum period and are planning to breast-feed, such mothers should be initiated on ART and their infants should receive extended NVP prophylaxis for 12 weeks.

l. Mothers who are diagnosed with HIV during labor or in the immediate post-partum period and are planning exclusive replacement feeding (ERF) should be referred for evaluation and treatment of HIV. Infants of these mothers should be given NVP prophylaxis for 6 weeks.

m. Mothers who are HIV-infected and insist on not breastfeeding and opt for exclusive replacement feeding (ERF) should be explained that they are doing so at their own risk and this is contrary to the WHO/NACO's guidelines of giving exclusive breastfeeds. When taking choice for exclusive replacement feeding, they should fulfill the AFASS (A – Affordable F – Feasible A – Acceptable S – Sustainable S – Safe) criteria.[21] Explain the advantages of ERF as (i) No risk of HIV transmission; and (ii) ERF milk can be given by other persons. Also enumerate the disadvantages like (i) Animal milk is not a complete food for baby; (ii) Formula milk may be complete but is expensive; (iii) Baby has more risk of infections—diarrhea, respiratory and ear infection and malnutrition; and (iv) Careful and hygienic preparation required each time to sterilize feeding cups, using boiled water and fresh preparation of all feeds 12–15 times in the first 4 months of baby's life.

n. Mother who is receiving ART but interrupts ART regimen while breastfeeding (due to toxicity, stock-outs or refusal to continue etc); determine an alternative ART regimen or solution for mother and counsel her regarding continuing ART

without interruption. NVP should be given to infant until 6 weeks after maternal ART is restarted or until 1 week after breastfeeding has ended.

o. The preferred feeding option for HIV-exposed infants <6 months of age is exclusive breastfeeding. However, in certain situations like maternal death and severe maternal illness breastfeeding may not be possible, in such cases ERF should be done only when AFASS criteria is fulfilled.

p. Breastfeeding should stop once a nutritionally adequate and safe diet without breast milk can be provided. Breastfeeding should not be stopped abruptly. Gradually wean from breast milk over a one month period.

q. Mothers known to be HIV infected may consider expressing and heat-treating breast milk as an interim feeding strategy in special circumstances such as:

- When the infant is born with low birth weight or is otherwise ill in the neonatal period and unable to breastfeed; or
- When the mother is unwell and temporarily unable to breastfeed or has a temporary breast health problem such as mastitis; or if antiretroviral drugs are temporarily not available.

r. Nevirapine should be given as prophylaxis for 6 weeks daily to infants of HIV-infected mothers who are receiving ART and are breastfeeding. Those infants who are receiving replacement feeding should be given four to 6 weeks of infant prophylaxis with daily NVP [or twice-daily Zidovudine (AZT)]. Infant prophylaxis should begin at birth or when HIV exposure is recognized postpartum.[20,21] The recommended dose of Nevirapine is shown in Table 28.3.

s. Infants who are identified as HIV–exposed after birth (through infant testing [at 6 weeks or after] or maternal HIV antibody testing) and are breastfeeding, in such cases maternal ART should be

TABLE 28.3: Doses of nevirapine

Infant age	Dose
Birth to 6 wks (Birth weight 2000–2499 g)	10 mg once daily
Birth to 6 wks (Birth weight ≥2500 g)	15 mg once daily
>6 wks to 6 mo	20 mg once daily
>6 mo to 9 mo	30 mg once daily
>9 mo to end of breastfeeding	40 mg once daily

initiated and the infant should receive NVP prophylaxis. Perform infant DNA/PCR test if child is 6 weeks or older, immediately initiate 6 weeks or longer of NVP and strongly consider extending this to 12 weeks. The treatment options and baby's HIV status is discussed in Table 28.4.

t. Infant identified as HIV-exposed after birth (through infant or maternal HIV antibody testing) and are not breastfeeding. Refer mother to ART Centre after CD4 tests and baseline test and treatment should be started. No NVP needs to be given to infants. Do HIV DNA/PCR test in accordance with national recommendations on early infant diagnosis and initiate treatment if the infant is infected.

u. For breastfeeding infants who have been diagnosed HIV positive, pediatric ART should be started and breastfeeding to be continued ideally until the baby is 2 years old.[25]

v. For breastfeeding infants, diagnosed HIV-negative, breastfeeding should be continued until 12 months of age ensuring the mother is on ART as soon as possible. The Early Infant diagnosis (EID) is repeated for the 3rd time (when previous 2 EIDs have been negative) after 6 weeks of stopping breast feeds. If rapid test is positive, then do Dried Blood Spot (DBS). If DBS is positive, then do, Whole Blood Sample (WBS) test. If WBS test is positive, Pediatric ART should be initiated. However, confirmation test for HIV has to be done at 18 months using 3 rapid antibody tests for all babies irrespective of the earlier EID status or the fact that Pediatric ART has already been initiated.

Concept and Need of Human Milk Banks in India

a. Human Milk Banks should be promoted considering the large number of babies needing pasteurized donor human milk when mother's own milk is not available. In 1980 the WHO and UNICEF jointly declared: "Where it is not possible for the biological mother to breastfeed, the first alternative, if available, should be the use of human milk from other sources".[26]

TABLE 28.4: Options for HIV exposed babies after birth

	HIV negative	HIV positive
Breastfeeding	Exclusive breastfeeding for six months Continue breastfeeding for one year. The stoppage of breastfeeding after one year should be gradual and not abruptly	Exclusive breastfeeding for six months Continue breastfeeding for two years The stoppage of breastfeeding should be gradual and not abruptly
Complementary	At six months	At six months feeding
NVP Prophylaxis	NVP for 6 weeks extending to twelve weeks if breastfeeding	NVP for 6 weeks if breastfeeding No NVP if not breastfeeding
ART	ART to mother only and NVP prophylaxis to they baby	ART to mother and start Pediatric ART also

ART: antiretroviral treatment; NVP: Nevirapine

b. Cost effectiveness of using banked human milk in neonatal intensive care units has been documented in Western countries, largely due to reduction in rates of necrotizing enterocolitis,[27,28] reduction in severe infections[29,31] and decreased length of hospital stay.[32] Given the high incidence of sepsis and a large burden of premature births, this intervention has a potential to result in substantial saving for the nation in terms of finances and human capital.

c. Presence of human milk bank is also a factor promoting breastfeeding.

- Use of pasturized donor human milk in NICU is associated with increased breastfeeding rate at discharge from the hospital for very low birth weight (VLBW) infants.[33]
- The novel approach of promoting human milk banks through mode of collecting breast milk donations in form of camps can be a strong means of promoting breastfeeding in the society.

d. It is recommended that there should be a human milk bank in each sick newborn care units (SNCU) and neonatal ICU initially preferably in government set-up, and subsequently in private and corporate sectors.

Feeding in Other Specific Situations

a. Feeding during sickness is important for recovery and for prevention of under nutrition. Even sick babies mostly continue to breastfeed and the infant can be encouraged to eat small quantities of nutrient rich food more frequently and by offering foods that the child likes to eat.

b. Infant feeding in maternal illnesses

- Painful and/or infective breast conditions like breast abscess, mastitis and psychiatric illnesses which pose a danger to the child's life, e.g. postpartum psychosis, schizophrenia may need a temporary cessation of breastfeeding.
- Chronic infections like tuberculosis, leprosy, or medical conditions like hypothyroidism need treatment of the primary condition and do not warrant discontinuation of breastfeeding.

- Breastfeeding is contraindicated when the mother is receiving certain drugs like anti-neoplastic agents, immuno-suppressants, antithyroid drugs like thiouracil, amphetamines, gold salts, etc. Breastfeeding may be avoided or continued with caution when the mother is receiving following drugs–atropine, reserpine, psychotropic drugs. Other drugs like antibiotics, anesthetics, antiepileptics, antihistamines, digoxin, diuretics, prednisone, propranolol etc. are considered safe for breastfeeding.[34]

c. Infant feeding in various conditions related to the infant

- Breastfeeding on demand should be promoted in normal active babies. However, in difficult situations like VLBW, sick, or depressed babies, alternative methods of feeding can be used based on neuro-developmental status. These include feeding expressed breastmilk through intra-gastric tube or with the use of cup and spoon. For very sick babies, expert guidance should be sought. If the baby is transferred to SNCU/NICU, mothers should be supported to start breastmilk expression within initial hours, continue at least 3 hourly during the day time and at least once at night.

- Ensure early transfer of mothers with the baby in SNCU/NICU and that has arrangement to accommodate the mothers in the immediate vicinity and that mothers are permitted to visit, hold and touch the baby at will if the baby's condition permits.

- Ensure that majority of babies are on exclusive breastfeeding or on breastfeeding plus expressed breastmilk at discharge from the SNCU/NICU.

- Gastro-Esophageal Reflux Disease (GERD) is often treated conservatively when it is mild, through thickening of the complementary foods, frequent small feeds and upright positioning for 30 minutes after feeds.

- Primary Lactose Intolerance is congenital and may require long term lactose restriction. Secondary Lactose Intolerance is usually transient and resolves after the underlying condition has remitted. Most of the cases of diarrhea do not require stoppage of breastfeeding.

- Various Inborn Errors of Metabolism warrant restriction of specific offending agent and certain dietary modifications e.g. in galactosemia, dietary lactose and galactose should be avoided. This is probably the only absolute contraindication to breastfeeding.

- During emergencies, priority health and nutrition support should be arranged for pregnant and lactating mothers. Donated or subsidized supplies of breastmilk substitutes (e.g. infant formula) should be avoided, must never be included in a general ration distribution, and must be distributed, if at all, only according to well-defined strict criteria. Donations of bottles and teats should be refused, and their use actively avoided.

Micronutrient in Infant Feeding

a. Breastmilk has usually adequate amount of iron, calcium, phosphorus and vitamin A for a normal newborn. Preterm infants who are breastfed should receive 2 mg of supplemental iron per kg of body weight each day after one month of age.[35] Preterm and low birth weight infants may also need calcium and multivitamin supplements.

b. Breastfed infants can maintain normal vitamin D status in the early post-natal period only when their mother's vitamin D status is normal and/or the infants are exposed to adequate amount of sunlight. Corroborative evidences of high prevalence of vitamin D deficiency in Indian infants suggest that they should be given routine vitamin D supplementation of 400 IU daily, especially in those with higher risk of getting less of vitamin D. Even those on formula feed needs supplementation unless they consume more than 1000 mL of formula daily.[36,37] VLBW infants should be given vitamin D supplements at a dose ranging from 400 to 1000 IU per day until six months of age.[38]

c. Food items that supply micronutrients should be encouraged like GYOR (green, yellow, orange and red) vegetables and fruits, Use of food fortification like iron-fortified foods, iodized salt, vitamin A enriched food etc. are to be encouraged.

Junk Food and Infant Feeding

a. Consumers are often bewildered by nutritive and health claims, while children are highly influenced by advertisements enticing them to buy a product which may be unhealthy or in fact detrimental.[39]

b. The parents should understand that though the companies are promoting many foods as "Magic food" in reality such products do not exist.

c. Avoid Junk and Commercial food which are high in SSFAP (sugar, salt, fat, additives/preservatives and pesticides). Avoid giving ready-made, processed commercial food from the market.

d. Junk foods are one of the important reasons for the increasing incidence of childhood obesity. There is need to restrict consumpion of junk food especially in and around educational institutions and remote areas of the country.

e. The provisions of The Food Safety and Standards Act 2006 should be implemented and monitored regularly.[40]

Maternal Nutrition

a. In India, 22% babies born each year have low birth weight (LBW), which has been linked to maternal under-nutrition and anemia among other causes. Half of adolescents (boys and girls) have below normal body mass index (BMI) and almost 56% of adolescent girls aged 15–19 years have anemia.

b. Optimal nutrition of adolescent girls, pre-pregnant women and pregnant mothers is critical to intrauterine growth, fetal well-being and to prevent malnutrition in the postnatal period.[41]

c. There is growing evidence that maternal nutritional status can alter the epigenetic state (stable alterations of gene expressions through DNA methylation and histone modifications) of the fetal genome. This may provide a molecular mechanism for the impact of maternal nutrition on both fetal programming and genomic imprinting. Just as the damaging effects of malnutrition, pass from one generation to the next, so can benefits of good nutrition.[42]

d. The maternal nutrition should also be balanced, fresh and preferably home-made and there should not be any unscientific restrictions.

OPERATIONAL GUIDELINES

Recommendations for Governmental and International Agencies

a. Global legislation, binding to all states and private organizations including labor benefits, 6 months maternity and appro-priate paternity leave is strongly recom-mended. Maternity leave, day care facilities and paid breastfeeding breaks should be available to all employed women in all sectors including those engaged in atypical forms of dependent work.

b. Breastfeeding is a human right both for the mother as well as baby. With due weightage and respect to National Family Planning Policies and Program, the benefits should be given to mother and the child (even after 2 issues) born out of unplanned pregnancy (Family planning method failure) or as a result of accidental death of previous child.

c. Scientific and unbiased IYCF practices must be promoted through regular advertise-ments in state, public or private owned audiovisual and print media. Public should be made aware that artificial, junk or packaged food can be injurious to the health of the children.

d. Necessary and adequate arrangements should be made for propaganda and implementation of the provisions of Infant Milk Substitute (IMS) Act which prevents advertising or promoting infant milk substitutes, feeding bottles and teats. In addition, further strengthening of the existing Act must be tried.

e. Adopt a National policy to avoid conflict of interests in the areas of child health and nutrition. Popularization of "unscientific health claims" by commercial ads through media needs to be restricted. UN agencies shall help in promoting the home made/available food (especially through various media) with the help of their brand ambassadors/endorsers.

f. There should be a board, commission or committee to monitor, evaluate and censor food product before it is released in the market. Such board or committees shall have a sensitized pediatrician and/or other equivalent health care expert/ nutrition expert. A pediatrician shall also be involved in the commission/committee/board entrusted with drafting of any code, bill, laws, rules/regulations related to food, nutrition, drinks, food products, etc.

g. Human milk banks shall be promoted, established and maintained at least in District/Civil hospitals and Medical colleges.

Role of Non-Government Organizations

a. Various programs or community projects should be initiated to provide home care and counseling on IYCF through formation of mother support groups especially by women's organizations.

b. The voluntary organizations should understand and advocate important recommendations at all levels. Various like-minded organizations should work preferably on the same platform and co-ordinate with each-other in promoting the IYCF practices.

Recommendations for Media

The media can have a vital role to play in strengthening the knowledge chain, serving as a link between the stakeholders and the community as community is exposed to images, articles and ideas in innumerable ways from television, newspaper headlines, magazine covers, movies, websites, video games and road side signboards. Media has a great power but it is high time that it recognizes its responsibility towards child nutrition:

a. Media has to take concrete steps to avoid directly or indirectly glamorizing/promoting bottle feeding, artificial, commercial and ready to use food. Instead, the risks involved in artificial feeding and other suboptimal feeding practices should be advertised prominently in bold prints.

b. Media support is even more important on certain occasions, celebrations, and social mobilization activities such as World Breastfeeding Week and Nutrition Weeks.

c. The companies and media should have self-regulatory pledge for responsible advertising/marketing. They should help in promoting healthier dietary choices and a more active life style for Indian children.

d. Sportsman, celebrities should not promote various nutritional products; only evidence-based scientifically sound and authentic information shall be provided.

Recommendations for Training

a. It is recommended that all the community health workers, PPTCT counselors, and other personnel caring for children including doctors should undergo three days skill training on IYCF (including IMS Act). In situations where three day training is not feasible, some impact can be made with short duration sensitization programs of half day or one day.

b. IYCF should also be included in the curriculum of undergraduate and postgraduate medical education, nursing education, home science, child nutrition courses etc.

c. State, National and International level workshops on IYCN should be organized at regular intervals for capacity building of IYCN Resource Personnel.

d. In addition to above measures dedicated skilled breastfeeding (IYCN) support is critical to achieve IYCF goals. Hence there is a need to launch an ambitious program to create a spectrum of such resources (Lactation consultants, IYCF counselors and Peer counselors).

Baby Friendly Concepts

Baby Friendly Hospitals Initiatives (BFHI) is recommended to be spread to all especially medical college hospitals departments. The revised and expanded version of BFHI has been implemented by UNICEF and WHO in 2009.[43] BFHI was implemented partially in some states of India in 1992 but over the years it has not been reinforced or reevaluated. Strengthening of this initiative in the community would lead to better child survival.

Box 28.2 Summarises key recommendations related to infant and young child feeding.

Box 28.2: Key messages related to infant and young child nutrition

- Initiation of breastfeeding as early as possible after birth, preferably within one hour.
- Exclusive breastfeeding in the first six months of life and no other foods or fluids.
- Appropriate and adequate complementary feeding after completion of six months. Complementary foods should not be confused with supplementary foods.
- Hand washing with soap and water at critical times – including before eating or preparing food and after using the toilet.
- Avoid junk food. Home food should be preferred over artificial, commercial, tinned or packaged food.
- Promote and establish Human Milk Banks.
- Full immunization and Vitamin-A supplementation with deworming.
- Effective home based care and treatment of children suffering from severe acute malnutrition.
- Adequate nutrition and anemia control for adolescent girls, pregnant and lactating mothers.
- Effective implementation and monitoring of IMS Act and other laws related to child nutrition.

REFERENCES

1. C-14 Population in five year age-group by residence and sex. New Delhi; Office of the Registrar General and Census Commissioner, Ministry of Home Affairs, Government of India; 2011. Available from: http://www.censusindia.gov.in/2011census/C-series/C-14.html. Accessed July 11, 2015.

2. Improving Child Nutrition. The achievable imperative for global progress. New York: United Nations Children's Fund (UNICEF); c 2013. Available from: www.unicef.org/publications/index.html. Accessed July 11, 2015.

3. Arnold F, Parasuraman S, Arokiasamy P, Kothari M. Nutrition in India. National Family Health Survey (NFHS-3), India, 2005-06. Mumbai. Available from: hetv.org/india/nfhs/index.html. Accessed September 15, 2015.

4. Presentation on Annual Health Survey Fact Sheet Key Findings. New Delhi; Office of the Registrar General and Census Commissioner, Ministry of Home Affairs, Government of India; 2011. Available from: http://www.censusindia.gov.in/2011-Common/AHSurvey.html. Accessed July 11, 2015.

5. Ten steps to successful Breastfeeding- UNICEF/WHO Baby Friendly Hospital Initiative (BFHI). Initiation of breastfeeding by breast crawl. Available from: http://breastcrawl.org/10steps.shtml. Accessed September 15, 2015.

6. World Health Organization. Kangaroo Mother Care: A Practical Guide. Geneva: Department of Reproductive Health and Research, World Health Organization; 2003. Available from: http://www.who.int/maternal_child_adolescent/documents/9241590351/en/. Accessed Sept 15, 2015.

7. WHO. Relactation: review of experience and recommendations for Practice. Available from: http://www.who.int/maternal_child_adolescent/documents/who_chs_cah_98_14/en/. Accessed July 21, 2015.

8. Kesaree N. Drop and Drip method. Indian Pediatr 1993;30:277–8.

9. Auerbach KG, Avery JL. Induced Lactation: A study of adoptive nursing by 240 women. Am J Dis Child 1981;135:340–3.

10. Kramer P. Breastfeeding of adopted infants. Br Med J 1995:310:188.

11. Banapurmath CR, Banapurmath S, Kesaree N. Successful induced non-puerperal lactation in surrogate mothers. Indian J Pediatr 1993;60: 639–43.

12. WHO Child Growth Standards: Methods and Development: Length/height-for-age, weight-forage, weight-for-length, weight-for-height and body mass index-for-age. Geneva: World Health Organization; 2006. Available from: http://www.who.int/childgrowth/en/. Accessed Sept 15, 2015 .

13. Infant and Young Child Feeding: Model Chapter for Textbooks for Medical Students and Allied Health Professionals, Geneva: World Health Organization; 2009. Available from: http://www.ncbi.nlm.nih.gov/books/NBK148955/. Accessed September 15, 2015.

14. Dewey K, Lutter C. Guiding Principles for Complementary Feeding of the Breastfed Child. Washington DC, USA: PAHO/WHO, Division of Health Promotion and Protection/Food and Nutrition Program; 2003. Accessed September 15, 2015.

15. Report of the Expert Consultation of the Optimal Duration of Exclusive Breastfeeding. Geneva: World Health Organization; 2001.

16. Family Nutrition Guide. Burgess A, Glasauer P. Rome: Publishing Management Service, Information Division, Food and Agriculture Organization, Viale delle Terme di Caracalla; 2004.

17. Saadeh R, Martines J. Complementary Feeding: Family foods for Breastfed Children. Geneva: World Health Organization; 2000.

18. Teacher's Guide. Complementary Feeding Counseling: A Training Course. Geneva: World Health Organization; 2004.

19. Complementary Feeding: Report of the Global Consultation and Summary of Guiding Principles for Complementary Feeding of the Breastfed Child. Geneva: World Health Organization; 2002.

20. World Health Organization, Consolidated Guidelines on the Use of Antiretroviral Drugs for Treating and Preventing HIV Infection. Recommendations for a Public Health Approach, June 2013.

21. NACO-Updated Guidelines for Prevention of Parent to Child Transmission (PPTCT) of HIV using Multi Drug Anti-retroviral Regimen in India December, 2013.

22. World Health Organization (WHO) PMTCT Guidelines for Pregnant and Breastfeeding Women Living with HIV. Available from: www.avert.org/world-health-organisation - who-pmtct-guidelines.htm. Accessed September 15, 2015.

23. Global update on HIV treatment 2013: Results, Impact and Opportunities: WHO Report in Partnership with UNICEF and UNAIDS: June 2013.

24. NACO-ART guidelines for HIV-Infected Adults and Adolescents: May 2013.

25. Pediatric NACO Guidelines 2013. Available from: http://naco.gov.in/upload/2014%20mslns/CST/Pediatric_14-03-2014.pdf. Accessed Sept 15, 2015.

26. WHO/UNICEF meeting on infant and young child feeding. J Nurse Midwifery 2015;25:31–9.

27. Arnold LDW. The cost-effectiveness of using banked donor milk in the neonatal intensive care unit: prevention of necrotizing enterocolitis. J Hum Lact 2002;18:172-7.

28. Lucas A, Cole TJ. Breast milk and neonatal necrotizing enterocolitis. Lancet 1990;336:1519–23.

29. Hylander MA, Strobino DM, Dhanireddy R. Human milk feedings and infection among very low birth weight infants. Pediatrics 1998;102:E38.

30. El-Mohandes AE, Picard MB, Simmens SJ, Keiser JF. Use of human milk in the intensive care nursery decreases the incidence of nosocomial sepsis. J Perinatol 1997;17:130–4.

31. Narayanan I, Prakash K, Bala S, Verma RK, Gujral VV. Partial supplementation with expressed breast-milk for prevention of infection in low-birth-weight infants. Lancet 1980;2:561–3.

32. Schanler RJ, Shulman RJ, Lau C. Feeding strategies for premature infants: Beneficial outcomes of feeding fortified human milk versus preterm formula. Pediatrics 1999;103:1150–7.

33. Arslanoglu S, Moro GE, Bellu R, Turoli D, De NG, Tonetto P, et al. Presence of human milk bank is associated with elevated rate of exclusive breast-feeding in VLBW infants. J Perinat Med 2013;41: 129–31.

34. American Academy of Pediatrics. The transfer of drugs and other chemicals into human milk. Pediatrics 2001;108;776–89.

35. Armstrong C. Practice Guidelines, AAP Reports on Diagnosis and prevention of Iron deficiency anemia. Am Fam Physician 2011;83:624.

36. Jain V. Vitamin D deficiency in healthy breastfed term infants at 3 months and their mothers in India; seasonal variation and determinants. Indian J Med Res 2011;133;267–73.

37. Balasubramanian S, Vitamin D deficiency in breastfed infants and the need for routine vitamin D supplementation. Indian J Med Res 2011;133; 250–2.

38. Guidelines on Optimal Feeding of Low Birth Weight Infants in Low and Middle Income Countries. WHO 2011.

39. Tiwari S. Legislations and infant feeding. In: Gupte S, Editor; Text Book of Nutrition. New Delhi: Peepee brothers 2006;126–134.

40. Mallick MR. Food safety and Standards Act, 2006. In: Criminal Minor Acts. 1st edition New Delhi, Professional book publishers 2006;1549–80.

41. Sethi GR, Sachdev HPS, Puri RK. Women's health and fetal outcome. Indian Pediatr 1991;28: 1379–92.

42. Kuthe A, Shah PK, Patil V. Maternal nutrition and fetus. In: Bharadva K, Tiwari S, Chaturvedi P, Bang A, Agarwal RK (Eds). Feeding Fundamentals: A handbook on Infant and Young Child Nutrition. First edition, Jaipur Pedicon 2011; 27– 32.

43. Baby-Friendly Hospital Initiative. Revised Updated and Expanded for Integrated Care. Geneva: World Health Organization; 2009.

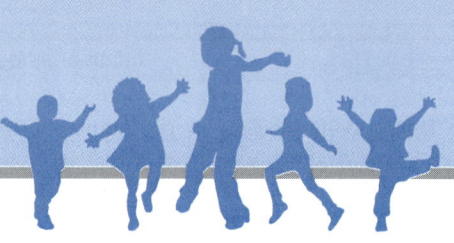

Human Milk Banking Guidelines

SKetan Bharadva, Satish Tiwari, Sudhir Mishra, Kanya Mukhopadhyay, Balraj Yadav,
RK Agarwal, Vishesh Kumar

Breastfeeding is the best method of infant feeding because human milk continues to be the only milk which is tailor-made and uniquely suited to the human infant. All mothers should be encouraged to breast-feed their infants. When a mother, for some reason, is unable to feed her infant directly, her breastmilk should be expressed and fed to the infant. If mother's own milk is unavailable or insufficient, the next best option is to use pasteurized donor human milk (PDHM). India faces its own unique challenges, having the highest number of low birth weight babies, and significant mortality and morbidity in very low birth weight (VLBW) population. In our country, the burden of low birth weight babies in various hospitals is about 20% with significant mortality and morbidities.[1,2] Feeding these babies with breastmilk can significantly reduce the risk of infections. Hence the Government, health experts and the civil society must join hands to propagate the concept of human milk banking for the sake of thousands of low birth weight and preterm babies.

Though wet nursing had been in practice since mythological ages, modern human milk banking is in its infancy in India. Lack of awareness, leadership deficit, infrastructural and maintenance costs, and fewer neonatal setups are some reasons for the same. The first milk bank in Asia under the name of Sneha, founded by Dr. Armeda Fernandez, was started in Dharavi, Mumbai on November 27, 1989. Currently, the number of human milk banks (HMB) has grown to nearly 14 all over India but the growth of human milk banks has been very slow as compared to the growth of neonatal intensive care units. One of the major reasons for loss of interest in human milk banking was the promotion of formula milk by the industry. Keeping in mind the complications associated with formula feeding to the sick, tiny preterm neonates and mothers' inability to breastfeed in the initial period, there is a need to establish human milk banks in all level II and level III facilities. It was with this objective that a need to formulate guidelines for establishment and operation of human milk banks in our country was felt. These guidelines do not intend to present detailed scientific literature but are an attempt to back-up the establishment and operation of human milk banking with scientific methods.

LOCATION OF HUMAN MILK BANKS

Human milk banks are primarily focused to provide donor milk to high risk newborns admitted in the neonatal unit. Therefore, a location in close proximity or even inside the boundaries of neonatal unit is desirable. This also helps in administrative supervision by medical staff. Presence of human milk banks in the neonatal units is associated with elevated rates of exclusive breastfeeding rates in VLBW babies.[3] Postnatal wards or Well Baby clinics of large hospitals are most suited for the purpose as donors are likely to be found in large numbers where medical and nursing staffs can encourage them to donate milk. Certain non-government organizations (NGOs) taking care of abandoned babies can also have a human milk bank in their facility.

THE RECIPIENTS

PDHM can be prescribed on priority for preterm babies and sick babies, babies of mothers with postpartum illnesses, and babies whose mothers have lactation failure, till their milk output improves.

Therapeutic benefits of breastmilk are noted in short gut syndrome, sepsis, and post-surgical gut healing in omphalocele, gastro-schisis, bowel obstruction and intestinal fistulas. In extremely preterm infants given exclusive diets of preterm formula versus human milk, there was a significantly greater duration of parenteral nutrition and higher rate of surgical necrotizing enterocolitis (NEC) in infants receiving preterm formula.[4] It is possible to administer trophic feeds (gut priming by early enteral feeds) exclusively with human milk in VLBW infants with banked human milk.[5]

If PDHM supplies are sufficient donor milk may be supplied for:
- Absent or insufficient lactation: Mothers with multiple births, who can not secrete adequate breastmilk for their neonates initially.
- For babies of non-lactating mothers, who adopt neonates and if induced lactation is not possible.
- Abandoned neonates and sick neonates.
- Temporary interruption of breastfeeding.

- Infant at health risk from breastmilk of the biological mother.
- Babies whose mother died in the immediate postpartum period.

INFRASTRUCTURE

There are no standard recommendations or specific guidelines mentioned regarding the space requirements for creation of human milk banks The minimum requirement is a partitioned room of 250 square feets that can comfortably lodge at least the equipment required for milk banking, a work area for the technician as well as some storage space for records, administration and area for counselling donors etc.

Privacy is of paramount importance for area of breastmilk expression. Provision of music/television and a crèche helps in reducing stress of donors. Teaching videos of Kangaroo Mother Care (KMC), expression of breastmilk and advantages of breastmilk feeding can be shown under supervision of milk bank staff.

EQUIPMENT

Pasteurizer/Shaker-water bath: It is essential to have a device to carry out heat treatment of donor milk at the recommended temperature of 62.5°C for a period of 30 minutes (Pretoria Holder pasteurization method) prior to its use. A conventional pasteurizer is expensive and generally of dairy-industry size and is often not suitable for the quantity of milk to be pasteurized in a human milk bank. A well accepted alternative is the use of a shaker water bath with a micro-processor controlled temperature regulator, an electronic timer device and a shaker speed controller. The milk in the container is boiled through the steam and hot water in the water shaker bath. To avoid coagulation of the milk and to distribute heat evenly, the tray on which the milk containers are placed is shaken/wobbled. This shaker water bath should be double walled and made of steel. Its size varies according to the need of the milk bank, with the tray capacity varying from 9 to 24 containers of 200 to 400 mL capacity.

Use of other safer methods of pasteurization with better preservation of nutrients and other properties, like flash heat treatment, HTST (High Temperature Short Time; 72°C for 16 seconds) and ultra violet irradiation are still not being used in human milk banks routinely.[6,7]

Deep freezer: A deep freezer to store the milk at –20°C is essential in the milk bank. It is desirable to order a deep freezer with a digital display of the temperature inside it with an alarm setting. It is desirable to have two deep freezers for processed milk. First for storage of the milk till the post-pasteurization milk culture reports are available. This freezer should be locked at all times with access only to the technician, so that no milk is accidentally used till the culture reports are available. The second deep freezer is used for storage of the pasteurized milk once the culture reports are negative and the milk is considered safe for disbursement.

Refrigerators: These are required to store the milk till the whole day's collection is over and the milk is ready to be mixed and pooled for further processing. It is also required for thawing the milk before being dispatched. Preferably two different units should be used for these purposes. If not possible, then strictly earmarked areas should be kept in one unit for each purpose.

Hot air oven/Autoclave: A hot air oven/auto-clave in the milk bank or centralized sterile service department is essential for sterilizing the containers used for collection from donors, containers for pasteurization and the test tubes needed for sending milk culture samples to the microbiology laboratory.

Breastmilk pumps: For milk banking, hospital grade electric pumps are preferred as they result in better volumes of expressed milks and are relatively painless and comfortable to use. There is no major difference in the types of electrical breast pumps.[8] Manually operated breastmilk pumps designed to operate more physiologically by simulating the infant's compressive action on the areola during breastfeeding can be used with lower cost implications.[9] They can be reused with chemical disinfection/sterilization. Breast pumps can be a source of infection,[10] and hence they should be cleaned properly.[11] Pump and its parts should be sterilized/disinfected as per manufacturer's instructions.

Containers: For collection and storing the milk, single use hard plastic containers of polycarbonates, pyrex or propylene are used across the world. However, in Indian experi-ence, cylindrical, wide-mouthed stainless steel containers of about 200 ml capacity with tight fitting/screwed caps are equally effective. They are easily available, and are durable, easy to clean and autoclave. There is no significant decrease in nutrient composition on storage; however, cellular components are reduced. Polythene milk bags are not suitable as they are fragile, associated with loss of lipids and vitamins and there is a risk of contamination, although some studies have challenged the loss of lipids.[12]

Generator/Uninterrupted power supply: Every milk bank should have a dedicated centralized source of uninterrupted power supply backup to run the deep freezers and refrigerators in case of electricity failure.

Milk analyzer: It is desirable to have macro-nutrient analysis of breastmilk to estimate the calorie, protein and fat of a milk sample, using infra-red spectroscopy technology, in teaching hospitals as a step towards lacto-engineering.

ADMINISTRATIVE STAFF

Human milk banks should have a panel of consultants to guide overall development and functioning. It can include representatives from the areas of pediatrics/neonatology, lactation, microbiology, nutrition, public health and food technology. It should consist of a Director (for planning, implementing and evaluating the services), milk bank officer (usually a doctor, for day-to-day running of the bank and training), Lactation management nurses (for counselling mothers and assisting expression of breastmilk), milk bank technician (for pasteurization of breastmilk and microbiological surveillance), Milk bank attendant (for collecting, sterilization of the containers and maintaining hygiene), receptionist (for record keeping and public relations) and a microbiologist (for micro-biology testing and infection control policies). General guidelines for staff are outlined in Box 29.1.

DONOR POPULATION

The donor population is formed by healthy lactating mothers with healthy babies, who are voluntarily willing to give their extra breastmilk for other babies without compromising the nutritional needs of their own baby. The donors can include mothers attending well baby clinics, mothers whose babies are in neonatal intensive care units, those who have lost their babies but are willing to donate their milk, or lactating working staff in the hospital, and motivated mothers from the community. Donors are not paid for their donations.

Try to reach maximum donor population using variety of avenues. Spreading awareness about possibility of breastmilk donation in

---

Box 29.1: General guidelines for staff of the human milk bank

- Standard operating procedures (SOP) of the bank (which should be displayed at proper places) should be adhered to.
- Hygienic practices like proper hand wash, donning gowns, mask, gloves, trimming nails, locking long hairs should be maintained.
- Gloves should be worn and changed between handling raw and heat-treated milk.
- Staff should undergo regular health checks and be immunized against Hepatitis B.
- There should be a program for ongoing training of the staff.

Box 29.2: Criteria for breastmilk donors

Who can donate?
A lactating woman who:
- is in good health, good health-related behavior, and not regularly on medications or herbal supplements (with the exception of prenatal vitamins, human insulin, thyroid replacement hormones, nasal sprays, asthma inhalers, topical treatments, eye drops, progestin-only or low dose estrogen birth control products);
- is willing to undergo blood testing for screening of infections; and
- has enough milk after feeding her baby satisfactorily and baby is thriving nicely.

Who cannot donate?
A donor is disqualified who:
- uses illegal drugs, tobacco products or nicotine replacement therapy; or
- regularly takes more than two ounces of alcohol or its equivalent or three caffeinated drinks per day; or
- has a positive blood test result for HIV, HTLV, Hepatitis B or C or syphilis; or
- is herself or has a sexual partner suffering from HBV, HIV, HCV and venereal diseases OR either one has high risk behavior for contracting them in last 12 months; or
- has received organ or tissue transplant, any blood transfusion/blood product within the prior 12 months.
- is taking radioactive or other drugs or has chemical environmental exposure or over the counter prescriptions or mega doses of vitamins, which are known to be toxic to the neonate and excreted in breastmilk; or
- has mastitis or fungal infection of the nipple or areola, active herpes simplex or varicella zoster infections in the mammary or thoracic region.

---

society by various means including mass communication can help in motivating donors. NGOs, social clubs and college students can play a good role in it. Criteria for breast milk donors[11] are outlined in Box 29.2.

COLLECTION OF BREASTMILK

After proper counselling, checking suitability for donation, getting written informed consent, history taking, physical examination and sampling for laboratory tests, the donor is sent to designated breastmilk collection area in the milk bank or in the milk collection center. Breastmilk is collected by trained staff with hygienic precautions, after method of breastmilk expression is chosen by the donor. Home collection of breastmilk is better avoided at present in our country due of the risk of contamination. Washing the breast with water before expression is as good as washing with disinfectant.[14] There is no rationale in discarding foremilk. Drip milk (the milk that drips from the non-feeding breast in some of lactating mothers) collected with the help of breastmilk shells has been found to be nutritionally inferior with lower fat content,[15] and is not recommended for banking.

The breastmilk may be expressed manually (hand expression) or with breast pumps. Manual expression is a low cost and effective method of expression, and associated with less risk of contamination. Simultaneous breast expression in breastfeeding women is more efficacious than sequential breast expression.[16] Milk should be collected in properly labeled sterile container and transported to HMB under cold storage condition.

Processing

All batches of collected raw breastmilk should be refrigerated immediately till the serological report comes negative. Fresh raw milk should not be added to the frozen milk since this can result in defreezing with hydrolysis of triglycerides.[17] While mixing fresh raw breastmilk to frozen raw breastmilk previously collected from same donor, it should be chilled before adding to frozen milk.[18] For sick or preterm babies, it is advisable to use a new container for each pumping.

Before pasteurization, pooling and mixing may be carried out from multiple donors to ease the process of processing and storage. Pasteurization is carried out by Holder's method.

Microbiological screening of donor milk is done before (if there is no cost constraint), and as soon as possible after pasteurization. Pre-pasteurization micro-biology can result in wastage of milk to the tune of about 30% in some cases.[19] Even after pasteurization, the endotoxins of organisms are still present in the milk in some cases but they have not been found to have any clinical effect on the baby. A bacterial count of 105 CFU/mL or more in raw breastmilk can be considered as an indicator of the poor quality of milk. Based on this and on the theoretical concern that heavily contaminated milk with specific bacteria (e.g. S. aureus, E.coli) may contain enterotoxins and thermostable enzymes even after pasteurization, expert panel selected 105 CFU/mL for total bacterial count, 104 CFU/mL for Enterobacteriaceae and S. aureus as threshold values, which are in consonance with milk banks operating in other parts of the world.[13,20] No growth is acceptable in post-pasteurization microbiology cultures. Whole batch of culture positive container of pasteurized milk should be discarded.

Storage

Pasteurized milk awaiting culture report should be kept in dedicated freezer/freezer area taking precaution not to disburse it till the culture is negative. Storage should be done in the same container that is used for pasteurization. It is advisable not to transfer processed milk in other containers as it has risk of contamination. Culture negative processed milk should be kept at –20°C in tightly sealed container with clear mention of expiry date and other relevant data on the label. It can be preserved for 3 to 6 months. Random cultures of preserved milk before disbursal can aid quality assurance.

Disbursal

PDHM should be disbursed at physician's requisition from NICU physician after informed consent from the parents of the recepient. Preterm baby should preferably get

PDHM from preterm donors. It should be done on First-in-first-out basis from the storage. Transport of PDHM should be done under cold storage in the same pasteurized container till its use.

Frozen PDHM should be thawed by either defrosting the milk rapidly in a water bath at a temperature not exceeding 37°C, or under running lukewarm water taking care that the cap of the container does not come in contact with the water as it is likely to get contaminated.[21] It should never be thawed in a microwave as this results in reduction in the IgA content of the milk and there is a risk of burns if the milk is used too soon.[18] Milk should not be refrozen after being thawed as this increases the hydrolysis of the triglycerides in the milk. While bringing to room temperature, it should be gently agitated to make a homogenous mixture before use and should be used preferably within 3 hours to prevent contamination.

Labeling and Record Keeping

HNB should have an operational objective of ensuring full traceability from individual donation to recipient, and maintaining a record of all storage and processing conditions. Written standard operating procedures should be followed. Confidentiality of records should be maintained by the milk bank. Proper labeling at all levels is mandatory; from sterile container for collection of donation, pooling vessel and pasteurization container to storage containers. Labels should be water resistant and names and identifying details of donors, dates of pasteurization, batch numbers and expiry date should be clearly readable. Record keeping at all levels should be meticulous for Donor Record File containing consent form, donor's and her child's data, screening reports, pasteurization batch files, and for PDHM Disbursal Record File containing relevant data, including recipient consent form. Though rarely required, complications can be prevented with appropriate labeling and record keeping.

As incubation period for most infection varies from a few weeks to 6 months and appearance of symptoms is faster in infants and children, there seems to be no rationale for keeping records beyond 5 years, unless one is working in an area where milk kinship issue is of paramount importance.

ECONOMIC IMPLICATIONS

Cost effectiveness of using banked human milk in neonatal intensive care units has been documented in Western countries, largely due to reduction in the rate of NEC.[22] In a country like ours, the cost of running a milk bank with potential cost-saving due to reduction in NEC, sepsis and duration of hospital stay have not been evaluated. Given the high incidence of sepsis and a large burden of premature births, this intervention may have the potential to result in substantial saving for the nation.

CONCLUSION

It is clear that artificial formula will never provide the broad range of benefits of human milk. Given the high rate of preterm births in the country and level of malnutrition that ensues in the postnatal growth in such babies after birth, there is an urgent need to establish milk banks across the country, especially in the large neonatal units of all hospitals. This document aims at providing expert opinion regarding the feasibility and operational guidelines for establishing milk banks in the country.

Note: This document is the abridged version of detailed guidelines. The detailed guidelines are available with IAP IYCF Chapter (www.iycfchapteriap.org).

REFERENCES

1. Das BK, Mishra RN, Mishra OP, Bhargava V, Prakash A. Comparative outcome of low birth weight babies. Indian Pediatr 1993;30:15–21.

2. Bharati P, Pal M, Bandyopadhyay M, Bhakta A, Chakraborty S, Bharati P. Prevalence and causes of low birth weight in India. Malayasian J Nutr 2011;17:301–13.
3. Arslanoglu S, Moro GE, Bellu R, Turoli D, De NG, Tonetto P, et al. Presence of human milk bank is associated with elevated rate of exclusive breast-feeding in VLBW infants. J Perinat Med 2013;41:129–31.
4. Cristofalo EA, Schanler RJ, Blanco CL, Sullivan S, Trawoeger R, Kiechl-Kohlendorfer U, et al. Randomized trial of exclusive human milk versus preterm formula diets in extremely premature infants. J Pediatr 2013;163:1592–5.
5. De NG, Berti M, De NM, Bertino E. Early enteral feeding with human milk for VLBW infants. J Biol Regul Homeost Agents 2012;26:69–73.
6. Israel-Ballard K, Donovan R, Chantry C, Coutsoudis A, Sheppard H, Sibeko L, et al. Flash-heat inactivation of HIV-1 in human milk: a potential method to reduce postnatal transmission in developing countries. J Acquir Immune Defic Syndr 2007;45:318–23.
7. Terpstra FG. Antimicrobial and antiviral effect of high-temperature short-time (HTST) pasteurization applied to human milk. Breastfeed Med 2007;2:27–33.
8. Burton P, Kennedy K, Ahluwalia JS, Nicholl R, Lucas A, Fewtrell MS. Randomized trial comparing the effectiveness of 2 electric breast pumps in the NICU. J Hum Lact 2013;29:412–9.
9. Fewtrell MS, Lucas P, Collier S, Singhal A, Ahluwalia JS, Lucas A. Randomized trial comparing the efficacy of a novel manual breast pump with a standard electric breast pump in mothers who delivered preterm infants. Pediatrics 2001;107:1291–7.
10. Gransden WR, Webster M, French GL, Phillips I. An outbreak of Serratia marcescens transmitted by contaminated breast pumps in a special care baby unit. J Hosp Infect 1986;7:149–54.
11. Breast Pumps. US FDA, Heal. Cent. Devices Radiol. Center for Devices and Radiological Health; 2013 Available from: http://www.fda.gov/MedicalDevices/ProductsandMedical Procedures/HomeHealthandConsumer/ Consumer Products/BreastPumps/ucm 061950.htm. Accessed November 14, 2013.
12. Janjindamai W, Thatrimontrichai A, Maneenil G, Puwanant M. Soft plastic bag instead of hard plastic container for long-term storage of breast milk. Indian J Pediatr 2013;80:809–13.
13. National Institute for Health and Care Excellence. Donor Breast Milk Banks: the Operation of Donor Milk Bank Services. NICE Clinical Guideline 93. Available from: http://guidance.nice.org.uk/cg93. Accessed October 17, 2013.
14. N Pickler RH, Munro C, Shotwell J. Contamination in expressed breast milk following breast cleansing. J Hum Lact 1997;13:127–30.
15. Arnold LD. A brief look at drip milk and its relation to donor human milk banking. J Hum Lact 1997;13:323–4.
16. Prime DK, Garbin CP, Hartmann PE, Kent JC. Simultaneous breast expression in breastfeeding women is more efficacious than sequential breast expression. Breastfeed Med 2012;7:442–7.
17. Morera PS, Castellote Bargallo AI, Lopez Sabater MC. Evaluation by high-performance liquid chromatography of the hydrolysis of human milk triglycerides during storage at low temperatures. J Chromatogr A 1998;823:467–74.
18. CDC. Proper Handling and Storage of Human Milk. Recommendations. Breastfeeding. Available from: http://www.cdc.gov/breastfeeding/recom mendations/handling_breastmilk.htm. Accessed Oct 17, 2013.
19. Simmer K, Hartmann B. The known and unknowns of human milk banking. Early Hum Dev 2009;85:701–4.
20. Hartmann BT, Pang WW, Keil AD, Hartmann PE, Simmer K. Best practice guidelines for the operation of a donor human milk bank in an Australian NICU. Early Hum Dev 2007;83:667–73.
21. ABM Clinical Protocol #8: Human Milk Storage for home use for full term infants. Revision March 2010. Breastfeed Med 2000;5.
22. Arnold LD. The cost-effectiveness of using banked donor milk in the neonatal intensive care unit: prevention of necrotizing enterocolitis. J Hum Lact 2002;18:172–7.

30 Consensus Guidelines on Evaluation and Management of a Febrile Child Presenting to the Emergency Department in India

Prashant Mahajan, Prerna Batra, Neha Thakur, Reena Patel, Narendra Rai, Nitin Trivedi, Bernhard Fassl, Binita Shah, Marie Lozon, Rockerfeller A Oteng, Abhijeet Saha, Dheeraj Shah, Sagar Galwankar

All over the world, fever in children is one of the most common reasons for parents to seek medical care. It is estimated that approximately 20% of all pediatric emergency department (ED) visits in the United States (US) are for evaluation of fever.[1] In recent decades, an extensive amount of literature and evidence has led to a consensus approach to the evaluation and management of febrile children; which has evolved secondary to its changing epidemiology. The change in epidemiology of the febrile child is the result of the substantial impact of conjugate vaccines against capsulated bacterial pathogens including *H. influenzae* and *S. pneumoniae*.[1]

To reduce variation, multiple guidelines have been proposed including those from academic societies such as the American Academy of Pediatrics (AAP) and American College of Emergency Physicians (ACEP).[2] Despite some differences, most guidelines advocate a comprehensive evaluation of the very young febrile infant (28 days and younger) and a less conservative approach for older infants. Febrile infants undergo invasive procedures such as lumbar puncture, complete blood counts and urinalysis. Most febrile infants, especially those less than 28 days of age, are routinely hospitalized and treated empirically with broad spectrum antibiotics

such as third generation cephalosporins along with ampicillin.

There continues to be practice variation also, when applying evidence and consensus-based guidelines.[3-5] Depending upon clinician suspicion, clinicians may evaluate for etiologies as variable as bacterial pneumonia and bacterial enteritis. Currently available "standardized" approaches, regardless of practice variation, remain problematic for various reasons: (i) prediction rules and/or guidelines have not been validated across cultural, geographic, socio-economic environments and may not be applicable in all clinical settings; (ii) the epidemiology of pathogens causing Serious Bacterial Infection (SBI) has changed due to the impact of conjugate vaccines; (iii) clinicians are not confident about the test characteristics of various screening tools, especially the discriminatory abilities of the complete blood counts, and finally; (iv) newer screening tools such as procalcitonin have not been studied or integrated into clinical decision making in a robust manner.

Evaluation and management of the febrile child in India: Children may present with fever as an initial/isolated symptom of a yet undifferentiated illness or with localizing signs that suggest an etiology such as pneumonia. A majority of children with fever without localizing signs will have a viral etiology which does not warrant laboratory evaluation and can often be managed with instructions for ensuring adequate hydration and use of antipyretics.[6] In one study it is estimated that up to 10% of febrile children, especially those 3 months of age and younger will have bacterial illnesses in the form of occult bacteremia, septicemia, bacterial meningitis, pneumonia, UTI, bacterial gastroenteritis, osteomyelitis, septic arthritis, and other general endemic tropical diseases.[7] However, etiologies of fever in the Indian ED context could vary from benign viral illnesses, commonly reported in US and Europe (e.g. respiratory syncytial virus (RSV), Enterovirus infections) to illnesses by organisms uncommon in industrialized countries: bacteria (e.g. *S. typhi*), viruses (e.g. measles, dengue, chikungunya) and parasites (e.g. malaria, kala azar) as well as endemic illness outbreaks due to meningococci and leptospira.

India is a tropical country with a distinct spectrum of common tropical illnesses particularly seen in post-monsoon season such as dengue, rickettsial infections, scrub typhus, malaria (usually due to Plasmodium falciparum), typhoid and leptospirosis.[8] Thus, the algorithmic approach utilized in the US and Europe is not applicable in Indian EDs, especially when evaluating a child with fever without source.

Emergency medicine is a growing medical specialty as evidenced by the rising number of publications appearing in the peer-reviewed literature demonstrating its growth and influence on healthcare delivery in India.[9] In conjunction with emergency medicine, as well as independently, pediatric emergency medicine is rapidly evolving as a sub-specialty and efforts are underway for its formal specialty status recognition.[10] Development of a consensus statement that is relevant to the epidemiology of illness in the Indian context will help reduce practice pattern variation, optimize resource allocation as well as education, training and decision-making by

both policy makers and health care administrators in the federal, public and private sectors. Moreover, evaluation and management of the febrile child, continues to remain a clinical challenge in the Indian ED context and the development of a consensus based practice guideline will serve as a valuable resource.

Process

We held two consensus meetings of Pediatric Emergency Medicine (PEM) Section of Academic College of Emergency Experts in India (ACEE-INDIA) in Delhi (October 2015) and in Pune (March 2016). An exhaustive literature review was performed and ongoing web-based discussions were held to arrive at a consensus on the proposed evaluation and management of febrile infants and children. We provide a pragmatic and simple to use algorithm that will assist, but not replace, clinician decision making for the ED evaluation and management of the febrile child.

We have identified the key concerns regarding a standardized approach to the evaluation and care of the febrile child in an ED in India (Box 30.1).

Literature review: Following the initial consensus meeting, an exhaustive review of available literature pertaining to each component was identified. We used structured queries including terms such as fever, febrile child, febrile infant, fever without source, serious bacterial infection, bacteremia, to search databases including Pubmed, Google scholar to develop a comprehensive database of peer reviewed literature in an Endnote file. These manuscripts along with textbook chapters on the febrile child in commonly accepted textbooks of pediatrics and pediatric emergency medicine were reviewed. The literature review included topics unique to the India based ED setting: fever in immuno-compromised and/or severely malnourished children, fever with localization, fever without localization and etiologies specific to our country like malaria, dengue, and enteric infections. A drafting committee was selected to synthesize the literature and key concerns outlined at the initial in-person meeting. Drafts were circulated electronically to engage and further solicit input. This process resulted in specific evaluation and management recommendations for each condition.

RECOMMENDATIONS

Considering the available literature and the needs identified by the expert panel, we created an algorithm for the evaluation and management for a febrile child presenting to the ED within the context of healthcare in India (Fig. 30.1). This algorithmic approach incorporated the following: localizing symptoms, epidemiologic evidence, physiologic state (i.e. immunocompromised or not;

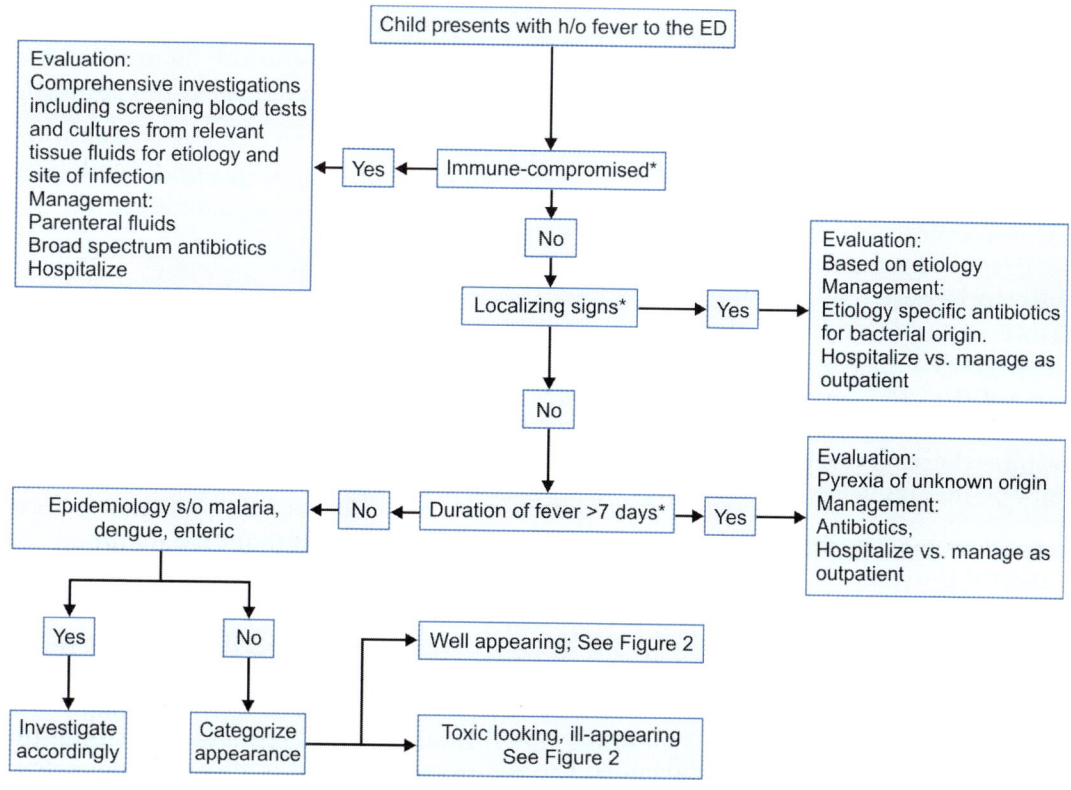

Fig. 30.1: Algorithm for evaluation and management for the febrile child presenting to emergency department within the context of health care in India

well appearing or ill appearing), duration of fever, and age of the child. For the purposes of algorithm application, we have outlined terms, definitions and categories below.

Definition of fever: Fever is defined as a rectal temperature ≥38.0°C or ≥100.4°F.[1,11] Axillary temperature is 0.3–0.6°C lower than the rectal temperature. Patients often present to the ED with subjective fever at home, felt by tactile assessment only. In this scenario, we suggest that clinicians obtain a detailed history including association with lethargy, perspiration, irritability or other concerning symptoms for ascertainment of clinically relevant fever and before providing a disposition.

Method of temperature assessment: Axillary thermometry is the most widely used method in clinical practice; however, axillary thermometers are not reliable with regards to measuring body temperature in infants and children.[12] Rectal temperature was identified as the most accurate measurement as it is closest to the core body temperature[1,13] and is the preferred method of temperature determination in very young children. Temporal artery and tympanic membrane thermometers can be used for quick assessment of temperature,[14] provided the clinician is aware of the limitations and performance characteristics of each method. Further, based on the clinical situation, one must confirm the core temperature by the rectal route. No definite cut-offs have been given for defining fever using tympanic and temporal thermometers.

Triage: A prompt and rapid clinical assessment by trained providers should be performed at triage.[15,16] Vital signs (temperature, heart rate, respiratory rate, blood pressure, and pulse oximetry) measurement along with the use of pediatric assessment triangle and/or Pediatric Early Warning Scores (PEWS) to quantify severity of illness is highly recommended to help categorize the febrile child as well-appearing or ill-appearing.[17] Providers (health workers, nurses and physicians) should be trained in performance of these assessments reliably and perform them in a timely manner. All febrile children who appear to be at risk for cardio-pulmonary compromise and septic shock should have life-saving resuscitative procedures performed regardless of etiology of fever. These include obtaining vascular access (either intravenous or intraosseous), managing the airway with provision of oxygenation and placing the child on a cardiac monitor. If such resources are available, a bedside glucose test along with a capillary blood gas, point-of-care serum electrolytes, ionized calcium and lactate levels should be performed to guide resuscitation. Provision of broad-spectrum antibiotics to treat suspected bacterial pathogens should also be provided as rapidly as possible. If patient is in shock, management with rapid and adequate amounts of isotonic fluids should be initiated. Table 30.1 summarizes the identification and immediate management of emergent patients. Immediate treatment steps should be initiated by healthcare personnel and often can be initiated at triage.

Evaluation of the febrile child: After initial stabilization, patient's evaluation and management should be done as per the algorithm described in Fig. 30.1.

Immunocompromised Children

Immunocompromised children are at high risk of serious infections, with grave prognosis. Thus, it becomes important to identify this group in ED at triage itself and have an aggressive approach. Children with neutropenia, with malignancy on chemo-therapy, those on long term oral steroids like nephrotic syndrome, with human immuno-deficiency virus (HIV infection), and with primary immunodeficiency states are the children at high risk and need extensive evaluation in febrile state.[18] Fever in a neutropenic patient is always an emergency, regardless of triage status and should be categorized as a life-threatening event (E).

TABLE 30.1: Identification and immediate management of emergent/life-threatening conditions

Symptoms/signs	Immediate treatment	After stabilization
Airway and breathing • Airway obstruction • Cyanosis • Respiratory distress • Respiratory failure	1. Secure and clear airway 2. Provide bag and mask ventilation 3. Intubate if ongoing respiratory support is needed. 4. Give oxygen: Nasal Cannula 2–3 LPM or Face Mask 5 LPM	1. Blood glucose – correct immediately with D25 2cc/kg 2. Hemogram 3. Blood gas 4. Electrolytes 5. Peripheral smear for malaria parasites if indicated
Circulation • Heart rate • Capillary refill time • Pulses(bounding or weak) • Blood pressure • Urine output • Level of consciousness *CNS* • Unconscious or convulsions	1. Establish intravenous (IV) or intraosseous line (IO) line 2. Give isotonic fluid bolus if clinically indicated 3. Continued assessment for signs of shock and cardiovascular compromise	6. Specific investigatons as indicated for instance blood group type and cross match, toxicologic screens in blood and urine.

Fever With Focus or Localization

When a child presents to ED with fever and a localizing symptom/sign, specific management becomes easier. Some of the common localizing signs are seizures, cough, ear discharge, loose stools, dysuria and rashes. History and evaluation in the ED to determine the focus should be done after triage and initial stabilization. Management depends upon the common organisms that prevail in that particular age group. Many of these infections have viral etiologies, which need only supportive treatment and a follow up. Emerging antimicrobial resistance is a global health problem and rational use of antibiotics in ED will go a long way in ameliorating this issue.

Fever Without Localization

In a tropical country like India, it is not uncommon to have febrile children without any localization, with epidemiological evidence suggestive of a particular infectious etiology. These include conditions like malaria, dengue, and enteric fever. Due to the overlapping clinical presentation, it becomes difficult to pin point the diagnosis in ED itself. Such children should be investigated for the conditions with high index of suspicion and supportive therapy should be provided.

Fever without localization is a short duration febrile illness of 5 to 7 days without an identifiable cause after performance of history and examination.[19-21] ACEE recommends child to be categorized into well- or ill-/toxic-appearing. Emergent hospitalization and comprehensive evaluation is recommended in such a child at any age (Fig. 30.2). Further, evaluation and management of a well-looking child is based on the defined age groups i.e., neonates (28 days and less), young infant (29–90 days); older infant and young children (91 days – 2 years), and children more than 2 years (Fig. 30.2). There is no consensus among experts regarding optimal cut-offs for evaluation of fever without focus. Most have either used anecdotal or observational data as well as empiric data to arrive at cut-offs. Furthermore, the physiologic rationale is often missing. We chose the cut-offs as listed below:

28 days and less–most algorithms use this as a cut-off and is a category of the febrile infants that probably has the most consensus in the evaluation and management.

29-90 day cut-off – because this age group has probably been the least studied as well has

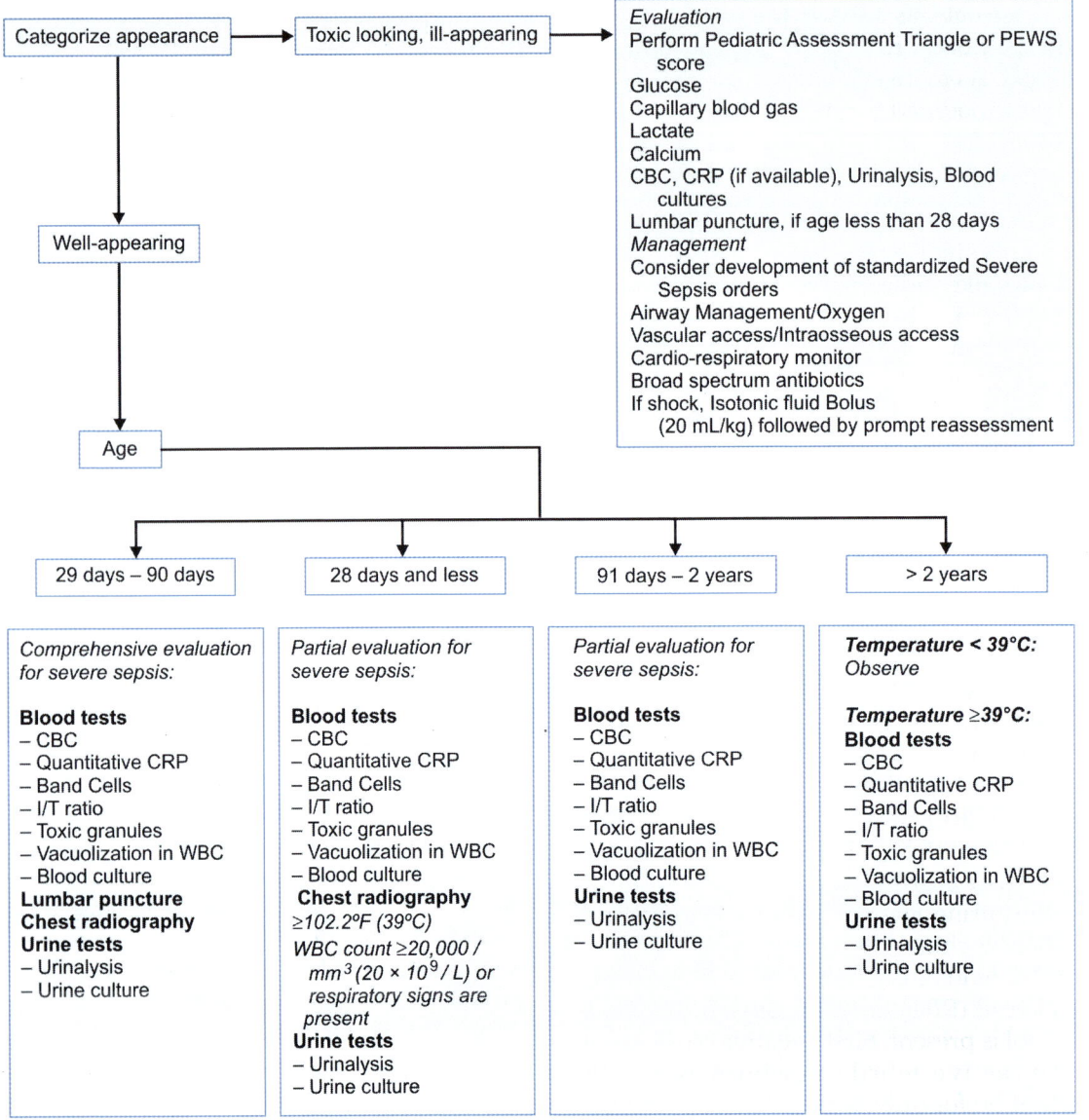

Fig. 30.2: Management of the febrile child based on appearance in the emergency department

the most variation with regards to a comprehensive evaluation, especially with relation to performance of lumbar punctures. In addition, this is also the age cut-off that is used in some febrile infant management algorithms.

91 days to 2 years – this is because most febrile infants beyond 90 days will have a positive impact of vaccinations as well as have a clinical examination that will allow the clinician to selectively evaluate for fever instead of a comprehensive evaluation that includes blood, urine and CSF studies. Specifically, the consensus chose to limit the upper age to 2 years because UTI risk drops substantially after the age of 2 years in female children.

These cut-offs are provided as a guide and also as a basis to collect data in the Indian context. As more evidence is generated, these may be modified further.

Evaluation

Evaluation should include a complete history and physical examination. In a tropical country like India, dehydration fever may be seen in newborns and young infants. Vaccination history could avoid unnecessary investigation. Signs like irritability; poor feeding, poor activity, and child not appearing well are subtle markers for serious underlying illness.[22] Pulse rate and volume, pulse oximetry, temperature, capillary refill time, respiratory rate (RR) and type should be documented. A complete head to toe exam with all clothes removed will help to find an occult cause of fever.

Newborns (< 28 days): All newborns with fever should be admitted. A complete investigative workup which includes complete blood count (CBC), C-reactive protein (CRP), peripheral blood smear (PBS) (band form, toxic granules, vacuolization, immature/total ratio), blood and urine culture, urine analysis (UA), lumbar puncture (LP), and chest X- ray (CXR) is mandatory. Stool should be examined for pus cell and red blood cell (RBC) only if change in frequency of stool is present. First negative septic screen in an active febrile newborn is not the indication for discharge.

Young infants (29 to 90 days): Active young infant between 29–90 days of age with fever should be observed in the ED with vital sign measurement. Complete blood count (CBC), peripheral blood smear (PBS), urine analysis (UA), and blood and urine culture is necessary. Chest radiography is indicated if temperature ≥102.2°F (39°C), leucocyte count ≥20,000 per mm3 or respiratory signs are present.[23] Urine tests recommended are microscopy and culture from urine obtained by catheterization.

91 days to 2 years: In some instances, lumbar puncture may be deferred in this age group. Investigative workup which include complete blood count (CBC), C-reactive protein (CRP), peripheral blood smear (PBS) (band form, toxic granules, vacuolization, immature/total ratio), blood and urine culture, and urinanalysis.

Children above 2 years: If temperature <39°C, only observation is recommended. If temperature is 39°C or more, investigative workup, which includes CBC, CRP, PBS (band form, toxic granules, vacuolization, immature/total ratio), blood and urine culture, Urinanalysis needs to be done.[23] PBS and rapid tests for malaria, dengue and enteric may be done in endemic areas. Blood culture may be taken in typhoid-endemic areas.

Sepsis Screen Parameters and Serious Bacterial Infection

Various sepsis screen parameters have been used with different permutations and combinations to rule in and rule out SBI. Markic, et al.[24] observed CBC, PCT, CRP and lab score ≥3 as useful markers for serious bacterial infections. Sensitivity and specificity was better in age group of ≤90 days when compared with age group of ≤180 days. In another large study, both CRP (area under the receiver operating curve-ROC 0.77, 95% CI 0.69–0.85) and PCT (ROC area 0.75, CI 0.67–0.83) were found to be strong predictors of serious bacterial infection.[24] Absolute band cells and PCT were reported as the best markers of SBI in children less than 36 months of age in another study, with PCT having the largest ROC (0.80, 95% CI 0.71–0.89).[25,26] The high cost and limited availability of PCT preclude its use as a screening tool in Indian EDs.

Management

In ill-appearing neonates and young infants, intravenous (IV) access should be established and empiric antibiotics should be started in the

ED. Up to 28 days of age, ampicillin 100 to 200 mg/kg/day divided 8 hourly and gentamicin 7.5 mg/kg/day divided 8 hourly should be started, whereas in older infants, intravenous Ceftriaxone 100 mg/kg/day or 75 mg/kg/day divided 12 hourly is given, depending on presence or absence of meningeal involvement.

Patient disposition from the ED: After initial stabilization and management in the ED, the patient may either be hospitalized or be discharged home. Box 30.2 gives indications for hospitalization and discharge of a febrile child from ED. Patiet's stable condition, definite follow up plan and compliance become important while discharging the patient home. Table 30.2 provides broad guidelines for admission in pediatric floor or intensive care unit (ICU).

Some patients may need transfer to another health facility, due to non-availability of appropriate resources or services. Box 30.3 summarizes the guidelines for referral that should be stringently followed.

Summary

The outlined algorithmic approach on management of fever in the ED is the first step of its kind initiated by the PEM Chapter of ACEE-India under the aegis of INDO-US Emergency and Trauma Collaborative. This approach is based on the current literature search and available evidence pertaining to Indian context, aiming to familiarize the emergency physicians to a stepwise approach

---

Box 30.2: Indications for hospitalization and discharge from emergency department

Indications for Hospitalization
- All emergency patients in need for airway stabilization, ventilation or continued O_2 requirement
- Age < 28 days
- Prolonged seizure/status epilepticus
- Altered sensorium
- Electrolyte imbalance
- Signs of Severe Dehydration
- Not feeding well
- Respiratory distress
- SPO_2 < 90% in room air
- Drug toxicity or drug reaction
- Unknown or undetermined cause
- Concern for non-compliance or inability to follow-up

Indications for Discharge
- No emergent need for airway, ventilation or circulatory support
- Vitals stable
- Child accepting
- Definitive management plan has been worked out
- Compliance ensured
- Follow up ensured

---

for evaluation and management of fever. This approach also includes focused triage and patient disposition guidelines. Further steps are intended to:

- Obtain input from experts in pediatrics, EM, PEM, infectious diseases, epidemiologists to modify the algorithm
- Create a robust database to collect retrospective and prospective data to elucidate

---

TABLE 30.2: Patient disposition guidelines

Disposition	Action
Observation in ED	Reassess patient frequently, review and document vital signs hourly
Discharging home	Provide appropriate counseling and a follow-up plan. Elicit understanding of care plan by caretakers
Admission/transfer to pediatric floor	Hemodynamically and respiratory stable patient, needs ongoing treatment, monitoring and workup;
Transfer to ICU	Patient remains in critical condition, warrants ongoing cardio-respiratory support to sustain life

ED: Emergency department; ICU: Intensive care unit

Box 30.3: Guiedelines for transfer* to another health facility

- Transfer, only when it is stable to transfer.
- Appropriate stabilization before transportation:
  - Secure airway
  - Intravenous or intraosseous access
  - Place on cardiac monitor
- Discuss transfer options with the patients' primary caregiver if available. Transfer is dependent upon patient's current status, the clinical concerns of the provider, the best place for receiving adequate care, and if caregiver/family is willing to transfer.
- Directly communicate with receiving hospital regarding that transfer is required.
- Transport with person(s), capable of managing any emergency en-route.

Due to non-availability of appropriate resources or services

the epidemiology of the febrile child across various settings.

- Modify the algorithm based on epidemiological evidence.
- Implement the algorithm and monitor compliance as well as measure impact on practice pattern variation, clinical outcomes and resource burden.

This algorithmic approach will require ongoing, periodic revision(s) as new research emerges and is established in the field.

REFERENCES

1. Balmuth F, Henretig FM, Alpern ER. Fever. In: RG Bachur& KN Shaw (eds.) Fleisher & Ludwig's Textbook of Pediatric Emergency Medicine, 7th edition. Lippincott Williams and Wilkins. Philadelphia, PA, USA.2016. p. 176–85.

2. ACEP Clinical Policies Committee and Clinical Policies Subcommittee on Pediatric Fever. Clinical Policy for Children Younger than Three Years Presenting to the Emergency Department with Fever. Ann Emerg Med. 2003;42:530–45.

3. Seow VK, Lin AC, Lin IY, Chen CC, Chen KC, Wang TL, et al. Comparing different patterns for managing febrile children in the ED between emergency and pediatric physicians: impact on patient outcome. Am J Emerg Med. 2007;25: 1004–8.

4. Phillips B, Selwood K, Lane SM, Skinner R, Gibson F, Chisholm JC; United Kingdom Children's Cancer Study Group. Variation in policies for the management of febrile neutropenia in United Kingdom Children's Cancer Study Group centres. Arch Dis Child.2007;92:495–8.

5. Aronson PL, Thurm C, Williams DJ, Nigrovic LE, Alpern ER, Tieder JS, et al.; Febrile Young Infant Research Collaborative. Association of clinical practice guidelines with emergency department management of febrile infants ≤56 days of age. J Hosp Med. 2015;10:358–65.

6. Harper MB. Update on the management of the febrile infant. Clin Pediatr Emerg Med. 2004;5: 5–12.

7. Abrahamsen SK, Haugen CN, Rupali P, Mathai D, Langeland N, Eide GE, et al. Fever in the tropics: Aetiology and case-fatality-A prospective observational study in a tertiary care hospital in South India. BMC Infect Dis. 2013;13:355.

8. Singhi S, Rungta N. Tropical fever: Management guidelines. Ind J Crit Care Medicine. 2014;18: 62–9.

9. Jatana SK. Pediatric emergencies in office practice—an overview. Med J Armed Forces India. 2012; 68:4–5.

10. Mahajan P, Batra P, Shah B, Saha A, Galwankar S, Aggrawal P, et al. The 2015 Academic College of Emergency Experts in India's INDO-US Joint Working Group white paper on establishing an academic department and training pediatric emergency medicine specialists in India. Indian Pediatr. 2015;52:1061–71.

11. Niven DJ, Gaudet JE, Laupland KB, Mrklas KJ, Roberts DJ, Stelfox HT. Accuracy of peripheral thermometers for estimating temperature: a systematic review and meta-analysis. Ann Intern Med. 2015;163:768–77.

12. Brown PJ, Christmas BF, Ford RP. Taking an infant's temperature: Axillary or rectal thermometer? N Z Med J. 1992;105:309–11.

13. Batra P, Goyal S. Comparison of rectal, axillary, tympanic, and temporal artery thermometry in the pediatric emergency room. Pediatr Emerg Care. 2013;29:63–6.

14. Batra P, Saha A, Faridi MM. Thermometry in children. J Emerg Trauma Shock. 2012;5:246–9.

15. Pocketbook of Hospital Care for Children: Guidelines for the Management of Common Childhood Illnesses – Second Edition. WHO 2013. Available from: http://apps.who.int/iris/bitstream/

10665/81170/1/9789241548373_eng.pdf. Accessed August 25, 2016.

16. WHO Emergency Triage and Treatment (ETAT). Manual for Participants. WHO Press. Geneva, Switzerland. 2005. Available from: http://apps.who.int/iris/bitstream/10665/43386/1/9241546875_eng.pdf. Accessed August 25, 2016.

17. Seiger N1, Maconochie I, Oostenbrink R, Moll HA. Validity of different pediatric early warning scores in the emergency department. Pediatrics. 2013;132:e841–50.

18. Holtzclaw BJ. Managing fever and febrile symptoms in HIV: Evidence-based approaches. J Assoc Nurses AIDS Care. 2013;24: S86–102.

19. Jhaveri R, Byington CL, Klein JO, Shapiro ED. Management of the nontoxic-appearing acutely febrile child: a 21st century approach. J Pediatr. 2011;159:181–5.

20. Brown L, Shaw T, Moynihan JA, Denmark TK, Mody A, Wittlake WA. Investigation of afebrile neonates with a history of fever. Canad J Emerg Med. 2004;6:343–8.

21. Ishimine P. Fever without source in children 0 to 36 months of age. Pediatr Clin North Am. 2006; 53:167–94.

22. Care Process Model. Emergency Management of the well-appearing febrile infant age 1–90 days.

Intermountain Health Care. May 2013. Available from: https://intermountain healthcare.org/ext/Dcmnt%3Fncid%3D520441555. Accessed August 25, 2016.

23. Bressan S, Andreola B, Cattelan F, Zangardi T, Perilongo G, Da Dalt L. Predicting severe bacterial infections in well-appearing febrile neonates: laboratory markers accuracy and duration of fever. Pediatr Infect Dis J. 2010;29: 227–32.

24. Markic J, Kovacevic T, Krzelj V, Bosnjak N, Sapunar A. Lab-score is a valuable predictor of serious bacterial infection in infants admitted to hospital. Wien Klin Wochenschr. 2015;127:942–7.

25. Nijman RG, Moll HA, Smit FJ, Gervaix A, Weerkamp F, Vergouwe Y, et al. C-reactive protein, procalcitonin and the lab-score for detecting serious bacterial infections in febrile children at the emergency department: a prospective observational study. Pediatr Infect Dis J. 2014; 33:e273–9.

26. Mahajan P, Grzybowski M, Chen X, Kannikeswaran N, Stanley R, Singal B, et al. Procalcitonin as a marker of serious bacterial infections in febrile children younger than 3 years old. Acad Emerg Med. 2014;21:171–9.

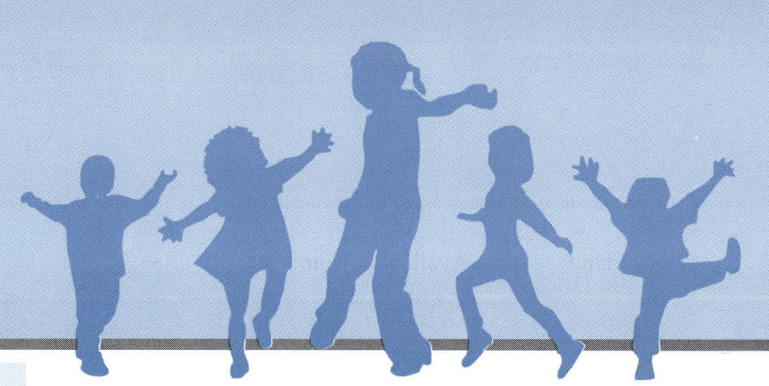

The Fifth Edition of Diagnostic and Statistical Manual of Mental Disorders (DSM-5)

Neetu Sharma, Ruchi Mishra, Devendra Mishra

The Diagnostic and Statistical Manual of Mental Disorders (DSM) is the most important resource for the purpose of psychiatric diagnoses, whether by the psychiatrist or the general practitioner. The American Psychiatric Association published the fifth edition of DSM (DSM-5),[1] containing significant changes in the diagnostic criteria for certain disorders from those in DSM-IV, which had been in widespread clinical use for nearly two decades.[2] DSM-5 was developed over a six-year official process utilizing the contributions of more than 400 multi-disciplinary professionals from varied specialties from across the world.

Pervasive developmental disorders (autism spectrum disorder), attention-deficit/hyperactivity disorder and Global developmental delay/mental retardation are common childhood neurodevelopmental disorders and comprise the bulk of referrals to Child Development Centers.[3] We herein enlist the major diagnostic changes in DSM-5 (Table 31.1).

AUTISM

Autism is now being increasingly recognized to be a common neurodevelopmental disorder, with prevalence approaching 1% of the population.[1] In DSM-IV, deficits in three core domains were required for the diagnosis of Autism, *viz.* Reciprocal social interactions, Restricted and repetitive behaviors or interests, and Verbal and nonverbal communication. As per DSM-5, deficits in only the first two core domains are required for diagnosis, *viz.* Deficits in social communication and social interaction (as manifested by deficit in social-emotional reciprocity, deficit in nonverbal communicative behavior used for social interaction, and deficit in developing, maintaining, and understanding relationships); and, Restrictive, repetitive pattern of behavior, interest, or activities (as manifested by at least two of: stereotyped or repetitive motor movements, use of objects, speech; insistence on sameness, inflexible adherence to routines, or ritualized patters of verbal or nonverbal behavior; highly restricted, fixated interests that are abnormal in intensity or focus; hyper- or hypo-reactivity to sensory input or unusual interest in sensory aspects of the environment).[1] Thus delay in language development is no longer required for diagnosis.

Another important change has been that Autism spectrum disorder (ASD) has been introduced as a new term in DSM-5 and covers all the previous four DSM-IV diagnoses, *viz.* Autistic disorder (autism), Asperger's disorder, Childhood disintegrative disorder, and Pervasive developmental disorder-NOS.[2]

TABLE 31.1: Change in DSM-5 from DSM-IV-TR	
DSM-IV	*DSM-5*
Autism	
• *Category* Four subcategories: Autistic disorder; Asperger syndrome; Pervasive developmental disorder– not otherwise specified; and disintegrative disorder.	All are combined into one term–Autism spectrum disorders
• *Case symptoms/areas of impairement* Social reciprocity; communicative intent; and restricted repetitive behaviors.	Deficits in social communication and social interaction; and restricted, repetitive patterns of behavior, interests, or activities
• Symptom severity: Not specified.	Defined for each area of diagnostic criteria.
• Sensory behaviors: Not included in criteria.	Added in the criteria
• Appearance of symptoms: Requires that symptoms begin prior to the age of 3 years; and symptoms must cause functional impairment.	Symptoms begin in early childhood, with the clause that "symptoms may not be fully manifest until social demands exceed capacity"
Attention deficit/Hyperactivity disorder	
• Age of diagnosis: arbitrarily set at 7 yrs	"Several inattentive or hyperactive-impulsive symptoms were present prior to age 12"
• Number of criteria for diagnosis: Six for both hyperactivity and impulsivity	Reduced to 5 for both hyperactivity and impulsivity
• Exemplification of criteria: criteria just mentioned, not exemplified.	Examples of all the 18 symptoms have been described for all age ranges.
• Pervasive disorders were previously an exclusion criterion.	Co-morbid diagnosis with ASD is now allowed.
• Subtyped into predominantly hyperactive, predominantly impulsive or both types co-existing.	Subtyping has been replaced by variable presentation.

Sensory behaviors, which were not a part of the diagnostic criteria in DSM-IV, have now been added. The previous classification did not specify symptom severity, which has now been defined for each area of the diagnostic criteria. A new entity, Social Communication Disorder has been introduced for children who fulfill all three social criteria of ASD but do not have any features of the repetitive and restrictive behavior criteria.[1] Rett's disorder is now considered as an associated known genetic condition. The requirement for appearance of symptoms prior to the age of three years, as given in DSM-IV[2] has now been replaced with "symptoms begin in early childhood", with the clause that "symptoms may not be fully manifest until social demands exceed capacity".[1] It has also been emphasized that those already diagnosed as per DSM-IV do not require any re-evaluation.

ATTENTION-DEFICIT/HYPERACTIVITY DISORDER

Attention-deficit hyperactivity disorder (ADHD) is also a common disorder, with population surveys suggesting that it occurs in about 5% of children and 2.5% adults across the globe.[1] In DSM-5, the text description of all the symptoms has been retained, but it has been suggested that ADHD is not limited to childhood and may extend across the whole life span causing impairment even later in life. The age of diagnosis of ADHD, which was previously set at seven years[2] has been changed to the description "several inattentive or hyperactive-impulsive symptoms were present prior to age 12".[1] This has been done because it was found that many children had onset of symptoms even after the age of seven years. Moreover, a good recall by adult of the childhood symptoms at less than seven years is often unreliable. It was recently shown that if the age of recall of symptoms was increased from 7 years to 12 years, the percentage of people who could recollect their symptom onset increased from 50% to 95%.[4] Concurrently, the number of criteria for the diagnosis in adolescents and adults has been lowered to five symptoms both for inattention as well as for hyperactivity and impulsivity (as opposed to six in DSM-IV). This has been done as there is research evidence for clinically significant impairment due to ADHD with the cut-off at five symptoms.[4] Pervasive disorders were previously an exclusion criterion, but a co-morbid diagnosis with ASD is now allowed.

MENTAL RETARDATION/INTELLETUAL DISABILITY

Reflecting the increasing use of the term in professional and lay literature, Intellectual disability is the new term in DSM-5 replacing the term Mental retardation in DSM-IV. The previous version classified the severity on the basis of the cognitive capacity (Intelligence quotient, IQ), but DSM-5 specifies that severity is to be determined by adaptive functioning rather than by IQ score.[1] Global developmental delay is diagnosed in "individuals who are unable to undergo systematic assessment of intellectual functioning" including children younger than five years, when clinical severity cannot be reliably assessed during early childhood.[1]

DSM-5: ADVANTAGES AND PITFALLS

International Classification of Diseases (ICD-11) is likely to be introduced next year, and DSM-5 has been developed to have a greater harmony with ICD-11, though that needs to be confirmed after widespread clinical and research use. DSM-5 has also given more emphasis to issues important to diagnosis and clinical care like gender and culture on the presentation of the disorder.[1] The multi-axial

diagnosis, a characteristic feature of earlier editions has also been given the go by, as this was incompatible with the diagnostic system in rest of medicine.

There has been some concern in recent publications on the implications of these changes, especially related to the more stringent ASD diagnostic criteria,[5] but some positive aspects have also been identified.[6] Field studies have shown that for autism and ADHD, clinicians in general agree with which patients meet DSM-5 diagnostic criteria; though, for some other conditions there is less agreement.[7] Those interested in more details of DSM-5 can refer to the full document,[1] or to an online resource with an extended description of all changes (*www.psychiatry. org/dsm5*).[1] However, the major hindrance to the immediate application of these criteria in clinical practice will probably be the availability of diagnostic tools in agreement with the new criteria. The recently developed Indian tools for ASD[8] and ADHD[9] will also need to measure up.

REFERENCES

1. American Psychiatric Association. Diagnostic and Statistical Manual of Mental Disorders, 5th ed. Arlington, VA American Psychiatric Publishing; 2013.
2. American Psychiatric Association. Diagnostic and Statistical Manual of Mental Disorders (4th ed., Text Revision). Washington, DC: 2000.
3. Jain R, Juneja M, Mishra D. Referral profile of a child development clinic in Northern India. Indian J Pediatr. 2012;79:602–5.
4. Barkley RA, Brown TE. Unrecognized Attention-deficit/hyperactivity disorder in adults presenting with other psychiatric disorders. CNS Spectr. 2008;13:977–84.
5. Frazier TW, Youngstrom EA, Speer L, Embacher R, Law P, Constantino J, et al. Validation of proposed DSM-5 criteria for autism spectrum disorder. J Am Acad Child Adolesc Psychiatry. 2012; 51:28–40.
6. McPartland JC, Reichow B, Volkmar FR. Sensitivity and specificity of proposed DSM-5

diagnostic criteria for autism spectrum disorder. J Am Acad Child Adolesc Psychiatry. 2012;51: 368–83.

7. Kupfer DJ, Kuhl EA, Regier DA. DSM-5—the future arrived. JAMA. 2013;309:1691–2.

8. Juneja M, Mishra D, Russell PSS, Gulati S, Deshmukh V, Tudu P, et al. INCLEN diagnostic tool for Autism Spectrum Disorder (INDT-ASD): Development and validation. Indian Pediatr. 2014;51:359–65.

9. Mukherjee S, Aneja S, Russell P, Gulati S, Deshmukh V, Sagar R, et al. INCLEN diagnostic tool for Attention Deficit Hyperacticity Disorder (INDT-ADHD): Development and validation. Indian Pediatr. 2014;51: 457–62.

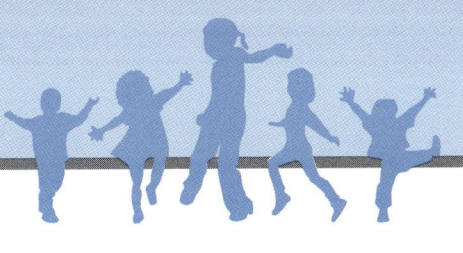

Updated Neonatal Resuscitation Guidelines 2015 — Major Changes

Satvik C Bansal, Somashekhar M Nimbalkar

The latest guidelines on neonatal resuscitation from American Heart Association (AHA)[1] and European Resuscitation Council (ERC)[2] were released in October 2015. There have been slight variations between these guidelines; although they use nearly identical literature for evidence evaluation. We present here the major changes in the recent guidelines,[3,4] and comparison between the ERC and AHA guidelines of 2015. The major changes are detailed in Table 32.1. Some of the major recommendations of previous AHA guidelines are continued without reviews and are elaborated in Table 32.2. The major recommendations are summarized in Box 32.1.

IMPLICATIONS FOR RESOURCE-LIMITED SETTINGS

With the emergence of scientific evidence from developing countries, these studies from resource-limited countries are forming the basis of major changes in clinical practice guidelines. Also, specific and separate recommendations are being made for resource-limited settings, as many of the standard recommendations may not be feasible in these settings.

We discuss some of the points below to put things into perspective:

- Therapeutic hypothermia has been recommended in resource-limited setups. The cost is still forbidding for those in need as well as the availability of centers that can provide it. Newer phase-change material based devices are available and evidence is increasing of its safety for use in Indian conditions.[7]
- Skin-to-skin contact has been stressed as a method for maintaining newborn temperature in the peri-partum period based on evidence drawn from India and other resource-limited countries.[8]
- The evidence for delayed cord clamping has grown stronger as well as the evidence for cord milking. The guidelines caution against cord milking below 29 weeks. This has great relevance to neonatal management and is a significant change.
- Removal of routine tracheal suction in non-vigorous neonates is a welcome change, leading to uniformity of the guidelines in all the scenarios. This significant change is contributed by evidence drawn from India.[9]
- The routine use of ECG and pulse oximeters, might find little practical use in resource-limited settings. There is still no

TABLE 32.1: Comparison of the 2015 Neonatal Resuscitation Guidelines Changes with the 2010 Guidelines

Resuscitation step	AHA 2010 recommendations	AHA 2015 recommendations	ERC 2015 recommendations	Remarks
Umbilical cord management	No recommendation given	• Delayed Cord Clamping (DCC) for >30 • No recommendation for infants resuscitated at birth. • Cord milking - Routine use is not recommended.	• DCC for ≥1 min is recommended. • No recommendation for infants resuscitated at birth. • Cord milking–Routine use is not recommended.	Delayed cord clamping is recommended, however wait for the minimum wait for clamping is different in both the . newer guidelines
Normal temperature of newborn in the delivery room	No temperature range specified	The temperature of non-asphyxiated infants should be maintained between 36.5–37.5°C	The temperature of non-asphyxiated infants should be maintained between 36.5–37.5°C	The newer guidelines specifically mention the range of temperature, which was missing till now.
Interventions to maintain normal temperature	In VLBW (<1500) pre-term babies- • Delivery room temp to 26°C • Plastic wrap • Exothermic mattress • Radiant heat.	In infants <32 wk various combinations of following strategies should be used: • Radiant warmers and plastic wrap with a cap. • Increased room temperature. • Thermal mattress. • Warmed humidified resuscitation gases.	In infants <32 wk various combinations of following strategies should be used: • Radiant warmers and plastic wrap with a cap. • Increased room temperature. • Thermal mattress. • Warmed humidified resuscitation gases.	Additional strategies to maintain temperature are recommended for <32 weeks rather than the weight criteria of <1500 g. Use of warm humidified resuscitation gases is introduced.
Warming of unintentionally hypothermic new-borns (i.e. hypothermic after resuscitation)	No recommendation given	Either rapid (0.5°C/h or greater) or slow rewarming (less than 0.5°C/h).	No recommendations given	There has always been debate on how to rewarm newborns. The AHA 2015 recommends both methods.
Maintaining normo-thermia in resource-limited settings	No specific recommendation	• Covering the newborn in a clean food-grade plastic bag up to the level of the neck and swaddle them after drying. • Skin-to-skin contact or kangaroo mother care.	For babies born outside hospital setup • Placement in food grade plastic bag after drying and then swaddling. • Skin to skin contact care (in >30 wk).	AHA has separately introduced recommendations for maintaining normal newborn temperature in resource-limited countries. The ERC gives similar recommendations for babies born outside ideal

Contd....

TABLE 32.1: Comparison of the 2015 Neonatal Resuscitation Guidelines Changes with the 2010 Guidelines (*Contd...*)

Resuscitation step	AHA 2010 recommendations	AHA 2015 recommendations	ERC 2015 recommendations	Remarks
				delivery environment and thus can be applied to resource-limited countries
Clearing the airway when meconium is present	Endotracheal suctioning in non-vigorous babies.	• Routine intubation for tracheal suction in non-vigorous babies is not suggested. • Initial steps followed by positive pressure ventilation (PPV) should be done as per routine indications	• Routine intubation for tracheal suction in non-vigorous babies is not suggested. • Initial steps followed by PPV be done as per routine indications. For suctioning use of 12–14 FG catheter, connected to a suction source ≤50 mmHg. • Routine surfactant is not recommended.	This major change has wide implications for developing countries and it puts emphasis on earlier initiation of PPV in non-vigorous babies with meconium stained liquor. ERC 2015 also recommends against the routine use of surfactant in babies delivered through meconium stained liquor (MSL).
Assessment of heart rate	No specific recommendation for heart rate measurement	Use of 3-lead electrocardiograpm (ECG) for measurement of the newborn's heart rate.	Use of 3-lead ECG for measurement of the newborn's heart rate.	It is doubtful if this will be utilized in resource-limited settings.
Administration of oxygen in preterm infants	No earlier recommendation	• In newborns <35 wk of gestation begin resuscitation with low oxygen (21% to 30%). • Titrate according to the pre-ductal oxygen saturation.	• In newborns < 35 wk of gestation begin resuscitation with low oxygen (21% to 30%). • Titrate according to the pre-ductal oxygen saturation.	A major change for preterms and reduces the complexity for the resuscitation team.
Positive pressure ventilation (PPV)	Positive and expiratory pressure (PEEP) with PPV can be used at birth if suitable equipment is available.	• Routine application of sustained inflation >5 secs is not recommended. • Effectiveness of respiratory mechanics monitors and exhaled CO_2 monitors not established. • In preterm newborns, along with PPV use approximately 5 cm H_2O PEEP.	• Routine application of sustained inflation >5 secs is not recommended. • For first 5 positive pressure breaths, maintain the initial inflation pressure for 2–3s. • Effectiveness of respiratory mechanics monitors and exhaled	Both ERC and AHA latest guidelines also talk about application of sustained inflation in initial few breaths. However, the recommended rate of

Contd....

TABLE 32.1: Comparison of the 2015 Neonatal Resuscitation Guidelines Changes with the 2010 Guidelines (Contd...)

Resuscitation step	AHA 2010 recommendations	AHA 2015 recommendations	ERC 2015 recommendations	Remarks
		• For PPV- Ventilate at a rate of about 40–60 breaths per minute.	CO_2 monitors not established. • In preterm newborns, along with PPV use approximately 5 cm H_2O PEEP. • For PPV-ventilate at a rate of about 30 breaths per minute allowing 1 second for each inflation.	PPV is different in both the guidelines.
Spontaneously breathing preterm infants with respiratory distress	Either Continuous positive airway pressure (CPAP) or intubation with mechanical ventilation	CPAP is preferred than routine intubation	CPAP is preferred than routine intubation	Most resuscitation teams would be comfortable with CPAP in a controlled setting. Initiating it in the delivery room will require a paradigm change.
Chest compressions	No specific recommendations were provided for oxygen use during chest compressions. However, it mentioned providing 100% oxygen, in newborns with bradycardia even after 90 seconds of resuscitation with lower concentration of oxygen.	• Give 100% oxygen with chest compression. • Routine use of End tidal carbon dioxide (ETCO$_2$) monitors or pulse oximeters for detection of return of spontaneous circulation is not recommended.	Recommends giving 100% oxygen with chest compressions, although mentions lack of evidence for the same.	The 2010 AHA guidelines based, AAP-AHA Neonatal Resuscitation Textbook, mentioned 100% oxygen with chest compressions,[5], regardless of time of resuscitation, despite not being in the guidelines released in 2010.
Induced therapeutic hypothermia	Only under clearly defined protocols and in places with multi-disciplinary care.	Recommends use also in resource-limited settings (i.e., lack of qualified staff, inadequate equipment)	• Only under clearly defined protocols and in places with multi-disciplinary care. • Whole body cooling and selective head cooling are appropriate.	Again taking into consideration the emerging evidence from developing countries, AHA recommends therapeutic hypothermia in resource-limited settings also.
Sodium bicarbonate infusion	No recommendation	No recommendation	• During prolonged arrests unresponsive to other therapies.	Usage of sodium bicarbonate in

Contd....

TABLE 32.1: Comparison of the 2015 Neonatal Resuscitation Guidelines Changes with the 2010 Guidelines (*Contd...*)

esuscitation step	AHA 2010 recommendations	AHA 2015 recommendations	ERC 2015 recommendations	Remarks
Prognostic tools	No recommendation given	No recommendation given	• Dosage 1–2 mmol/kg; slow intravenous injection. Combined APGAR appears to be a better predictor of outcome than routinely used APGAR score. In Combined APGAR, the interventions needed to achieve the particular score are scored as well and a combined score is generated.[6]	prolonged arrests doesn't find any mention in AHA guidelines More studies are required to form a universal recommendation
Guidelines for withholding resuscitation	*Not indicated*- Conditions with almost certain early death and or with high morbidity. *Nearly always indicated*- Conditions with a high rate of survival and acceptable morbidity. *Borderline:* In conditions with uncertain prognosis in which survival is borderline, and morbidity is high.	Prognosis for < 25 weeks consider: • accuracy of gestational age assessment. • Chorioamnionitis. • Available facilities. • Region-specific guidelines to be followed.	*Not indicated*—Conditions with almost certain early death and or with high morbidity. *Nearly always indicated*— Conditions with a high rate of survival and acceptable morbidity. *Borderline:* In conditions with uncertain prognosis in which survival is borderline, and morbidity is high. • Comfort and dignity of the baby and family should not be ignored.	AHA 2015 introduces regard for region specific guidelines. ERC 2015 mentions fixed criteria similar to AHA 2010.
*Structure of educational programs and instructors	No recommendation	Instructors to be trained using timely, objective, structured, and individually targeted verbal and/or written feedback	No recommendation	
$Structure of educational programs – Providers	Simulation, briefing, and debriefing techniques should be used.	Training should occur more frequently than the current 2-year interval.	No recommendation	

*AHA guidelines mention recommendations for training of instructors; $AHA 2015 recommends increase in frequency of provider courses, for better retention of skills

TABLE 32.2: Recommendations that remain unchanged	
Temperature control	Resuscitation should be performed with temperature-controlling interventions.
Clearing the airway when amniotic fluid is clear	Routine suctioning is not recommended.
Assessment of need of oxygen therapy	Oximetry should be used to monitor if any neonate needs PPV, with persistent and monitoring of oxygen therapy central cyanosis persists and with the use of supplementary oxygen.
Administration of oxygen in term infants	Initiate resuscitation with room air. Supplementary oxygen may be administered to achieve appropriate pre-ductal oxygen saturation.
Initial breaths and assisted ventilation	An initial inflation pressure of 20 cm water is adequate; some term babies may require up to $\geq$30 to 40 cm water. Rate of giving PPV–40 to 60 per minute.
Endotracheal tube placement	Exhaled CO_2 detection is most reliable.
Chest compressions	Coordinated chest compressions and PPV should be done if heart rate <60 per minute after establishing effective ventilation.
Epinephrine	IV dose–0.01 to 0.03 mg/kg of 1:10 000 epinephrine. For an endotracheal route - 0.05 to 0.1 mg/kg.
Volume expansion	Volume expansion when blood loss is known/suspected. Dose–10 mL/kg of isotonic crystalloid solution or blood, may be repeated.

data available of widespread use of pulse oximeters in India and given the resource constraints, this change may not be practiced uniformly.

• Similarly, use of exhaled CO_2 monitors, oxygen blenders, and laryngeal mask airways will remain out of reach in most resuscitation situations in resource limited settings

• Decreased usage of oxygen in preterm newborns, and preference CPAP over mechanical ventilation might contribute to the decentralization of newborn care and better care at level 1 or level 2 setups.

• While earlier there was a mandate for training all health personnel involved in neonatal care every two years in neonatal resuscitation, the committees have recommended more frequent trainings without stipulating, a duration between trainings. The evidence is rising for 'Low Dose High Frequency' trainings for neonatal resuscitation.

CONCLUSION

There are critical changes in updated resuscitation guidelines of 2015 with subtle differences between the AHA and ERC. The authors believe that the Indian Academy of Pediatrics and the National Neonatology Forum of India will bring out India-specific recommendations to guide the resuscitation methods to be followed in India. This will ensure that the clinicians practicing resuscitation on a daily basis have some basis for their variance from International Guidelines.

Box 32.1: Major changes in updated guidelines

- Delayed cord clamping for both term and preterm infants who do not require resuscitation at birth. Routine use of cord milking (outside of a research setting) for infants born at less than 29 weeks of gestation is not recommended
- Temperature should be recorded as a predictor of outcomes and as a quality indicator. It is recommended that the temperature of newly born non-asphyxiated infants be maintained between 36.5°C and 37.5°C after birth
- Strategies (radiant warmers, plastic wrap with a cap, thermal mattress, warmed humidified gases, and increased room temperature plus cap plus thermal mattress) are advocated to prevent hypothermia in preterm infants. In resource-limited settings, simple measures to prevent hypothermia in the first hours of life (use of plastic wraps, skin to-skin contact, and even placing the infant after drying in a clean food-grade plastic bag up to the neck) may reduce mortality.
- Neonates born through meconium-stained amniotic fluid and who are non-vigorous at birth, should be placed under a radiant warmer and PPV should be initiated if needed. Routine intubation for tracheal suction is no longer recommended. Intubation and suction of the airway may be used as needed for ensuring oxygenation and ventilation.
- Use of a 3-lead ECG for assessment of heart rate in first minute may be used. However, the use of the ECG should not replace the need for pulse oximetry to evaluate the newborn's oxygenation.
- Resuscitation of preterm newborns of less than 35 weeks of gestation should be initiated with low oxygen (21% to 30%) and the oxygen titrated to achieve pre-ductal oxygen saturation approximating the range achieved in healthy term infants.
- CPAP may be offered to spontaneously breathing preterm infants with respiratory distress in place of routine intubation for administering PPV.
- Recommendation to use of 100% oxygen whenever chest compressions are provided.
- In resource-limited settings, use of therapeutic hypothermia may be considered under clearly defined protocols and in facilities with the capabilities for multidisciplinary care and follow-up.
- Neonatal resuscitation task training should be done more frequently than the current 2-year interval.

REFERENCES

1. Wyckoff MH, Aziz K, Escobedo MB, Kapadia VS, Kattwinkel J, Perlman JM, et al. Part 13: Neonatal Resuscitation: 2015 American Heart Association Guidelines Update for Cardiopulmonary Resuscitation and Emergency Cardiovascular Care. Circulation. 2015;132:S543–60.

2. Wyllie J, Bruinenberg J, Roehr CC, Rüdiger M, Trevisanuto D, Urlesberger B. European Resuscitation Council Guidelines for Resuscitation 2015. Resuscitation. 2015;95:249–63.

3. Kattwinkel J, Perlman JM, Aziz K, Colby C, Fairchild K, Gallagher J, et al. Neonatal Resuscitation: 2010 American Heart Association Guidelines for Cardiopulmonary Resuscitation and Emergency Cardiovascular Care. Pediatrics 2010;126:e1400–13.

4. Roehr CC, Hansmann G, Hoehn T, Bührer C. The 2010 Guidelines on Neonatal Resuscitation (AHA, ERC, ILCOR): similarities and differences—what progress has been made since 2005? Klin Padiatr. 2011;223:299–307.

5. Kattwinkel J, ed. Textbook of Neonatal Resuscitation. 6th ed. Elk Grove Village, IL: American Academy of Pediatrics, American Heart Association, 2010. p.146

6. Dalili H, Nili F, Sheikh M, Hardani AK, Shariat M, Nayeri F. Comparison of the four proposed Apgar scoring systems in the assessment of birth asphyxia and adverse early neurologic outcomes. PloS One. 2015;10:e0122116.

7. Thomas N, Chakrapani Y, Rebekah G, Kareti K, Devasahayam S. Phase changing material: an alternative method for cooling babies with hypoxic ischaemic encephalopathy. Neonatology 2015;107:266–70.

8. Nimbalkar SM, Patel VK, Patel DV, Nimbalkar AS, Sethi A, Phatak A. Effect of early skin-to-skin contact following normal delivery on incidence of hypothermia in neonates more than 1800 g: randomized control trial. J Perinatol. 2014;34:364–8.

9. Chettri S, Adhisivam B, Bhat BV. Endotracheal suction for nonvigorous neonates born through meconium stained amniotic fluid: a randomized controlled trial. J Pediatr 2015;166:1208–13.

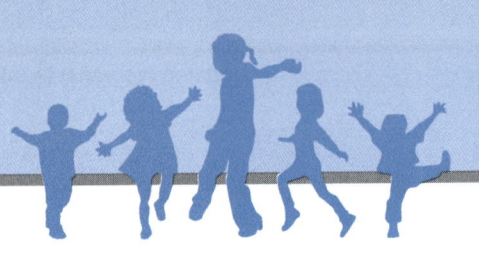

What is New in the 2015 PALS Update?

Shalu Gupta, Muralidharan Jayashree

The past decade has seen a marked improvement in the survival to discharge rates from pediatric in-hospital cardiac arrest (IHCA). Rates of return of spontaneous circulation (ROSC) from IHCA has increased significantly from 39% to 77%, and survival to hospital discharge improved from 24% to 36-43%, for the period from 2001 to 2013.[1] However, the same survival benefit has not been reported for out-of-hospital cardiac arrest (OHCA); 8.3% survival to hospital-discharge across all age-groups.[2]

The American Heart Association (AHA) Guidelines for Cardiopulmonary resuscitation (CPR) and Emergency cardiovascular care (ECC) for Pediatric Advanced Life Support (PALS) are updated every five years based on the body of evidence that has accumulated over this period. The current update (2015) to the 2010 AHA Guidelines focuses on certain key areas related to pediatric resuscitation.[3,4]

The questions to be addressed in PICO format (population, intervention, comparator, and outcome) were identified and prioritized by seven task forces. These questions pertained to three core areas, *viz.* pre-arrest, intra-arrest, and post-resuscitation care. The patient outcomes studied were short term, *i.e.* beyond ROSC or discharge from the pediatric intensive care unit (PICU) and long term survival with favorable neurologic/functional status at 30, 60 and 180 days, and 1 year.

A detailed search for relevant articles was performed in all the three online databases (PubMed, Embase, and the Cochrane Library) following which each task force carried out a detailed systematic review based on the recommendations of the Institute of Medicine of the National Academies.[5]

Each recommendation is labeled with a Class of Recommendation (COR) and a Level of Evidence (LOE).The quality of the evidence was categorized into high, moderate, low, or very low, based on the study methodologies and the five core GRADE domains of risk of bias, inconsistency, indirectness, imprecision, and publication bias.[6] This update used the most recent AHA COR and LOE classification system that is a modification of the Class III recommendation and introduces LOE B-R (randomized studies) and B-NR (non-randomized studies) as well as LOE C-LD (limited data) and LOE C-EO (consensus of expert opinion).[3] Based on the above, the task force then formulated 18 questions in the following areas and critically appraised the available evidence. The same is summarized in the accompanying tables (Tables 33.1–33.3).

A. ***Pediatric pre-arrest care:*** In pre-arrest scenario, the following five areas were considered important so as to prevent a cardiac or respiratory arrest (Table 33.1).

TABLE 33.1: Pediatric pre arrest[3,4]

S. No	Target population	Questions	Treatment recommendations
1.	Infants and children hospitalized in non intensive care unit (ICU) wards	Whether the use of pediatric RRT/MET, changes the • Frequency of cardiac or pulmonary arrest and • Overall hospital mortality	May be considered for admitted high risk children. Emphasis here is on the potential to recognize and intervene for patients with deteriorating illness so as to prevent them from progressing to cardiac/respiratory arrest
2.	Infants and children hospitalized in non ICU wards	Whether the use of a PEWS changes • Overall hospital mortality, and • Cardiac arrest frequency	Very-low-quality evidence from one pediatric observational study Hence no recommendation possible
3.	Infants and children with myocarditis/ dilated cardiomyo-pathy with imminent cardiac arrest	Whether a specific approach like ECMO changes • Cardiac arrest frequency • Return of spontaneous circulation • Survival to hospital discharge • Survival with favorable neuro-logic/ functional outcome at discharge, 30,60,180 days, and/or 1 year	No evidence in favor, though veno-arterial ECMO may be considered in acute fulminant myocarditis with imminent arrest (very-low-quality evidence)
4.	Emergency tracheal intubation	Whether premedication with atropine changes • Survival with favorable neurologic/functional outcome at discharge, 30, 60, 90, 180 days, an/or 1 year after event • Incidence of cardiac arrest • Incidence of arrhythmias and peri-intubation shock	Not recommended for routine use. May be used in situation where risk of brady-cardia is high (e.g. succinyl choline use) Atropine to be given as 0.02 mg/kg with no minimal dose concept
5.	Infants and children with septic shock	Whether the use of restrictive volumes of resuscitation fluid (<20 mL/kg) or the use of non-crystalloid fluids, change • Time to resolution of shock • Need for ventilation or vasopressor support • Frequency of complications • Total intravenous (IV) fluids administered • Length of hospital stay • Ventilator-free days • Survival to hospital discharge	Routine use of bolus intravenous fluids (crystalloids or colloids) for infants and children with a "severe febrile illness" and who are not in shock in not recommended Initial bolus of 20 ml/Kg is indicated in shock associated with severe sepsis, severe malaria, dengue shock syndrome with emphasis on frequent reassessments to detect deterioration at an early stages No advantage of non crystalloids except in dengue shock syndrome (time to resolution of shock)[7]

RRT: Rapid response team; MET: Medical emergency team; PEWS: Pediatric early warning score; ECMO: Extra-corporeal membrane oxygenation

1. Rapid response team (RRT)/medical emergency team (MET).
2. Pediatric early warning score (PEWS).
3. Specific management in dilated cardiomyopathy (DCMP)/mycarditis.
4. Use of atropine as premedication.
5. Use of restrictive volumes and non-crystalloids in septic shock.

B. *Intra-arrest:* Advanced life support: Seven aspects during advanced life support delivery were looked at to improve outcomes (Table 33.2).
1. Energy dose for initial and subsequent defibrillation.
2. Use of invasive hemodynamic monitoring for systolic and diastolic BP titration.
3. Chest compression techniques to achieve a specific $ETCO_2$ threshold.
4. Use of amiodarone for shock-refractory VF or pulseless VT (pVT).
5. Use of vasopressor/s during cardiac arrest, e.g. epinephrine/vasopressin.
6. Use of ECMO for resuscitation (ECPR).
7. Significance of any intra-arrest prognostic factors.

C. *Post arrest care:* Six key areas in post arrest management were reviewed to give recommendations (Table 33.3).

TABLE 33.2: Intra arrest-Advanced life support[3,4]

S. No	Target population (infants & children)	Questions	Treatment recommendations
1.	With VF or pVT	Whether any specific energy dose/s for defibrilation attempt(s) changes • Termination of arrhythmia • ROSC • Survival to hospital discharge, survival with favorable neurological/functional outcome at discharge, 30, 60, 180 days, amd/or 1 year	For initial dose use of monophasic/biphasic shock at 2 to 4 J/kg For further shock use escalating doses of ≥4J/kg. Should not exceed 10 J/kg or maximum dose in adults
2.	Requiring CPR	Whether use of invasive hemodynamic monitoring targeting specific blood pressure values for both systolic and diastolic, changes • Likelihood of ROSC • Survival to hospital discharge • Survival to hospital discharge, 60 days and 180 days after event with favorable neurologic outcome	Invasive blood pressure monitoring to guide CPR quality may be used (very-low-quality evidence) No specific target values of BP are available
3.	With cardiac arrest	Whether chest compression technique to achieve a specific $ETCO_2$ threshold, changes • ROSC	The quality of chest compression, may be evaluated by capnography (very low) Specific target values to guide chest compression have not been established

(Contd...)

TABLE 33.2: Intra arrest-Advanced life support[3,4] (*Contd...*)

S. No	Target population (infants & children)	Questions	Treatment recommendations
		• The likelihood of survival on discharge • Survival at 180 days with good neurologic outcome	
4.	With refractory VF/pVT	Whether use of amiodarone versus lidocaine, changes • Termination of arrhythmias • ROSC • Recurrence of VF • Risk of complications (e.g. need for tube change, airway injury, aspiration) • Survival at hospital discharge	For shock-refractory VF or pVT, either of the drugs amiodarone or lidocaine may be used
5.	With cardiac arrest	Whether the use of vasopressor (epinephrine, vasopressin, combination of vasopressors) changes • ROSC • Survival at hospital discharge • Survival to 180 days with good neurologic outcome	No pediatric studies that demonstrate the effectiveness of any vasopressors or its combination Give standard-dose epinephrine for pediatric cardiac arrest, which is mainly based on one adult OHCA RCT[8] (very-low-quality evidence)
6.	In hospital cardiac arrest	Whether use of eCMO for resuscitation (ECPR), changes • Survival to intensive care discharge • Survival at hospital discharge • Survival to 180 days with good neurologic outcome	In settings with protocols, expertise and equipment for ECMO, ECPR might be considered in patients with underlying cardiac disease.
7.	With cardiac arrest	Whether presence of any specific intra-arrest prognostic factor, changes • Survival to hospital discharge with good neurologic outcome • Survival at discharge, 30 days, 60 days, 180 days, and/or one year • Survival to 30, 60, days with good neurologic outcome • Survival to 180 dyas with good neurologic outcome	For OHCA, age <1 year, longer durations of cardiac arrest and non-shockable rhythm are poor prognostic markers[9] In IHCA, positive predictors are age <1 year and initial presence of a shockable rhythm

CPR: Cardiopulmonary resuscitation; ROSC: Return of spontaneous circulation; VF: Ventricular fibrillation; pVT: Pulseless ventricular tachycardia

TABLE 33.3: Pediatric post cardiac arrest care[3,4]

S. No.	Target population (infants & children)	Questions	Treatment recommendations
1.	ROSC post cardiac arrest	Whether use of therapeutic hypothermia (TTM) changes • ICU length of stay • Survival to hospital discharge	For persisting coma after OHCA, TTM be used. However, ideal target temperature range and duration are unknown, use either hypothermia (32°–34°C) or normothermia (36°C–37.5°C)[10] For pediatric survivors after IHCA insufficient data exists Temperature ≥38°C should not be allowed after ROSC
2.	Post cardiac arrest ROSC	Whether use of targeted PaO_2 target, changes • Survival at ICU discharge • Survival at 6 months • Survival at 6 months • Survival at 180 days with good neurologic outcome	Target normoxemia (PaO_2 ≥60 and <300 mmHg) after ROSC Wean O_2 to target SpO_2 <100%, but >94%
3.	Post cardiac arrest ROSC	Whether ventilation to a specific $PaCO_2$ target, change • Survival to ICU discharge • Survival to 30, 60 days, 6 months with good neurologic outcome • Survival to 180 days with good neurologic outcome	The limits of $PaCO_2$ (both upper and lower) are unknown and no specific $PaCO_2$ in pediatric patients with ROSC has been demonstrated to have better outcomes Worse survival outcome was associated with $PaCO_2$ ≥50 mmHg.[11] Avoid hypercapnia
4.	Post arrest ROSC	Whether use of intravenous fluids and inotropes and/or vasopressors to maintain blood pressure, changes • Patient satisfaction • Survival to hospital discharge • Survival with favorable neurologic/functional outcome at discharge, 30, 60, 180 days, and/or 1 year	Parenteral fluids, inotropes/vasoactive drugs are recommended to maintain SBP >5th percentile for age Continuous BP monitoring is desirable
5.	Post cardiac arrests	Whether use of neuroelectrophysiology information (EEG), predict • Survival to hospital discharge with without good neurologic outcome • Survival at 6 months • Survival with favorable neurologic outcome at 30, 60, 180 days and 1 year	On hospital discharge EEG within first 7 days showing discontinuous/isoelectric line predicts poor neurologic outcome
6.	After ROSC	Whether presence of any specific prognostic factors, changes • Survival at hospital discharge with good neurologic outcome • Survival at discharge, 30, 60, 180, and/or 1 year • Survival to 30, 60, 180 days with good neurologic outcome	Multiple factors should be taken into account while predicting outcome (e.g. pupillary size at 12–24 hrs, serum neurologic markers, and lactate)

OHCA and IHCA: Out-of-hospital and in-hospital cardiac arrest

1. Role of targeted temperature management (TTM).
2. Use of targeted PaO_2.
3. Ventilation to targeted PCO_2.
4. Targeted perfusion and BP with fluids, inotropes and/or vasopressors.
5. Use of EEG.
6. Role of any prognostic factors.

REFERENCES

1. Girotra S, Spertus JA, Li Y, Berg RA, Nadkarni VM, Chan PS, et al. American Heart Association Get With The Guidelines–Resuscitation Investigators. Survival trends in pediatric in-hospital cardiac arrests: an analysis from Get with the Guidelines– Resuscitation. Circ Cardiovasc Qual Outcomes. 2013; 6:42–49.
2. Sutton RM, Case E, Brown SP, Atkins DL, Nadkarni VM, Kaltman J, et al. A quantitative analysis of out–of–hospital pediatric and adolescent resuscitation quality. A report from the ROC Epistry–Cardiac arrest. Resuscitation 2015; 93: 150–157.
3. De Caen AR, Berg MD, Chameides L, Gooden Ck, Hickey RW, Scott HF, et al. Part 12: Pediatric Advanced Life Support: 2015 American Heart Association Guidelines Update for Cardiopulmonary Resuscitation and Emergency Cardiovascular Care. Circulation. 2015;132(suppl):S526–42.
4. Maconochie IK, De Caen AR, Aickin R, Atkins DL, Biarent D, Guerguerian AM, et al. on behalf of the Pediatric Basic Life Support and Pediatric Advanced Life Support Chapter Collaborators. Part 6: Pediatric Basic Life Support and Pediatric Advanced Life Support 2015 International Consensus on Cardiopulmonary Resuscitation and Emergency Cardiovascular Care Science with Treatment Recommendations. Resuscitation. 2015; 95: e147–68.
5. Institute of Medicine. Standards for Systematic Reviews. 2011. Available from: http:// www.iom.edu/Reports/2011/Finding-What-Works-in-Health-Care-Standards-for-Systematic-Reviews/Standards.aspx. Accessed August 15, 2015.
6. Schünemann HJ, Schünemann AH, Oxman AD, Brozek J, Glasziou P, Jaeschke R, et al. GRADE Working Group. Grading quality of evidence and strength of recommen-dations for diagnostic tests and strategies. BMJ. 2008; 336:1106–10.
7. Ngo NT, Cao XT, Kneen R, Wills B, Nguyen VM, Nguyen TQ, et al. Acute management of dengue shock syndrome: a randomized double-blind comparison of 4 intravenous fluid regimens in the first hour. Clin Infect Dis. 2001; 32:204–13.
8. Jacobs IG, Finn JC, Jelinek GA, Oxer HF, Thompson PL. Effect of adrenaline on survival in out-of-hospital cardiac arrest: a randomized double-blind placebo-controlled trial. Resuscitation. 2011; 82:1138–43.
9. Kitamura T, Iwami T, Kawamura T, Nagao K, Tanaka H, Nadkarni VM, et al. Conventional and chest-compression-only cardiopulmonary resuscitation by bystanders for children who have out-of-hospital cardiac arrests: a prospective, nationwide, population-based cohort study. Lancet. 2010; 375:1347–54.
10. Lin JJ, Hsia SH, Wang HS, Chiang MC, Lin KL. Therapeutic hypothermia associated with increased survival after resuscitation in children. Pediatr Neurol. 2013; 4:285–90.
11. Castillo DJ, López-Herce J, Matamoros M, Cañadas S, Rodriguez- Calvo A, Cechetti C, et al. Iberoamerican Pediatric Cardiac Arrest Study Network RIBEPCI. Hyperoxia, hypocapnia and hypercapnia as outcome factors after cardiac arrest in children. Resuscitation. 2012; 83:1456–61.

ILAE Classification of Seizures and Epilepsies, 2017

R Dhinakaran, Devendra Mishra

Seizures are a common pediatric problem, and of considerable interest to pediatricians.[1,2] Classification of seizures and epilepsy is the cornerstone in the evaluation and management of seizures. It helps in understanding the types of seizure, identifying and labeling the type of epilepsy, and grouping similar entities into specific syndromes—thereby guiding antiepileptic therapy and patient counseling. Epilepsy classification is primarily used for the diagnosis of patients, but it is also critical for research, communication among clinicians and researchers, and development of antiepileptic therapies.[3]

The International League Against Epilepsy (ILAE) has been playing a pivotal role in classification of epilepsy.[4–7] The 1981 and 1989 ILAE classifications were a major breakthrough in understanding the types and classification of seizures and epilepsy.[4,5] Since then, multiple modifications and revisions have been proposed.[6,7] In 2017, ILAE published an updated classifications of both seizures[8] and epilepsies,[3] these being the "first new official papers on classification from the ILAE since 1989".[9] With advancement in technology and research, new insight has been gained in understanding the phenotypic pattern and the basic mechanism of seizure, thus making revision a necessary process. The stated

purpose of revisions is to include new seizure types, have a better organized classification and to enable usage of appropriate terms for better understanding.[3]

We herein list some of the important aspects of the revised classification for the benefit of the readers—these include, among others, new focal seizure types which were earlier in generalized category alone (e.g., epileptic spasm could be focal as well as generalized), new generalized types (like myoclonic atonic and epileptic spasm), and classifying focal seizure by its "first clinical manifestation".[8] The full documents are available at the ILAE website (https://www.ilae.org/guidelines/definition-and-classification).

The new classification framework of epilepsy is a multilevel classification with four main components; three of them sequential *viz.*, (i) the seizure type, followed by (ii) the epilepsy type, and then (iii) the epilepsy syndrome. The fourth component, identifying etiology, is an overarching activity, continuing at each individual step (Fig. 34.1). The framework is designed to enable classification of epilepsy in different clinical settings implying that patient characterization will be possible at every level, depending on the resources available to the clinician making the diagnosis.[3] Supporting information *viz.*, Video

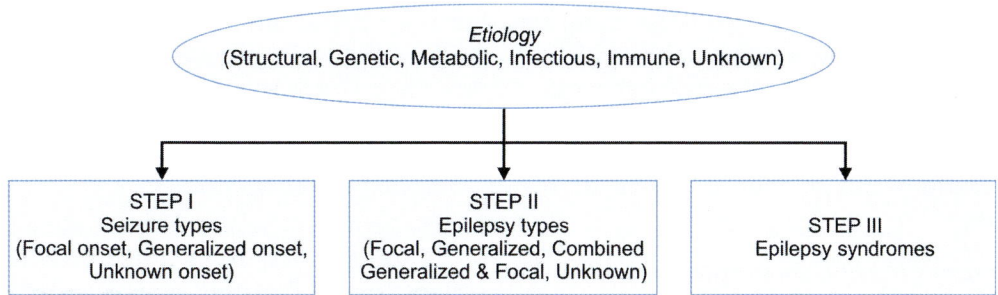

Fig. 34.1: Schematic representation of the multi-level classification of seizure and epilepsy (ILAE, 2017).

record, Electro-encephalography (EEG), neuroimaging, gene mutations and autoimmune panel, if available, are to be utilized in classifying epilepsy type and/or epilepsy syndrome.[3]

Classifying Seizures

The new basic 2017 classification of seizure is based on three key features *viz.*, (i) locus of seizure origin in brain; (ii) level of awareness during seizure; and, (iii) other features. The basic operational seizure type classification includes:[8] Focal onset seizures (Aware/ Impaired awareness; Motor/Non-motor onset; and Focal to bilateral tonic-clonic); Generalized onset (Motor/Non-motor (Absence)); and Unknown onset (Motor/Non-motor; Unclassified).

Inclusion of new seizure types: The new seizure types included in the classification are enlisted in Box 34.1.

Box 34.1: Newer terminologies for seizure type in ILAE seizure classification, 2017

Focal seizures
Motor: Epileptic spasms, myoclonic, tonic, tonic clonic, clonic, atonic, hyper-kinetic, automatism
Non-motor: Behavior arrest, emotional
Focal to bilateral tonic-clonic
Generalized seizures
Absence with eyelid myoclonia, epileptic spasms, myoclonic–atonic, and myoclonic–tonic–clonic

---

Clarification of impairment of consciousness: Consciousness is a complex phenomenon with both subjective and objective components. In the 2017 classification, awareness has been chosen to be the best surrogate marker of consciousness, and is simpler to evaluate.[8] Awareness is operationally defined as "knowledge of self and environment".[8]

Re-classification of certain seizure types into either focal or generalized onset: Seizures are classified by earliest prominent motor or non-motor features; even though, uncertainty is present in every seizure classification.[8] The term 'bilateral' is used for propagation patterns and 'generalized' for seizures that engage bilateral networks from onset. Few seizure types like epileptic spasms, myoclonic, tonic, tonic-clonic, clonic, atonic, which were previously included only in generalized-onset seizures are now also included in focal-onset seizures.[8]

Classification of seizure of unknown onset: Situations in which patient is alone or asleep or the attender is not able to describe the seizure onset clearly is classified as Seizure of unknown onset. If clinician is confident that an event is seizure but cannot classify it due to incomplete information, it is grouped under unclassified seizures. In the 2017 classification, Seizure of unknown onset is further classified as tonic-clonic, epileptic spasms or behavior arrest depending upon the predominant motor or non-motor activity noticed during the episode.[8] This is essential in guiding treatment, and for reclassification into focal or generalized onset with future episodes. In this regard, the term 'unknown onset' is a placeholder–not a characteristic of the seizure.[8]

New terms for old ones: Some of the terms used in seizure-classification lack community acceptance or public understanding. The terms dyscognitive, simple partial, complex partial, psychic, and secondarily generalized were eliminated. The term 'partial' was replaced by 'focal', as the term partial conveys a sense of part of a seizure, rather than a location or anatomic system. 'Focal to bilateral tonic-clonic' replaced 'focal seizure with secondary generalization,' as this term can better reflect the propagation pattern of a seizure (Table 34.1).[8]

Updated glossary of seizure terms: Glossary of seizure terms has also been updated and it includes new definition for terms like emotional seizure, eyelid myoclonia, myoclonic atonic,

TABLE 34.1: New terms introduced in the ILAE seizure classification, 2017

Old terms	New terms
Partial	Focal
Simple partial	Focal aware
Complex partial	Focal impaired awareness
Psychic	Cognitive
Secondary generalized	Focal to bilateral tonic-clonic tonic-clonic
Arrest, freeze, pause, interruption	Behavior arrest
Dyscognitive	Focal impaired awareness
Astatic	(Focal or generalized) atonic
Grand mal	Generalized tonic clonic, focal to bilateral tonic clonic, unknown onset tonic clonic
Infantile spasm	Epileptic spasm
Psychomotor	Focal impaired awareness

behavior arrest, unaware, and unclassified seizure.[10] Common descriptors used to describe seizures have also been standardized in the new 2017 classification.[10]

Classifying Epilepsy Types

A new group of combined generalized and focal epilepsy has been introduced in the epilepsy type. Idiopathic generalized epilepsy was renamed as Genetic generalized epilepsy, which includes Childhood absence epilepsy, juvenile absence epilepsy, Juvenile myoclonic epilepsy and Generalized tonic–clonic seizures alone.[3] The terms 'Epileptic encephalopathy' and 'Developmental encephalopathy' have been redefined, and 'malignant' and 'catastrophic' are omitted. The term 'benign' used in some epilepsy syndromes like BECTS (Benign epilepsy with centro-temporal spikes) is now replaced by 'self-limited' or 'pharmaco-responsive' depending on the situations.[3]

Epilepsy Syndromes

Diagnosis of an Epilepsy syndrome, if possible, is the third level of diagnosis.[10] An epilepsy syndrome is diagnosed on the basis of all or some of age at presentation, seizure type, EEG findings, etiological substrate, neuroimaging, genetic analyses, occurring in a typical pattern.[10] Recognition of a syndrome helps in determining etiology, evaluating for co-morbidity, deciding management, and conveying prognosis.

Labeling Etiology

This epilepsy classification lays stress on determining etiology at all stages along the diagnostic process, starting from the initial presentation and evaluation. Six major etiological categories have been recognized in the classification (Fig. 34.1), with an understanding that a patient's epilepsy may be classified into more than one etiological group. An example would be a 'structural' cause (cortical tuber) in a 'genetic' condition (tuberous sclerosis).

CONCLUSION

These new classifications of seizures and the epilepsies are likely to lead to improved understanding of seizure etiology, making appropriate diagnosis and will guide targeted therapies to the patient. This classification may also help in greater ease of communication about seizure types among clinicians, the non-medical community, and researchers. The simultaneously published instruction manual on applying the seizure classification terminology will immensely assist in everyday clinical practice.[9] A companion piece to present these concepts for people with epilepsy and their caregivers is also available.[10]

REFERENCES

1. Mishra OP, Upadhyay A, Prasad R, Upadhyay SK, Piplani SK. Behavioral problems in Indian children with epilepsy. Indian Pediatr. 2017;54:116–20.

2. Sajjan S, Jain P, Sharma S, Seth A, Aneja S. Injuries in children with epilepsy: A hospital-based study. Indian Pediatr. 2016;53:883–5.

3. Scheffer IE, Berkovic S, Capovilla G, Connolly MB, French J, Guilhoto L, et al. ILAE Classification of the epilepsies: Position paper of the ILAE commission for classification and terminology. Epilepsia 2017;58:512–21.

4. Commission on classification and terminology of the International League Against Epilepsy. Proposal for revised clinical and electroencephalographic classification of epileptic seizures. Epilepsia. 1981;22:489-501.

5. Commission on classification and terminology of the International League Against Epilepsy. Proposal for revised classification of epilepsies and epileptic synd-romes. Epilepsia. 1989;30:389-99.

6. Engel J Jr. A proposed diagnostic scheme for people with epileptic seizures and with epilepsy: Report of the ILAE Task Force on classification and terminology. Epilepsia. 2001;42:796-803.

7. Berg AT, Berkovic SF, Brodie MJ, Buchhalter J, Cross JH, van Emde Boas W, et al. Revised terminology and concepts for organization of seizures and epilepsies: Report of the ILAE Commission on Classification and Terminology, 2005–2009. Epilepsia. 2010;51:676-85.

8. Fisher RS, Cross JH, French JA, Higurashi N, Hirsch E, Jansen FE, et al. Operational classification of seizure types by the international league against epilepsy: Position paper of the ILAE commission for classification and terminology. Epilepsia. 2017;58:522-30.

9. Fisher RS, Cross JH, Souza CD, Higurashi N, Hirsch E, Jansen FE, et al. Instruction manual for the ILAE 2017 operational classification of seizure types. Epilepsia. 2017;58:531-42.

10. Brodie MJ, Zuberi SM, Scheffer IE, Fisher RS. The 2017 ILAE classification of seizure types and the epilepsies: What do people with epilepsy and their caregivers need to know? Epileptic Disord. 2018;20:77-87.